ANNALS *of* THE NEW YORK ACADEMY OF SCIENCES

T0179750

EDITOR-IN-CHIEF
Douglas Braaten

ASSOCIATE EDITOR
Rebecca E. Cooney

PROJECT MANAGER
Steven E. Bohall

Artwork and design by Ash Ayman Shairzay

The New York Academy of Sciences
7 World Trade Center
250 Greenwich Street, 40th Floor
New York, NY 10007-2157

annals@nyas.org
www.nyas.org/annals

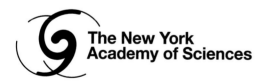

**The New York
Academy of Sciences**

Published by Blackwell Publishing
On behalf of the New York Academy of Sciences

Boston, Massachusetts
2012

ANNALS *of* THE NEW YORK ACADEMY OF SCIENCES

VOLUME
1274

ISSUE

Myasthenia Gravis and Related Disorders I

12th International Conference

ISSUE EDITORS

Gil I. Wolfe,[a] Matthew N. Meriggioli,[b] Emma Ciafaloni,[c] and Robert L. Ruff[d]

[a]University at Buffalo School of Medicine and Biomedical Sciences, [b]University of Illinois College of Medicine at Chicago, [c]University of Rochester Medical Center, and [d]Case Western Reserve University School of Medicine

TABLE OF CONTENTS

vii   Introduction for *Myasthenia Gravis and Related Disorders*
Gil I. Wolfe, Matthew N. Meriggioli, Emma Ciafaloni, and Robert L. Ruff

1   Biologics and other novel approaches as new therapeutic options in myasthenia gravis: a view to the future
Marinos C. Dalakas

Structure and function of the neuromuscular junction: recent advances

9   Myasthenogenicity of the main immunogenic region
Jon Lindstrom and Jie Luo

14   Structure of the neuromuscular junction: function and cooperative mechanisms in the synapse
Masaharu Takamori

24   Active zones of mammalian neuromuscular junctions: formation, density, and aging
Hiroshi Nishimune

Advances in immunology and their relationship to myasthenia gravis

33   The etiology of autoimmune diseases: the case of myasthenia gravis
Jean-François Bach

40   Defects of immunoregulatory mechanisms in myasthenia gravis: role of IL-17
Angeline Gradolatto, Dani Nazzal, Maria Foti, Jacky Bismuth, Frederique Truffault, Rozen Le Panse, and Sonia Berrih-Aknin

48   Targeting plasma cells with proteasome inhibitors: possible roles in treating myasthenia gravis?
Alejandro M. Gomez, Nick Willcox, Peter C. Molenaar, Wim Buurman, Pilar Martinez-Martinez, Marc H. De Baets, and Mario Losen

Academy Membership: Connecting you to the nexus of scientific innovation

Since 1817, the Academy has carried out its mission to bring together extraordinary people working at the frontiers of discovery. Members gain recognition by joining a thriving community of over 25,000 scientists. Academy members also access unique member benefits.

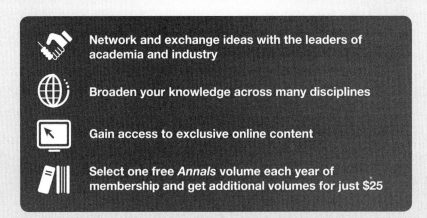

Network and exchange ideas with the leaders of academia and industry

Broaden your knowledge across many disciplines

Gain access to exclusive online content

Select one free *Annals* volume each year of membership and get additional volumes for just $25

Join or renew today at **www.nyas.org**.
Or by phone at **800.843.6927** (**212.298.8640** if outside the US).

60   The role of B cell–activating factor in autoimmune myasthenia gravis
Robert P. Lisak and Samia Ragheb

68   Functional defect in regulatory T cells in myasthenia gravis
Muthusamy Thiruppathi, Julie Rowin, Qin Li Jiang, Jian Rong Sheng, Bellur S. Prabhakar, and Matthew N. Meriggioli

Myasthenia gravis: clinical and laboratory developments

77   Jitter analysis with concentric needle electrodes
Erik Stålberg

86   Management challenges in muscle-specific tyrosine kinase myasthenia gravis
Amelia Evoli, Paolo E. Alboini, Ana Bisonni, Alessia Mastrorosa, and Emanuela Bartocccioni

92   Antibodies identified by cell-based assays in myasthenia gravis and associated diseases
Angela Vincent, Patrick Waters, M. Isabel Leite, Leslie Jacobson, Inga Koneczny, Judith Cossins, and David Beeson

Myasthenia gravis: outcome measurements and clinical trial development

99   The MG composite: an outcome measure for myasthenia gravis for use in clinical trials and everyday practice
Ted M. Burns

107   Patient registries: useful tools for clinical research in myasthenia gravis
Fulvio Baggi, Renato Mantegazza, Carlo Antozzi, and Donald Sanders

114   The Myasthenia Gravis-Specific Activities of Daily Living Profile
Srikanth Muppidi

Animal models of neuromuscular junction disease

120   Regulatory T cell–based immunotherapies in experimental autoimmune myasthenia gravis
Miriam C. Souroujon, Revital Aricha, Tali Feferman, Keren Mizrachi, Debby Reuveni, and Sara Fuchs

127   The role of complement in experimental autoimmune myasthenia gravis
Linda L. Kusner and Henry J. Kaminski

133   Novel animal models of acetylcholine receptor antibody–related myasthenia gravis
Erdem Tüzün, Windy Allman, Canan Ulusoy, Huan Yang, and Premkumar Christadoss

140   Animal models of antimuscle-specific kinase myasthenia
David P. Richman, Kayoko Nishi, Michael J. Ferns, Joachim Schnier, Peter Pytel, Ricardo A. Maselli, and Mark A. Agius

Ann. N.Y. Acad. Sci. ISSN 0077-8923

Introduction for *Myasthenia Gravis and Related Disorders*

Myasthenia gravis (MG) is an acquired autoimmune syndrome caused by the failure of neuro-muscular transmission, which results from the binding of autoantibodies to proteins involved in signaling at the neuromuscular junction (NMJ). Although the precise origin of the immune response in MG is not known, it remains one of the better characterized autoimmune disorders, and serves as a paradigm not only for understanding autoimmunity but also for the study of the NMJ and ion channels.

Earlier diagnosis and the availability of effective treatments have reduced the burden of high mortality and severe disability previously associated with myasthenia gravis. However, diagnosing the disease remains problematic and can be delayed because of its nonspecific and fluctuating symptoms. Furthermore, the management of MG is associated with considerable limitations. Treatment options in related myasthenic disorders are also inadequate. Present treatments for MG are either targeted toward symptoms or involve immunosuppressive therapies that have variable efficacy and that uniformly carry significant risk of infection or malignancy. Conventional treatments result in global, unfocused immunosuppression, rather than targeted inhibition of the autoreactive immune cells.

Myasthenia gravis and other disorders of the NMJ are relatively rare and are often neglected by national health authorities and the pharmaceutical industry. Held every five years, the International Conference on Myasthenia Gravis and Related Disorders attracts thought leaders in the field and provides a venue for researchers and clinicians to exchange ideas, establish collaborations, and continue to move the field forward. The international conferences also provide forums for younger investigators to communicate their recent findings.

The 12th International Conference on Myasthenia Gravis and Related Disorders was held on May 21–23, 2012 in New York City at the conference center at the New York Academy of Sciences. The meeting was cosponsored by the New York Academy of Sciences and the Myasthenia Gravis Foundation of America, with additional support provided by the NIH/NINDS/NCATS/ORD. Educational grants were received from Alexion Pharmaceuticals and BioMarin Pharmaceutical, Inc.; corporate sponsorships were received from CSL Behring, IBL International, KRONUS, Athena Diagnostics, and Terumo BCT. Nearly 300 scientists and clinicians from around the world attended the meeting.

The plenary sessions included 50 presentations. Over 100 abstracts were presented during two poster sessions. The keynote address by Marinos C. Dalakas summarized the evolution of biologics and other novel approaches in the treatment of MG and other immune-mediated neuromuscular disorders. Other highlights included latest developments pertaining to the structure of the NMJ; defects in regulatory T cells; the discovery of low-density lipoprotein receptor-related protein 4 as

doi: 10.1111/j.1749-6632.2012.06835.x

an autoimmune target in MG; stem cell–mediated immunomodulation of lymphocytes derived from MG patients; recent basic and clinical findings in MuSK MG; the creation of patient registries; and updates on clinical trials, including the international thymectomy trial, acute management of MG exacerbations, methotrexate in MG, and preliminary investigations using complement inhibitors.

The four organizers of the conference would like to thank Brooke Grindlinger of the New York Academy of Sciences and Samuel Schulhof of the Myasthenia Gravis Foundation of America for their support of the three-day conference. Others who played integral roles include Melinda Miller and Melanie Koundourou, the New York Academy of Sciences, and Tor Holtan, the Myasthenia Gravis Foundation of America. Finally, we would like to acknowledge Douglas Braaten, editor-in-chief, *Annals of the New York Academy of Sciences,* for his help in assembling these proceedings.

GIL I. WOLFE

University at Buffalo School of Medicine and Biomedical Sciences, Buffalo, New York

MATTHEW N. MERIGGIOLI

University of Illinois College of Medicine at Chicago, Chicago, Illinois

EMMA CIAFALONI

University of Rochester Medical Center, Rochester, New York

ROBERT L. RUFF

Case Western Reserve University School of Medicine, Cleveland, Ohio

Ann. N.Y. Acad. Sci. ISSN 0077-8923

ANNALS OF THE NEW YORK ACADEMY OF SCIENCES

Issue: *Myasthenia Gravis and Related Disorders*

Biologics and other novel approaches as new therapeutic options in myasthenia gravis: a view to the future

Marinos C. Dalakas[1,2]

[1]Thomas Jefferson University, Philadelphia, Pennsylvania. [2]Neuroimmunology Unit, Department of Pathophysiology, University of Athens Medical School, Athens, Greece

Address for correspondence: Professor Marinos C. Dalakas, M.D., F.A.A.N., Pathophysiology, University of Athens Medical School, 75 Mikras Asias Str., Athens Greece 1152 mdalakos@med.uao.gr or Thomas Jefferson Univerity, 901 Walnut Street, 4th floor, Philadelphia, PA 19107. marinos.dalakas@jefferson.edu

Myasthenia gravis (MG) is caused by complement-fixing antibodies against the acetylcholine receptors (AChR). Regulatory T cells (T_{reg} cells), Th17 cells, and recognition of AChR epitopes by $CD4^+$ T cells are fundamental. Novel biological agents now in the offing, offer the potential for specific treatment options in MG by targeting the following: (1) T cell intracellular signaling pathways, costimulation, and transduction molecules; (2) B cells, against CD20 molecules, or the B cell trophic factors BAFF and APRIL; (3) complement, against C5 that intercepts the formation of MAC; (4) cytokines and cytokine receptors targeting interleukin (IL)-6, IL-17, and the Janus tyrosine kinases (JAK)1 and JAK3; and (5) cellular adhesion and T cell migration molecules. Reengineering of pathogenic antibodies (i.e., molecular decoys) by constructing recombinant antibodies that block the complement binding of the pathogenic AChR antibodies is an additional approach. The promising therapeutic profile of these agents should be weighted against excessive cost and rare complications necessitating the need for controlled trials to secure efficacy and balance benefit against risks.

Keywords: myasthenia gravis; immunotherapy; monoclonal antibodies; immunobiologic therapies

Introduction

Myasthenia gravis (MG) is the prototypic autoimmune disease because the antigen, the acetylcholine receptor (AChR), is known; antibodies against the AChRs are detected and measured in the patients' serum; the patients' IgG binds to the AChRs at the postsynaptic region and, by fixing complement or cross-linking, results in internalization or degradation of the AChRs and simplification of the postsynaptic junctional folds; the IgG antibodies are pathogenic because they transmit the disease to experimental animals and cause destruction of the AChRs in cultured myotubes; immunization of healthy animals with AChRs leads to clinical signs of myasthenia that can be subsequently passed to other animals with purified IgG; and removal of the pathogenic autoantibodies results in clinical improvement.[1–3] Apart from the pathogenic antibodies, regulatory T cells (T_{reg} cells) and $CD4^+$ T cells also play a role because they recognize AChR epitopes in the context of MHC class II molecules and exert a helper function on B cells for the production of antibodies.[4]

All the above makes MG an attractive candidate disease for antigen-specific therapy. In spite of the advances in molecular immunology, however, such a specific therapy has been very challenging[4,5] and, at present impractical, because the autoimmune T cell and antibody responses are highly heterogeneous; it is not technically possible to target the discreet populations of sensitized T or B cells for immunomodulation; for the induction of tolerance there is a fundamental need to induce regulatory T cell subsets that recognize disease-inducing epitopes, a process with insurmountable difficulties; and there are safety concerns owing to the need to administer high doses of immunodominant (and potentially pathogenic) epitopes to induce T cell tolerance, without inducing T cell activation.[5] As a

doi: 10.1111/j.1749-6632.2012.06832.x

result, the current management of MG is based on drugs exerting a nonantigen-specific immunosuppression or immunomodulation.[6] Although MG is no longer "gravis," because it responds fairly well to the available therapies, we still do not have a cure for the disease. Furthermore, a number of patients do not respond sufficiently well to the available therapies or suffer severe side effects from the long-term use of steroids or immunosuppressants, necessitating the need for more effective therapies with long-term benefit and less severe side effects. This review is aimed to identify the targets of future immunotherapies in MG and elaborate on the available biological agents that might possibly offer more targeted therapies, based on the experience we have gained from their application in other autoimmune diseases.

Current immunotherapies in myasthenia gravis

Conventional, nonspecific therapies
Corticosteroids. Even after many years of progress in the therapy of the disease and our success in reducing mortality, corticosteroids remain the first-line drugs. High doses, even up to 100 mg daily prednisone, may be required to achieve remission.

Immunosuppressants. These drugs are aimed to reduce the prednisone to the lowest possible every-other day dose that controls the disease and prevent relapses. The choice of the immunosuppressant varies among practitioners because no controlled comparative studies are available. The most commonly used drugs are azathioprine, mycophenolate mofetil, and cyclosporine. Attention is now being received by the use of methotrexate and, for difficult cases, tacrolimus.[6]

Immunomodulating, nonspecific therapies (for transient benefit)
These modalities include immunoglobulin (IVIg) and plasmapheresis. Whenever patients with difficult disease need immediate help, especially during an acute worsening or a crisis, plasmapheresis or intravenous IVIg are the best treatment options.[6–9] Although never compared in a blinded controlled study, plasmapheresis seems to work faster than IVIg and might be preferable for managing a crisis but requires a hospital setting. Both of these therapies, however, are immunomodulating and offer transient benefits appropriate only for short-term peri-

ods. The disease is ultimately controlled either when the aforementioned immunosuppressive agents take effect or with the application of new and more targeted therapies, as outlined below.

Future immunotherapies in MG: the rationale for using newer agents and biologicals

New biological agents are currently on the market for a number of autoimmune disorders, offering a target-specific, "missile-like" therapy:

1. monoclonal antibodies. Depending on which portion of the IgG molecule is derived from humans, these are either chimeric, when only the Fc portion of the IgG is from human immunoglobulin, or humanized when the whole molecule is from human IgG, except for the hypervariable region, which is from the mouse;
2. therapeutic fusion proteins ("-cepts"). These are engineered when the Fc region of IgG1 is fused to the extracellular domain of certain key molecules, such as CTLA-4 (abatacept); LFA-3 (alefacept); VEGF-A (aflibercept), approved for wet macular degeneration; IL-1 receptor (rilonacept or IL-1 Trap), approved for CAPS; and most of the TNF-α inhibitors, approved for rheumatoid arthritis; and
3. reengineering of pathogenic antibodies (molecular decoys), which will be discussed below.

Specific therapeutic targets related to the pathogenesis of MG

To understand the rationale for using the new biological agents, it is useful to review the main immunopathogenetic network of MG and identify the implicated key molecules that we need to target to induce tolerance or restore immune balance.

It is unclear how MG begins but, like all the other autoimmune disorders, the process starts when tolerance is broken probably by infections or molecular mimicry (when the AChR protein shares sequence homologies with microbial antigens), resulting in cross-reactivity and autoimmunity. When this happens, AChR, the antigen, is presented via the antigen-presenting cells (APCs) in the periphery or the thymus to $CD4^+$ T cells via costimulatory molecules leading to upregulation of key cytokines, such as IL-4 and IL-6, that stimulate B

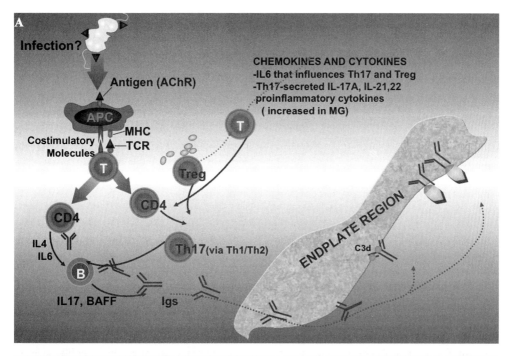

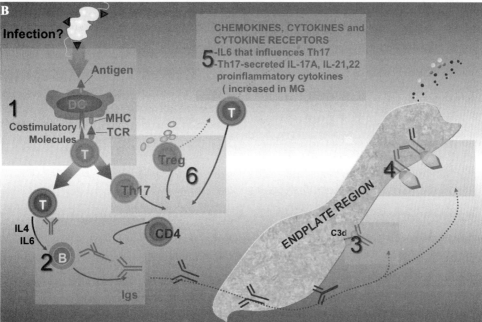

Figure 1. (A) The AChR is presented via the APCs (in the periphery or the thymus) to CD4[+] T cells via costimulatory molecules leading to upregulation of cytokines, such as IL-4 and IL-6, that stimulate B cells to produce anti-AChR antibodies that, by fixing complement at the endplate region, lead to destruction of the AChRs. T_{reg} and Th17[+] cells also play a critical role because they affect antibody production via Th1/Th2 cytokine balance. Cytokines, such as IL-6, that affect the induction of T_{reg} cells to pathogenic Th1 cells, and proinflammatory cytokines, such as IL-17A, IL-21, and IL-22, are increased in MG patients and maintain the immune imbalance. (B) The crucial targets of action of specific immunotherapeutic drugs in MG are directed against the following sequential targets (in boxes): (1) molecules involved in T cell activation and costimulation; (2) antibodies, B cells, and B cell–surviving factors; (3) complement; (4) FcR on Ig molecules that bind to targeted tissues; (5) CD4[+] T cells and cytokines that facilitate antibody production by B cells; and (6) T_{reg} and Th17 cells that affect production of antibodies via Th1/Th2 cytokine balance.

cells to produce anti-AChR antibodies, as depicted in Figure 1A. The antibodies, by fixing complement at the endplate region, lead to destruction of the AChRs (Fig. 1A). Treg and Th17 cells also play a critical role because they affect antibody production via Th1/Th2 cytokine balance.[10,11] In addition, cytokines such as IL-6 that affects the induction of Tregs to pathogenic Th1 cells, and other proinflammatory cytokines, such as IL-17A, IL-21, IL-22, are increased in MG patients enhancing further the immune process and maintaining the immune imbalance.[4,10,11] Accordingly, as depicted in Figure 1B, the crucial targets of action of specific immunotherapeutic drugs in MG are those directed against the following: (1) molecules involved in T cell activation and costimulation; (2) antibodies, B cells, and B cell–surviving factors; (3) complement; (4) FcR on Ig molecules that bind to targeted tissues; (5) CD4$^+$ T cells and cytokines that facilitate antibody production by B cells; and (6) T_{reg} and Th17 cells that affect production of antibodies via Th1/Th2 cytokine balance. Agents against these targets, also proposed for other autoimmune neuromuscular disorders,[12–18] are sequentially discussed below as potential future treatment options in MG.

Agents targeting T cell intracellular signaling pathways, antigen recognition, and costimulation

The T cell receptor (TCR) interaction with antigen/MHC complex activates intracellular phosphotyrosine kinases that mediate signaling via phosphorylation of immunoreceptor tyrosine-based activation motifs and transduction molecules such as CD52.[18,19] Blockade of the CD52 molecule can be accomplished using the specific monoclonal antibody alemtuzumab (Campath®) that causes a long-lasting lymphocyte depletion.[19,20] Alemtuzumab has been very promising in multiple sclerosis with almost 70% reduction of relapses and disability prevention in two large clinical trials.[21] It has been also promising in CIDP where a controlled trial is planned.[22]

T cell activation is mediated via costimulatory factors delivered by LFA$_1$/ICAM or LFA$_3$/CD2 interactions. These molecules can be blocked by two monoclonal antibodies, one against LFA3 (alefacept), that exerts a downregulatory role on memory T cells and cytokine production, and another against LFA-1 ([efalizumab] Raptiva®) that blocks

reactivation of memory T cells.[13–17,19] Both of these drugs were effective and approved in 2002 for the treatment of psoriasis but were withdrawn from the market a year ago because of association with PML. Monoclonal antibodies against the costimulatory molecules CTLA-4 and CD40 have been also aggressively pursued for various autoimmune disorders and transplantation with promising results in experimental animals, but rather disappointing in humans. Most notable among them were the anti-CTLA-4 (abatacept) and anti-CD40/CD154 (toralizumab), both of which have been ineffective in SLE or had unacceptable side effects.[23] None of these anticostimulatory agents is currently on the market or have been approved for any indication.

The TCR engagement and costimulation activates downstream substrates, increasing the intracellular calcium concentration, which activates the phosphatase calcineurin. Calcineurin dephosphorylates the nuclear factor of activated T cells (NFAT) and enables it to enter the nucleus where it binds to IL-2 promoter to induce specific gene transcription that leads to cell proliferation and differentiation.[13–17,19] The IL-2 receptors can be effectively inhibited by the monoclonal antibody daclizumab that binds to CD25 (IL-2 receptor antagonist) and inhibits T cell proliferation. Daclizumab is very well tolerated, has been approved for one form of leukemia, and has been very promising in patients with multiple sclerosis in at least two clinical trials.[24] Daclizumab is an excellent agent to consider for MG.

Agents targeting B cells, B cell trophic factors, and autoantibodies

B cells are not only involved in complement activation and antibody production but also play a major role as APCs and production of cytokines, such as IL-1, IL-6, IL-10, and TNF-α.[25,26] Targeting B cells, therefore, may be rewarding in restoring immune balance as they are involved in several areas of the immune activation processes. Not only B cells but also their trophic factors BAFF (B cell activating factor) and APRIL (a proliferating inducing ligand), both TNF-α ligands, are potential therapeutic targets in MG (reviewed in Ref. 25), especially since the level of BAFF was found to be increased in the serum of MG patients.[27] There are at least nine drugs in the form of monoclonal antibodies or fusion proteins targeting B cells or B cell growth factors that are currently undergoing clinical trials in autoimmune diseases or their experimental models.[25] Among those, only two are currently on the market, rituximab and ofatumumab (Arzera®), both of which target the CD20 molecule on B cells. Rituximab, a chimeric monoclonal antibody (and occrelizumab its humanized version, when becomes available), is directed against CD20, a 297 amino acid, nonsecreted, membrane-associated phosphoprotein of 33–37 kD that is present on all B cells except stem cells, pro-B cells, and plasma cells.[25,26] Ofatumumab targets different CD20 epitopes because it binds both the small and the large loops of CD20 closer to B cell membrane. These agents cause depletion of circulating B cells either by complement lysis or apoptosis. Based on a number of reports (but not controlled studies), rituximab at 375 mg/m^2 once a week for four weeks, or 2 g (divided in two, 1 g each, biweekly infusions) has been effective in patients with MG and seems especially promising in MuSK-positive MG.[28] In a recent study, improvement was noted in up to 96% (25/26) of MuSK-MG patients and 81% (30/37) of AChR-MG. More robust and long-lasting response was noted in IgG1 and IgG4-mediated antibodies such as those seen against MuSK.[28] Controlled studies are needed. Follow-up infusions are needed usually after 6–12 months. The timing of the second infusion may be dictated by the reappearance of CD20$^+$CD27$^+$ memory B cells, which are directly involved with antibody production, and usually re-emerge after six to eight months.[25,28] Experience with the use of rituximab in anti-MAG neuropathies has shown that the expansions of CDR3 sequences of memory B cells eight months after the infusion may be predictors of response to therapy as the nonresponders appear to have higher load of IgM memory B cell expansions that persist after the first series of infusions.[29] Because in this study, a low efficiency to reduce B cell expansions was associated with poor clinical response, patients who do not respond after one full series of rituximab infusions (total 2 g) may potentially benefit from repeated therapy to further reduce the clonally related autoreactive B cells.[29]

Agents targeting complement

A monoclonal antibody against C_5 (eculizumab) inhibits C_5 and intercepts the formation of membranolytic attack complex and the subsequent generation of proinflammatory molecules.[17] Eculizumab, approved for paroxysmal hemoglobinuria, is a suitable drug to test in difficult MG cases because the pathogenic AchR antibodies are fixing complement at the end plate region.[30] A randomized, double blind, placebo-controlled, crossover, multicenter, phase II study of eculizumab in patients with refractory generalized myasthenia gravis has now shown that the drug was effective, albeit very expensive. Another very effective agent in inhibiting complement activation, as demonstrated *in vitro*, in animal models and in patients, is IVIg that inhibits complement uptake and intercepts the formation and deposition of MAC on the targeted tissues.[7,31] Although IVIg has multiple actions,[7] one of the most likely mechanisms of effectiveness in MG is probably via complement inhibition and inhibition of antibody binding to the endplate by supplying idiotypic antibodies.

Modulation of the Fc receptors

Even though MG is an antibody-mediated disease and macrophages do not play a role as final effector cells at the endplate region, Fc receptors are important because they determine antibody-mediated effector functions, complement activation and antibody-dependent cell-mediated cytotoxicity.[32] In antibody-mediated animal models of autoimmune diseases, the Fc-linked sugar moiety is a molecular switch shifting IgG activity to anti-inflammatory pathways. An agent that is known to have an effect on Fc receptors is IVIg. Sialic acid–rich IVIg suppresses inflammation by upregulating the inhibitory Fcγ RIIB receptors.[33] Normally, 1–2% of the IVIg has the sialic acid containing anti-inflammatory glycoform but enriching it enhances the anti-inflammatory effect by 20%.[33] This implies that new IVIg products engineered to have increased sialic acid within the Fc portion may be a more effective form of IVIg in MG. Fcγ RIIB receptor is also the main inhibitory receptor expressed on B cells that play a role in B cell tolerance and could be a future therapeutic target in MG patients.

Agents targeting cytokines and cytokine receptors

Available anti-TNF-α agents such as etanercept (Embrel®), infiximab (Remicade®), and atalimumab (Humira®) have been approved for rheumatoid arthritis because of their established benefit based on controlled trials. These agents, however, are not indicated in MG because they not only can activate the production of AChR antibodies, they also can trigger full-blown clinical myasthenia gravis.[34] Resolution of symptoms and reduction of antibodies ensues after discontinuation of these agents. Among other promising anticytokine agents that can be relevant as future treatment options in MG are the following:

1. Tocilizumab, an IL-6 receptor antagonist, which is promising in SLE[35] and is relevant in MG because IL-6 affects the induction of Treg cells to pathogenic Th1 cells.
2. Brodalumab and inekizumab, both monoclonal antibodies directed against IL-17, which have been recently shown to be effective in psoriasis.[36,37] This is a relevant therapeutic target in MG because the balance of T helper type 1 (Th1), Th2, Th17, and T_{reg} cell subsets of $CD4^+$ helper T cells are redistributed during the development of experimental MG, indicating that Th17 cells drive the autoimmune responses by secreting IL-17.[38] Further, IL-17 is increased in MG and, alone or with BAFF, controls the survival and proliferation of B cells and their differentiation into Ig-producing cells.[39]
3. Tofacitinib, an oral Janus kinase inhibitor, is directed against JAK1 and JAK3 tyrosine kinases that mediate signal transduction activity involving the surface receptors of multiple cytokines, including IL-2, -4, -7, -9, -15, and -21.[40,41] These cytokines are integral to lymphocyte activation, function, and proliferation. *In vitro*, tofacitinib inhibits interleukin-2–dependent differentiation of type 2 and type 17 helper T cells and attenuates signaling by proinflammatory cytokines, such as IL-6 and IFN-γ.[40,41] Blockade of the Janus kinases results in suppression of both T and B cells while maintaining regulatory T cell function. The drug, which has been shown to be effective in ulcerative colitis and rheumatoid arthritis,[40–42] may be also a good candidate agent for trials in MG.
4. GM-CSF selectively activates certain DC subsets and can suppress ongoing anti-AChR immune responses by mobilizing antigen-specific T_{reg} cells capable of suppressing autoimmune MG.[43]

Agents targeting cellular adhesion and T cell migration

In this category of drugs belong natalizumab and fingolimod. Natalizumab, directed against the $\alpha_4\beta_1$ integrin (VLA4) on leucocytes, a fundamental molecule for adhesion and transmigration of T cells, is approved for multiple sclerosis and Crohn's disease.[44] It is a very reasonable drug to try in difficult MG cases in new trials. The same applies for fingolimod, an anti-T cell migration agent that traps lymphocytes in the lymphoid organs. The drug approved for multiple sclerosis, can be also considered in MG trials.

Re-engineering of pathogenic antibodies (molecular decoys)

These are recombinant antibodies that block binding of circulating Abs and eliminate complement and cell-mediated cytotoxicity. Because they do not block all B cells or inhibit the universal complement pathway, they are ideal for antibody-mediated disorders like MG because they are nonpathogenic.[45,46]

It was recently shown that these antibodies act like molecular decoys preventing the development of neuromyelitis optica (NMO) lesions, mediated by aquaporin-4 (AQP-4) antibodies without toxicity. Such recombinant monoclonal antibodies were produced from clonally expanded plasma blasts derived from the CSF of NMO patients by introducing amino acid mutations into the IgG1Fc sequences to generate constructs deficient in complement and antibody-dependent cytotoxicity (CDC and ADCC). These antibodies exert their action by blocking the binding of circulating Abs, thereby eliminating CDC and ADCC, due to steric competition owing to their large physical size compared to the native AQP4. In the reported series, the mutated recombinant antibody rAb-53 blocked binding of the nonmutated rAb-53 antibody to AQP4 and prevented complement-dependent cytotoxicity and ADCC in NMO-IgG-exposed AQP4-expressing cells.[45,46] It also reduced the NMO-like lesions in a mouse brain model of NMO IgG.[45,46]

Conclusion

Monoclonal antibodies offer guarded optimism as potential future therapies in autoimmune neuromuscular diseases and MG. Exciting new agents and molecular decoys are in the offing for experimental therapies, while biomarkers (i.e., B cell expansions) may help predict the patients more likely to respond. There are, however, two major concerns, excessive cost and long-term safety, necessitating the need to establish efficacy only with controlled trials.

Conflicts of interest

The author has received speaking honoraria or consultation fee for serving on the Steering Committees for Baxter, Octapharma, Grifols, Novartis, Dysimmune Foundation and Therapath.

References

1. Engel, A.G. 2006. Acquired autoimmune myasthenia gravis. In *Myology*. A.G. Engel & C. Frankni-Armstrong, Eds.: 1769–1792. McGraw-Hill. New York.
2. Drachman, D.B. 2008. Therapy of myasthenia gravis. *Handb. Clin. Neurol.* **91:** 253–272
3. Vincent, A. & P. Rothwell. 2004. Myasthenia gravis. *Autoimmunity* **37:** 317–319.
4. Meriggioli, M.N. *et al.* 2008. Strategies for treating autoimmunity: novel insights from experimental myasthenia gravis. *Ann. N.Y. Acad. Sci.* **1132:** 276–282.
5. Sabatos-Peyton, C.A., J. Verhagen & D.C. Wraith. 2010. Antigen-specific immunotherapy of autoimmune and allergic diseases. *Curr. Opin. Immunol.* **22:** 609–615.
6. Sanders, D.B. & A. Evoli. 2010. Immunosuppressive therapies in myasthenia gravis. *Autoimmunity* **43:** 428–435.
7. Dalakas, M.C. 2010. Evidence-based efficacy of intravenous immunoglogulin in human myasthenia gravis and mechanisms of action. In *Myasthenia Gravis: Mechanisms of Disease and Immune intervention*. Premkumar Christadoss, Ed.: 89–102. Linus Publication Inc. New York.
8. Dalakas, M.C. 2004. The use of intravenous immunoglobulin in the treatment of autoimmune neurological disorders: evidence-based indications and safety profile. *Pharmacol. Therap.* **102:** 177–193.
9. Gajdos, P., S. Chevret & K. Toyka. 2008. Intravenous immunoglobulin for myasthenia gravis. *Cochrane Database Syst. Rev.* **23:** CD002277.
10. Aricha R *et al.* 2011. Blocking of IL-6 suppresses experimental autoimmune myasthenia gravis. *J. Autoimmun.* **36:** 135–141.
11. Masuda, M. *et al.* 2010. Clinical implication of peripheral CD4+CD25+ regulatory T cells and Th17 cells in myasthenia gravis patients. *J. Neuroimmunol.* **225:** 123–131.
12. Dalakas, M.C. 2011. Immunotherapy of inflammatory myopathies: practical approach and future prospects. *Curr. Treat. Options Neurol.* **13:** 311–323.
13. Dalakas, M.C. 2006. Therapeutic targets in patients with inflammatory myopathies: present approaches and a look to the future. *Neuromusc. Disord.* **16:** 223–236.
14. Gold, R., M.C. Dalakas & K.V. Toyka. 2003. Immunotherapy in autoimmune neuromuscular disorders. *Lancet Neurol.* **2:** 22–32.
15. Hohlfeld, R. & M.C. Dalakas. 2003. Basic principles of immunotherapy in neurological diseases. *Sem. Neurol.* **23:** 121–132.

16. Dalakas, M.C. 2008. Immunotherapy of myositis: issues, concerns future prospects *Nature Rev. Rheumatol.* **2010:** 129–137.
17. Dalakas, M.C. 2011. Advances in the diagnosis, pathogenesis and treatment of CIDP. *Nat. Rev. Neurol.* **7:** 507–517.
18. Tak, P.L. & J.R. Kalden. 2011. Advances in rheumatology: new targeted therapeutics. *Arthritis Res. Ther.* **25**(Suppl 1): S5.
19. Peterson, E.J. & G.A. Koretsky, 1999. Signal transduction in T lymphocytes. *Clin. Exp. Rheumatol.* **17:** 107–114.
20. Flynn, J.M. & J.C. Byrd. 2000. Campath-1H monoclonal antibody therapy. *Curr. Opin. Oncol.* **12:** 574–581.
21. The CAMMS223 Trial Investigators. 2008. Alemtuzumab vs. interferon Beta-1a in early multiple sclerosis. *N. Engl. J. Med.* **359:** 1786–1801.
22. Marsh, E.A. *et al.* 2010. Alemtuzumab in the treatment of IVIG-dependent chronic inflammatory demyelinating polyneuropathy. *J. Neurol.* **257:** 913–919
23. Tsokos, G.C. 2011. Systemic lupus erythematosus. *N. Engl. J. Med.* **365:** 2110–2121.
24. Wynn, D. et al . 2011. Daclizumab in active relapsing multiple sclerosis (CHOICE study): a phase 2, randomised, double-blind, placebo-controlled, add-on trial with interferon beta. *Lancet Neurol.* **9:** 381–390.
25. Dalakas, M.C. 2008. Inhibition of B cell, functions: implications for Neurology. *Neurology* **70:** 2252–2260
26. Dalakas, M.C. 2008. B cells as therapeutic targets in autoimmune neurological disorders. *Nat. Clin. Pract. Neurol.* **4:** 557–567.
27. Ragheb, S. 2008. A potential role for B-cell activating factor in the pathogenesis of autoimmune myasthenia gravis. *Arch. Neurol.* **65:** 1358–1362.
28. Díaz-Manera, J. *et al.* 2012. Long-lasting treatment effect of rituximab in MuSK myasthenia. *Neurology* **78:** 189–193.
29. Maurer, M.A. *et al.* 2012. Rituximab induces sustained reduction of pathogenic B cells in patients with peripheral nervous system autoimmunity. *J. Clin. Invest.* **122:** 1393–1402.
30. Tüzün, E., R. Huda & P. Christadoss. 2011. Complement and cytokine based therapeutic strategies in myasthenia gravis. *J. Autoimmun.* **37:** 136–143.
31. Basta, M. & M.C. Dalakas. 1994. High-dose intravenous immunoglobulin exerts its beneficial effect in patients with dermatomyositis by blocking endomysial deposition of activated complement fragments. *J. Clin. Invest.* **94:** 1729–1735.
32. Dhodapkar, K.M. *et al.* 2007. Selective blockade of the inhibitory Fcgamma receptor (FcgammaRIIB) in human dendritic cells and monocytes induces a type I interferon response program. *J. Exp. Med.* **204:** 1359–1369.
33. Anthony, R.M. *et al.* 2008. Recapitulation of IVIG anti-inflammatory activity with a recombinant IgG Fc. *Science* **320:** 373–376
34. Fee, D.B. & E.J. Kasarskis. 2009. Myasthenia gravis associated with etanercept therapy. *Muscle Nerve* **39:** 866–870.
35. Tsai, C.Y. *et al.* 2000. Increased excretions of beta2-microglobulin, IL-6, and IL-8 and decreased excretion of Tamm-Horsfall glycoprotein in urine of patients with active lupus nephritis. *Nephron* **85:** 207–214.

36. Papp, K.A. *et al.* 2012. Brodalumab, an anti-interleukin-17-receptor antibody for psoriasis. *N. Engl. J. Med.* **366:** 1181–1189.

37. Leonardi, C. *et al.* 2012. Anti-interleukin-17 monoclonal antibody ixekizumab in chronic plaque psoriasis. *N. Engl. J. Med.* **366:** 1190–1199.

38. Mu, L. *et al.* 2009. Disequilibrium of T helper type **1**, **2** and **17** cells and regulatory T cells during the development of experimental autoimmune myasthenia gravis. *Immunology* **10:** 1365–2567.

39. Roche, J.C. *et al.* 2011. Increased serum interleukin-17 levels in patients with Myasthenia gravis. *Muscle Nerve* 44: 278–280.

40. van Vollenhoven, R.F. *et al.* 2012. Tofacitinib or adalimumab versus placebo in rheumatoid arthritis. *N. Engl. J. Med.* 367: 508–519.

41. Fleischmann, R. *et al.* 2012. Placebo-controlled trial of to-facitinib monotherapy in rheumatoid arthritis. *N. Engl. J. Med.* 367: 495–507.

42. Sandborn, W.J. *et al.* 2012. Tofacitinib, an oral Janus kinase inhibitor, in active ulcerative colitis. *N. Engl. J. Med.* **367:** 616–624.

43. Sheng, J.R. *et al.* 2008. Regulatory T cells induced by GM-CSF suppress ongoing experimental myasthenia gravis. *Clin. Immunol.* 128: 172–180.

44. Wanda, Castro-Borrero *et al.* 2012 Current and emerging therapies in multiple sclerosis: a systematic review. *Ther. Adv. Neurol. Disord.* **5:** 205–220.

45. Tradtrantip, L. *et al.* 2012. Anti-aquaporin-4 monoclonal antibody blocker therapy for neuromyelitis optica. *Ann. Neurol.* **71:** 314–322.

46. Steinman, L. & S.S. Zamvil. 2012. Re-engineering of pathogenic aquaporin 4-specific antibodies as molecular decoys to treat neuromyelitis optica. *Ann. Neurol.* **71:** 287–288.

Ann. N.Y. Acad. Sci. ISSN 0077-8923

Myasthenogenicity of the main immunogenic region

Jon Lindstrom and Jie Luo

Department of Neuroscience, Medical School of the University of Pennsylvania, Philadelphia, Pennsylavania

Address for correspondence: Jon Lindstrom, Department of Neuroscience, Medical School of the University of Pennsylvania, 217 Stemmler Hall, Philadelphia, PA 19104-6074. JSLKK@mail.med.upenn.edu

In myasthenia gravis (MG) and experimental autoimmune MG (EAMG), many pathologically significant autoantibodies are directed to the main immunogenic region (MIR) of muscle nicotinic acetylcholine receptors (AChRs), a conformation-dependent region at the extracellular tip of $\alpha 1$ subunits of AChRs. Human muscle AChR $\alpha 1$ MIR sequences were integrated into *Aplesia* ACh-binding protein (AChBP). The chimera potently induced EAMG, while AChBP induced EAMG much less potently. AChBP is a water-soluble protein resembling the extracellular domain of AChRs; yet, rats immunized with chimeras developed autoantibodies to both extracellular and cytoplasmic domains of muscle AChRs. We propose that an initial autoimmune response directed at the MIR leads to an autoimmune response sustained by muscle AChRs. Autoimmune stimulation sustained by endogenous muscle AChR may be a target for specific immunosuppression. These studies show that the $\alpha 1$ MIR is highly myasthenogenic, and that AChR-like proteins distantly related to muscle AChR can induce EAMG and, potentially, MG.

Keywords: nicotinic acetylcholine receptor; AChR; MG; EAMG; antigenic structure

Introduction

The main immunogenic region (MIR) is a conformation-dependent region at the extracellular tip of muscle acetylcholine receptor (AChR) $\alpha 1$ subunits.[1–3] It is defined by the competitive binding of monoclonal antibodies (mAbs). It is the target of half or more of autoantibodies in myasthenia gravis (MG) and its animal model experimental autoimmune myasthenia gravis (EAMG). EAMG is typically induced by immunization with muscle-like AChRs from the electric organs of *Torpedo californica*;[2] mAbs to the MIR made from rats and mice with EAMG have all of the pathological activities of serum antibodies to AChRs: they can bind to the extracellular surface of muscle AChRs *in vivo*, fix complement causing focal lysis and the acute form of EAMG, cross-link muscle AChRs triggering their lysosomal destruction (antigenic modulation), and passively transfer EAMG.[1–3]

MIR chimeras

Detailed antigenic structure of the MIR was determined using chimeras of human $\alpha 1$ subunit sequence in *Aplysia californica* acetylcholine-binding protein (AChBP) and human $\alpha 7$ AChR.[3] All AChR subunits have homologous structures. The muscle-like AChRs of the electric organ of *T. californica* have five subunits organized like barrel staves in the order $\alpha 1$, γ, $\alpha 1$, δ, $\beta 1$ to form a central cation channel across the membrane whose opening is controlled by two ACh binding sites at the interfaces of $\alpha 1$ with γ and δ subunits.[4] AChBP has five identical subunits with five ACh binding sites at their interfaces.[5] AChBP resembles the extracellular structure of an AChR. AChBP subunits lack the transmembrane and cytoplasmic domains of AChR subunits, consequently AChBPs are soluble proteins. They are secreted by mollusk glia to modulate cholinergic signaling. There is no vertebrate homologue. Because AChBPs are water soluble, they are easy to crystallize, so their structure is known in great detail from X-ray crystallography.[5] AChBPs provide a model for the extracellular domains of AChRs and related receptors that are very difficult to crystallize.

Chimeras in which human $\alpha 1$ subunit sequences replace homologous parts of the AChBP protein insure that the $\alpha 1$ sequences assume conformations similar or identical to their conformation in native $\alpha 1$ subunits.[3] To make chimeras with AChBP or $\alpha 7$

doi: 10.1111/j.1749-6632.2012.06766.x

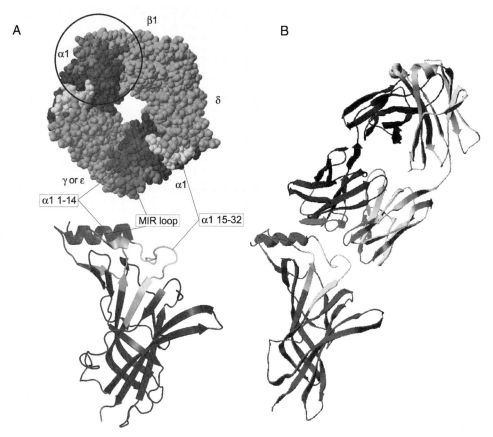

Figure 1. A model of the MIR α1(1–32, 60–81)/AChBP chimera and its interaction with an antibody to the MIR is shown. (A) MIR components are highlighted on a top view of the crystal structure of an *Aplysia* AChBP subunit.[6] Below, a front view ribbon diagram shows a single chimeric subunit. (B) The crystal structure of Fab 192[7] is accompanied by the structure of the mouse α1 extracellular domain.[8] Small differences in the sequences and conformation of the epitopes within the MIR profoundly influence the affinity with which antibodies are bound. The large size of bivalent IgG molecules with respect to the size of the MIR can result in competitive binding between different closely spaced epitopes within the MIR. The six hypervariable loops of the Fab, which form its antigen binding site are highlighted in cyan. This unusual mAb to the MIR does not appear to bind to the MIR loop per se, but competes for binding with mAbs that do. The Fab is angled to suggest this, but not actually docked on the subunit model. This is part of Figure 1 from Luo *et al.*[3]

AChRs that exhibited high affinity for four mAbs to the MIR derived from rats with EAMG and one mAb derived from a human with MG, it was necessary to include two α1 sequences: the N-terminal α helix (1–14) and the MIR loop (67–76).[3] The interaction between these two sequences accounts for the dependence of the antigenicity of the MIR on its native conformation. Some additional sequence was also required to provide additional components of the adjacent and overlapping epitopes that form the MIR or to permit its proper conformation in the chimera. The chimera α1 (1–30, 60–81)/AChBP exhibited K_D values for the mAbs of 0.075–2.5 nM and bound to serum autoantibodies from human,

canine, and feline MG patients.[3] The human MG mAb bound to native but unassembled human α1 subunits with a $K_D = 70$ nM, to assembled human muscle AChRs with a $K_D = 0.0068$ nM, and to the chimera with a $K_D = 0.075$ nM. Figure 1 depicts the structure of the chimera, a chimeric subunit, a model of the extracellular domain of the α1 subunit, and the structure of a Fab fragment of an MIR mAb.

Interaction between the N-terminal α helix and the MIR loop may be a critical step in the conformational maturation of AChR subunits that allows their assembly into mature AChRs. For example, α7 AChR subunits are efficiently synthesized in many cells, but their conformational maturation and consequent ability to assemble into mature AChRs depends on the chaperone Ric-3.[9] By contrast, $\alpha 1$ subunits efficiently mature in conformation. Replacing the N-terminal α helix of $\alpha 7$ with that of $\alpha 1$ prevented the expression of any mature $\alpha 7$ AChR, but replacing both the N-terminal α helix and the MIR loop of $\alpha 7$ with $\alpha 1$ increased expression of mature $\alpha 7$ AChRs on the cell surface 53-fold.[3] Deleting or mutating the N-terminal α helix of many types of AChR subunits prevents assembly of mature AChRs.[10] Mutations in or near the N-terminal α helix or MIR reduce expression of muscle AChRs causing myasthenic syndromes.[11]

Induction of EAMG

EAMG is usually induced by immunization of rats or mice with *Torpedo* electric organ AChR in adjuvant.[2] Syngeneic muscle AChR can also be used. There is an acute phase of weakness 7–10 days after immunization resulting from the sudden appearance of autoantibodies to AChRs. It begins when low levels of antibody are first present in the serum and bound to AChRs in muscle, is mediated by binding of complement to these antibodies and release of C3 fragments of complement that attract macrophages that disrupt the postsynaptic membrane, and ends when release of C3 is inhibited. There is a chronic phase of weakness starting about 30 days after immunization when high concentrations of autoantibodies develop in the serum and many of the AChRs in muscle are bound by antibodies. Then AChR loss is mediated by increased turnover due to endocytosis caused by cross-linking of the AChRs by antibody (termed antigenic modulation) and by focal lysis of the membrane due to complement cascades triggered by binding of antibodies. Complement-mediated disruption of synapse structure and the relationship between pre- and postsynaptic components further impairs synaptic transmission. Chronic EAMG closely resembles MG.

Denatured AChR is profoundly less potent at inducing EAMG than is native AChR, although repeated immunization with denatured $\alpha 1$ subunits can induce mild EAMG.[2,12] Passive immunization with MG patient autoantibodies or mAbs to the extracellular surface of muscle AChR can produce acute EAMG;[2] mAbs to the MIR are very potent at passively transferring EAMG.

Induction of EAMG with MIR chimeras

Female Lewis rats were immunized once at day 0 in TiterMax adjuvant at the base of the tail with *Torpedo* AChR, human $\alpha 1(1–32, 60–81)$/AChBP MIR chimera, or wild-type AChBP.[13]

Immunization with *Torpedo* AChR at a dose of 11 μg produced acute EAMG in 4/6 and fatal chronic EAMG in 6/6 rats.[13] The higher dose of 33 μg produced acute EAMG in 5/6 and chronic EAMG in 6/6, fatal in 5/6. Immunization with the MIR chimera produced acute EAMG in 3/6 at 11 μg, 5/6 at 33 μg, and 6/6 at 100 μg.[13] These doses of the chimera produced chronic EAMG in 3/6, 6/6, and 6/6 and fatalities in 2/6, 2/6, and 5/6. Thus, the MIR chimera potently induced EAMG, though this one small part of a single muscle-like AChR subunit was not quite as potent as native *Torpedo* AChR. Immunization with wild-type AChBP was much less potent than the MIR chimera, producing no acute EAMG, and producing EAMG slowly and less severely.[13] Chronic EAMG was 0/6 at 11 μg, 1/6 at 33 μg, and 3/6 at 100 μg with one fatality. The remarkable thing is that such a distantly related protein was able to induce EAMG at all. This implies that distantly related AChR-like proteins could, in principle, induce MG.

Properties of the antibodies induced

Immunization with *Torpedo* AChR produced large titers of antibody to itself after 120 days (750 nM at 11 μg and 2,500 nM at 33 μg) but virtually none to the MIR chimera or to AChBP.[13] It produced low levels to human muscle AChR (13 and 87 nM) and rat muscle AChR (1.4 and 13 nM).

Immunization with the MIR chimera produced substantial titers to the *Torpedo* AChR (550–750 nM).[13] The MIR cross-reacts relatively well between species, and the chimera has five $\alpha 1$ MIRs, whereas *Torpedo* AChR has two $\alpha 1$ MIRs, thus the chimera was more potent at making antibodies to *Torpedo* AChR than vice versa. The high intrinsic immunogenicity of the $\alpha 1$ MIR was demonstrated by the very high titers induced to the chimera (4,000–6,000 nM), as compared to AChBP (1,700–2,700 nM). The chimera also induced high titers to human muscle AChR (100–300 nM) and rat muscle AChR (18–55 nM). Immunization with AChBP produced very low titers to *Torpedo* AChR (≤ 67 nM), human muscle AChR (≤ 21 nM), or rat muscle AChR (≤ 2 nM).[13] Moderate titers induced to itself ($\leq$2,000 nM) or the chimera ($\leq$2,100 nM) emphasize the high intrinsic immunogenicity of the MIR.

All of the groups that developed EAMG developed similarly high titers to human AChR cytoplasmic domains, while those groups that did not develop EAMG developed no titers to cytoplasmic domains.[13] Since AChBP and the chimera have no cytoplasmic domains, the antibodies to cytoplasmic antibodies produced after immunization with these must be in response to rat muscle AChRs exposed to the immune system through disruption of the postsynaptic membrane by the autoimmune response to the MIR or other surface epitopes on the AChBP. The high levels of antibodies to cytoplasmic domains indicate that endogenous AChR stimulates a robust autoimmune response once EAMG is initiated. Immunization with the whole extracellular domain of human α1 subunits expressed in bacteria was very weak at inducing EAMG because it lacks a native conformation (500 μg initiated EAMG in only 7/24 rats), but all those rats that did develop EAMG developed antibodies to cytoplasmic domains.[14] Accounting for the fraction of α1 extracellular sequence used in the chimera and the dose necessary to produce EAMG in all of the immunized rats, the MIR/AChBP chimera is at least 200-fold more myasthenogenic than the bacteria-expressed α1 extracellular domain, providing an estimate of the benefit of expressing the α1 MIR in a nearly native conformation in an AChBP chimera.

Autoimmune stimulation by endogenous muscle AChR (as proven to occur by induction of antibodies to cytoplasmic domains by immunization with extracellular domains)[13,14] may be important for sustaining the autoimmune response in EAMG after the response to the initiating immunogen wanes. Evidence for this is a continued increase in the concentration of serum antibodies to rat muscle AChR 30 days following the initial immunization with electric organ AChR, a time when the concentration of antibodies to electric organ AChRs decreases.[15] Endogenous autoimmunization may also be important for sustaining MG. Specific immunosuppressive therapy of EAMG can be achieved by treatment for five weeks after the acute phase with a mixture of bacterially expressed human muscle AChR subunit cytoplasmic domains.[16] The mechanism of this therapy may involve antibody feedback, diversion, or other mechanisms. The target of this therapy may be the process of endogenous autostimulation of the response to muscle AChR, rather than suppression of the response to the initial immunogen.[13]

Antibodies from rats immunized with AChBP, the MIR chimera, or *Torpedo* AChR did not cross-react with human α3, α4, or α7 AChRs.[13] *Aplysia* AChBP has 20% sequence identity with α1, 23% with α3, and 24% with α7. Much of the antibody to α1 AChRs induced by AChBP may be a result of autostimulation by muscle AChRs subsequent to very limited initial cross-reaction. Lack of response to α3, α4, and α7 may reflect their lower antigenicity, immunogenicity, amount, concentration, or access to serum antibodies. Autonomic ganglia α3 AChRs can be the target of an antibody-mediated autoimmune attack, showing that they are accessible and vulnerable.[17] Muscle α1 AChRs may be intrinsically more vulnerable as a result of intrinsic immunogenicity of the MIR, the large amounts of AChR per synapse, their density in the synapse, or other factors.

Conclusions

The α1 MIR is a potent immunogen that can efficiently induce EAMG and be a primary target of the autoimmune response. AChBP chimeras are excellent as immunogens and antigens for conformation-dependent AChR epitopes. Proteins distantly related to muscle AChRs, such as AChBP, can induce EAMG. Thus, such proteins from microbial or other sources could, in principle, trigger MG. An autoimmune response to epitopes on the extracellular surface of muscle AChR results in high levels of autoimmune response to AChR cytoplasmic domains when EAMG is induced. This "epitope spreading" indicates that the autoimmune response to AChRs in EAMG, and perhaps MG, is sustained by muscle AChRs. This autostimulation by muscle AChRs may be a target for specific immunosuppression of EAMG or MG.

Acknowledgments

This research was supported by Grants from the NIH (NS11323 and NS052463) and the Muscular Dystrophy Association.

Conflicts of interest

The authors declare no conflicts of interest.

References

1. Tzartos, S. & J. Lindstrom. 1980. Monoclonal antibodies used to probe acetylcholine receptor structure: localization of the main immunogenic region and detection of similarities between subunits. *Proc. Natl. Acad. Sci. USA* **77:** 755–759.

2. Lindstrom, J. 2000. Acetylcholine receptors and myasthenia. *Muscle Nerve* **23:** 453–477.

3. Luo, J., P. Taylor, M. Losen, *et al.* 2009. Main immunogenic region structure promotes binding of conformation-dependent myasthenia gravis autoantibodies, nicotinic acetylcholine receptor conformation maturation, and agonist sensitivity. *J. Neurosci.* **29:** 13898–13908.

4. Unwin, N. 2005. Refined structure of the nicotinic acetylcholine receptor at 4Å resolution. *J. Mol. Biol.* **346:** 967–989.

5. Brejc, K., W. van Dyk, R. Klassen, *et al.* 2001. Crystal structure of an ACh-binding protein reveals the ligand-binding domain of nicotinic receptors. *Nature* **411:** 269–276.

6. Hansen, S., G. Sulzenbacher, T. Huxford, *et al.* 2005. Structures of *Aplysia* AChBP complexes with nicotinic agonists and antagonists reveal distinctive binding interfaces and conformations. *EMBO J.* **24:** 3635–3646.

7. Kontou, M., D. Leonidas, E. Vatzaki, *et al.* 2000. The crystal structure of the Fab fragment of a rat monoclonal antibody against the main immunogenic region of the human muscle acetylcholine receptor. *Eur. J. Biochem.* **267:** 2389–2397.

8. Delisanti, C., Y. Yao, J. Stroud, *et al.* 2007. Crystal structure of the extracellular domain of nAChR α1 bound to αbungarotoxin at 1.94 Å resolution. *Nature Neurosci.* **10:** 953–962.

9. Millar, N. 2008. RIC-3: a nicotinic acetylcholine receptor chaperone. *Brit. J. Pharmacol.* **153:** S177–S183.

10. Castillo, M., J. Mulet, M. Aldea, *et al.* 2009. Role of the N-terminal α helix in biogenesis of α7 nicotinic receptors. *J. Neurochem.* **108:** 1399–1409.

11. Engel, A.G., X.M. Shen, D. Selcen & S.M. Sine. 2010. What we have learned from congenital myasthenic syndromes. *J. Mol. Neuroscience* **40:** 143–153.

12. Lindstrom, J., B. Einarson & J. Merlie. 1978. Immunization of rats with polypeptide chains from Torpedo acetylcholine receptor causes an autoimmune response to receptors in rat muscle. *Proc. Natl. Acad. Sci. USA* **75:** 769–773.

13. Luo, J. & J. Lindstrom. 2012. Myasthenogenicity of the main immunogenic region and endogenous muscle nicotinic acetylcholine receptors. *Autoimmunity* **45:** 245–252.

14. Feferman, T., S.H. Im, S. Fuchs & M.C. Souroujon. 2003. Breakage of tolerance to hidden cytoplasmic epitopes of the acetylcholine receptor in experimental autoimmune myasthenia gravis. *J. Neuroimmunol.* **140:** 153–158.

15. Lindstrom, J., V. Lennon, M. Seybold & S. Whittingham. 1976. Experimental autoimmune myasthenia gravis and myastheniagravis: biochemical and immunochemical aspects. *Ann. N. Y. Acad. Sci.* **274:** 254–274.

16. Luo, J., A. Kuryatov & J. Lindstrom. 2010. Specific immunotherapy of experimental myasthenia gravis by a novel mechanism. *Ann. Neurology* **67:** 441–451.

17. Vernino, S., J. Lindstrom, S. Hopkins, *et al.* 2008. Characterization of ganglionic acetylcholine receptor autoantibodies. *J. Neuroimmunology* **197:** 63–69.

Ann. N.Y. Acad. Sci. ISSN 0077-8923

ANNALS OF THE NEW YORK ACADEMY OF SCIENCES
Issue: *Myasthenia Gravis and Related Disorders*

Structure of the neuromuscular junction: function and cooperative mechanisms in the synapse

Masaharu Takamori

Neurological Center, Kanazawa-Nishi Hospital and Kanazawa University, Kanazawa, Japan

Address for correspondence: Masaharu Takamori, M.D., Neurological Center, Kanazawa-Nishi Hospital, 6–15-41, Ekinishi-Honmachi, Kanazawa, Japan 920-0025. m-takamori@vanilla.ocn.ne.jp

As an overview of the structure of the neuromuscular junction, three items are described focusing on cooperative mechanisms involving the synapse and leading to muscle contraction: (1) presynaptic acetylcholine release regulated by vesicle cycling (exocytosis and endocytosis); the fast-mode of endocytosis requires a large influx of external Ca^{2+} and is promoted by the activation of G protein–coupled receptors and receptor tyrosine kinases; (2) postsynaptic acetylcholine receptor clustering mediated by the muscle-specific, Dok7-stimulated tyrosine kinase (MuSK) through two signaling mechanisms: one via agrin-Lrp4-MuSK (Ig1/2 domains) and the second via Wnt-MuSK (Frizzled-like cysteine-rich domain)-adaptor Dishevelled; Wnts/MuSK and Lrp4 direct a retrograde signal to presynaptic differentiation; (3) muscle contractile machinery regulated by Ca^{2+}-release and Ca^{2+}-influx channels, including the depolarization-activated ryanodine receptor-1 and the receptor- and/or store-operated transient receptor potential canonical. The first mechanism is dysfunctional in Lambert–Eaton myasthenic syndrome, the second in anti-acetylcholine receptor-negative myasthenia gravis (MG), and the third in thymoma-associated MG.

Keywords: neuromuscular junction; calcium channel; acetylcholine receptor; muscle-specific tyrosine kinase (MuSK); Wnt; transient receptor potential canonical (TRPC)

Introduction

Acetylcholine (ACh)-mediated signal transduction in the neuromuscular junction (NMJ) depends on coordinated interaction between the presynaptic active and periactive zones where synaptic vesicle exocytosis followed by endocytosis takes place, and the postsynaptic differentiation where ACh receptors (AChRs) are clustered by cytoskeletal dynamics centered on muscle-specific tyrosine kinase (MuSK). Synaptic signals are electrically and then chemically conducted to the highly specialized skeletal muscle where Ca^{2+}-mediated muscle contraction ensues. Retrograde signals from muscle to nerve participate in presynaptic differentiation. The various components of these regulated interactions include cooperative mechanisms to compensate for synaptic and contractile fatigue in normal state. These components, however, are immunologically targeted in Lambert–Eaton myasthenic syndrome

(LEMS), myasthenia gravis (MG), and thymoma-associated MG.

Synaptic vesicle cycling: exocytosis and two modes of endocytosis

At the presynaptic active zone and periactive zone, exocytosis and endocytosis operate on synaptic vesicle cycling. For exocytosis, synaptotagmins (1 and 2) participate in the evoked, synchronous ACh release by binding Ca^{2+}; complexin is required to clamp SNARE complexes (synaptobrevin, syntaxin, and SNAP-25), thereby positioning SNARE complexes for subsequent synaptotagmin action.[1] Another Ca^{2+}-binding protein, slow Ca^{2+} sensor, participates in spontaneous, asynchronous ACh release.[1] The endocytosis takes place through two modes of synaptic vesicle retrieval: one is the conventional slow, clathrin-dependent retrieval that operates at the intracellular Ca^{2+} concentration, which is much lower than that which

doi: 10.1111/j.1749-6632.2012.06784.x

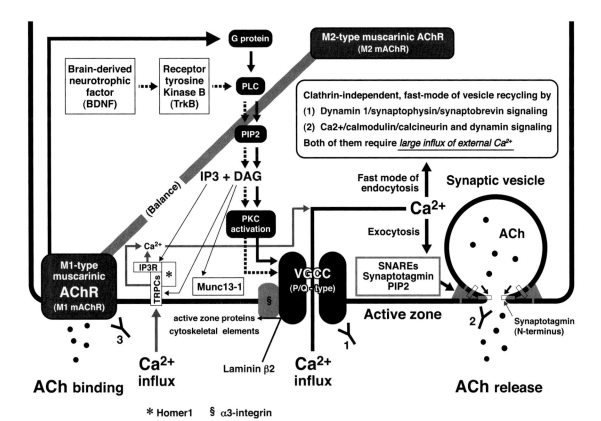

Figure 1. Presynaptic structure and targets of antibodies in Lambert–Eaton myasthenic syndrome. Signaling pathways modulate Ca^{2+} channels associated with exocytic and endocytic machineries, where synaptotagmins act as Ca^{2+} sensors and potentially compensate for defective acetylcholine (ACh) release. The compensatory mechanisms are triggered by M1 mAChR activation/BDNF-TrkB interaction leading to P/Q-type voltage-gated Ca^{2+} channel (VGCC) and non–voltage gated Ca^{2+} channels (transient receptor potential canonical, TRPCs) via the PLC-mediated signaling cascade. M1 mAChR maintains balance with M2 mAChR, which functions as an inhibitor of ACh release under physiological conditions. When neuromuscular transmission is defective, the balance between M1 and M2 mAChRs shifts in favor of M1 mAChR, and the compensatory mechanisms promote a large influx of external Ca^{2+} for the Ca^{2+}-triggered exocytosis and the fast-mode of endocytosis in clathrin-independent manners (1 and 2 shown in the figure). TRPCs also play a role in Ca^{2+} influx by way of IP3-IP3R interaction triggered by PLC-generated IP3-binding and followed by dissociation of TRPCs-Homer1-IP3R. ACh release upregulation can also be provided by the regulation of synaptic vesicle priming protein, Munc 13–1, by PLC-generated DAG, and by the stabilization of active zone structure by muscle-derived laminin β2–mediated retrograde signal. M1 mAChR, M1-type muscarinic acetylcholine receptor; BDNF, brain-derived neurotrophic factor; TrkB, receptor tyrosine kinase B; PLC, phospholipase C; PIP2, phosphatidylinositol 4,5-bisphosphate; DAG, diacylglycerol; PKC, protein kinase C; IP3, inositol triphosphate; IP3R, IP3 receptor; SNAREs, synaptobrevin, syntaxin and SNAP-25. Y marks indicate the targets of Lambert–Eaton myasthenic syndrome antibodies: (Y1), P/Q-type VGCC; (Y2) synaptotagmin (extracellularly exposed segment during exocytosis); (Y3) M1 mAChR.

triggers exocytosis; and the other is a fast, clathrin-independent retrieval.[2,3] The fast-mode of endocytosis operates by promoting recruitment of dynamin 1, synaptophysin, and synaptobrevin,[4,5] or by Ca^{2+}/calmodulin/calcineurin/dynamin signaling (endocytosis overshoot);[6] both of these mechanisms require a large influx of external Ca^{2+} (Fig. 1). Although the molecular basis of vesicle retrieval (including kiss-and-run recycling[7] and bulk endocy-

tosis[8]) remains debated, the synapse may use these two alternative or cooperative modes as an adaptive response to synaptic fatigue. The influx of external Ca^{2+} required for the Ca^{2+}-triggered exocytosis and the fast-mode of endocytosis is promoted by the activation of presynaptic M1-type muscarinic AChR (M1 mAChR)[9] as well as the interaction of brain-derived neurotrophic factor (BDNF) with receptor tyrosine kinase B (TrkB).[10]

They share a common pathway mediated by phospholipase C (PLC)-phosphatidylinositol 4,5-bisphosphate (PIP2)-diacylglycerol (DAG)-protein kinase C (PKC), leading to the modulation of P/Q-type voltage-gated Ca^{2+} channel (VGCC)[9,10] (Fig. 1). The influx of external Ca^{2+} is also promoted by the activation of non-VGCC (transient receptor potential canonical: TRPCs 3, 6, and 7) via PLC-generated PIP2/DAG[11] (Fig. 1). The TR-PCs may play an additional role in Ca^{2+} influx by way of inositol 1,4,5-triphosphate (IP3)-IP3 receptor (IP3R) interactions triggered by PLC-generated IP3-binding. This allows the TRPC-mediated Ca^{2+} influx to be free from inhibitory control by the scaffolding protein Homer1[12] (Fig. 1). Also, the PLC-generated DAG regulates vesicle priming protein, Munc13–1, to recruit ACh-containing vesicles for immediately releasable pool[13] (Fig. 1). In the skeletal NMJ, the M1 mAChR maintains balance with the M2 mAChR, which exists intracellularly and functions as a protein kinase A (PKA)-mediated inhibitor of ACh release under physiological conditions[9] (Fig. 1). This balance is modulated by ATP coreleased with ACh at the NMJ[14] and TrkB.[15] However, when neuromuscular transmission is defective, the balance between them shifts in favor of the M1 mAChR,[15,16] partly because of an M2 mAChR-mediated switch from PKA to PKC activation.[17]

The M1 mAChR is expressed in the mammalian peripheral nerve terminal and has an extracellularly exposed segment which could be accessible to antibodies.[18,19] It is proven that pharmacologically, AChR quantal release is enhanced by M1 mAChR activation via the activation of PKC and P/Q-type VGCC in voltage-clamped preparations of adult mouse muscle,[17] and also that the M1 mAChR is physiologically associated with TRPC-mediated Ca^{2+} influx.[20]

In view of these observations, we studied serum samples from LEMS patients by immunoblotting sera against human M1 mAChR fusion protein. We found that M1 mAChR antibodies were detected in 14 of 20 anti-P/Q-type VGCC-positive patients (70%) and in all five anti-P/Q-type VGCC-negative patients diagnosed with LEMS on a clinical basis and with electromyography; 10 anti-M1 mAChR-positive patients, 9 of whom were also positive for P/Q-type VGCC antibodies, which were associated with small-cell lung carcinoma.[21,22] Serum IgG from a patient positive for M1 mAChR anti-bodies but negative for antibodies against both P/Q-type VGCC and synaptotagmin1 produced electrophysiological features of LEMS in mice (reduced ACh quantal contents by microelectrode study).[22] The compensatory mechanism that activates M1 mAChR and modulates the fast-mode of synaptic vesicle recycling may frequently be restricted by coincident M1 mAChR antibodies in LEMS.[21,22]

Potential mechanisms that compensate for the presynaptic defect(s), such as that in LEMS include (1) a shift in dependence of ACh quantal release from the P/Q-type to other types of VGCC;[23] (2) the muscle-derived synaptic organizer laminin β2 tethering of P/Q- and N-type VGCCs and α3 integrin to the presynaptic active zone (including Bassoon, Piccolo, CAST/Erc2, and RIM1/2) and cytoskeletal elements (including spectrins, plectin1, AHNAK/desmoyokin, dystrophin, and myosin1), thereby stabilizing the active zone structure for transmitter release[24,25] (Fig. 1); and (3) RIM protein (Rab3 effectors) tethering of N- and P/Q-type VGCCs to the active zone, thereby enabling fast, synchronous triggering of transmitter release.[26]

Acetylcholine receptor clustering centered on MuSK and regulated by agrin/Lrp4 and Wnt signaling

In the postsynaptic membrane of the NMJ, AChRs aggregate at the crests of the junctional folds where they are clustered and stabilized by scaffolding components,[27] including the anchoring protein rapsyn. Rapsyn is immobilized by MuSK-linked heat-shock proteins[28,29] and contributes to MuSK-induced phosphorylation of AChR subunits.[30] MuSK is stimulated from "inside" the muscle cell by an adaptor protein Dok7[31,32] and from the "outside" by the low-density lipoprotein receptor-related protein 4 (Lrp4, agrin receptor) with and without agrin;[33–35] MuSK thereby contributes to AChR stabilization and clustering through various intracellular kinase cascades[27] (Fig. 2). Approximately 80% of MG patients have AChR antibodies; a proportion of anti-AChR-negative MG patients have antibodies against MuSK[36] and Lrp4.[37–39]

In addition to its interaction with agrin/Lrp4 signaling, MuSK contains the receptor for Wnts, which belong to a family of secreted glycoproteins.[27,40] There are 19 different Wnts in mice and humans, and recent studies highlight their involvement in critical aspects of NMJ function and

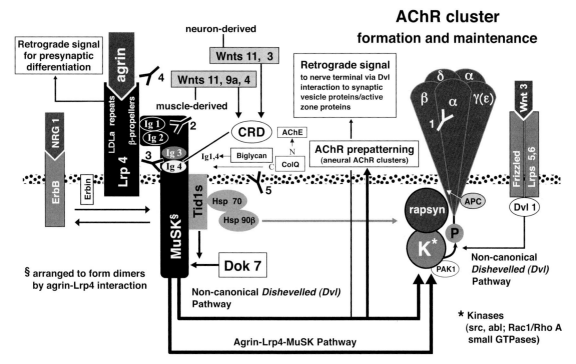

Figure 2. Postsynaptic structure and targets of antibodies in myasthenia gravis. Biosignals, centered on MuSK, contribute to AChR clustering and nerve terminal functions. MuSK is stimulated by Dok7; Dok7-binding to MuSK is regulated by Tid1s. The interacting sites of MuSK with the signals contributive to AChR clustering are the Ig1/2 domains for agrin-Lrp4 signaling, and the Frizzled-like cysteine-rich domain (CRD, Ig4 domain) for Wnt-noncanonical Dishevelled (Dvl) signaling. Small GTPase effector PAK1 serves as a bridge molecule linking two signalings. Lrp4 interacts with agrin at 3 of 8 low-density lipoprotein a (LDLa) repeats and at the first of 4 β-propeller domains on one hand, and with the MuSK Ig1 domain on the other hand. The neuron-derived Wnts11 and 3 and the muscle-derived Wnts11, 9a, and 4 contribute to AChR clustering. Wnts provide the signals to the noncanonical Dvl at agrin-independent (for AChR prepatterning) and agrin-dependent stages. Since it is not confirmed whether the Wnt3 receptor would be MuSK CRD or the Frizzled receptor, coreceptors of which are Lrps 5 and 6 (depicted in right edge), two possible pathways are depicted in the figure. The AChR clusters are formed and maintained at the postsynaptic membrane by rapsyn (stabilized by Tid1s via heat-shock proteins, Hsps 70 and 90β), collagen Q (ColQ: C-terminus interacts with MuSK; N-terminus interacts with acetylcholinesterase, AChE), and biglycan (interacts with the MuSK Ig1 domain and the MuSK Ig4 domain, CRD). Erbin is required for the crosstalk between the agrin-Lrp4 signaling and the neuregulin1 (NRG1)-ErbB receptor kinase signaling (depicted in left edge). Adenomatous poliposis coli (APC) acts as a Wnt downstream effector and participates in the agrin-induced AChR clustering. Wnts play a role in presynaptic ACh release by their retrograde signals acting on synaptic vesicle proteins and active zone proteins via Dvl. Muscle Lrp4 directs a retrograde signal to presynaptic differentiation. Lrp4, low-density lipoprotein receptor-related protein 4; Tid1s, tumorous imaginal disc-1, short form. Y marks indicate the targets of MG antibodies: (Y1) AChR α-subunit; (Y2) MuSK Ig1/2 domains; (Y3) MuSK CRD; (Y4) Lrp4; (Y5) interaction between MuSK and Collagen Q.

structure.[27,40] Wnts are either released from neurons and transported across the synapse by exosome-like, Evi (Evenness/Interrupted/Wntless/Sprinter)-containing vesicles requiring Rab11, syntaxin1A, and myosin5,[41] or are derived from muscle.[42,43] Wnts11[27,42] (similar to zebrafish Wnt11[44]), 9a[42], 4[43], and 3[45] bind to MuSK and contribute to AChR clustering via the pathway mediated by the non-canonical Dishevelled (Dvl, planar cell polarity) pathway (Fig. 2). It has not been confirmed whether the Wnt3 receptor is MuSK or the Wnt recep-

tor, Frizzled, but there is an extracellular similarity for both of them, and both contain a cysteine-rich domain (CRD)[27,40,42,45,46] (Fig. 2). Dvl is expressesd in skeletal muscles, interacts with kinase domains of MuSK independent of agrin, is increased in denervated muscles, and is essential for the noncanonical Wnt signaling cascade.[27,40,46] Reportedly, the reduced agrin-mediated AChR clustering by muscle-derived Wnt3a is mediated via the canonical Dvl pathway to β-catenin causing reduced rapsyn expression,[47] suggesting that this negative regulation maintains balance with the positive regulator neuron-derived Wnt3 and thereby helps to sculpt the mature synaptic architecture.[40,45,48]

In the MuSK ectodomain, its first and second immunoglobulin-like domains (Ig1/2) mediate agrin-Lrp4 signaling[49](via the MuSK Ig1 domain interacting with Lrp4, which forms tetrameric signaling complexes by dimerization of two agrin-Lrp4 binary complexes[50,51]), while its CRD (Ig4 domain) mediates the Wnt-Dvl signaling[52] (Fig. 2). The biosignal for AChR clustering by Wnts11 and 9a requires Lrp4 but not agrin;[42] the Wnt4-activated signal requires neither agrin nor Lrp4.[43] Wnt3 promotes the agrin/Lrp4-induced clustering of AChR.[45] Lrp4 is required for AChR clustering in association with MuSK and Wnts at both the agrin-independent (noninnervated) stage to form AChR microclusters (AChR prepatterning to form clusters in the central part of muscle and to guide incoming axons[44]) and the agrin-dependent (innervated) stage to form full-sized clusters of AChR.[27,33–35,45] Lrp4 is also believed to serve in muscle as a Wnt coreceptor in addition to functioning as the agrin receptor.[42,52] Disruption of the MuSK-Dvl interaction inhibits agrin/MuSK-induced AChR clustering.[46] Therefore, the Wnt-Dvl signaling via MuSK CRD contributes to AChR clustering in collaboration with the MuSK Ig1/2-mediated agrin-Lrp4 signaling in the NMJ. MuSK, Dvl, and small GTPase effector PAK1 (p21-activated kinase 1) form a ternary complex required for AChR clustering in muscle.[27,40,46] (Fig. 2).

Using the recombinant proteins expressed in HEK293F cells as antigens, we detected MuSK Ig1/2 antibodies in the serum samples from 33 of 43 anti-AChR-negative MG patients; 10 of these patients (30%) were additionally positive for MuSK CRD antibodies and therefore suspected of being involved in impairment of the Wnt-MuSK interaction. Although no statistical correlation was noted between the antibody specificity and clinical features in these 33 MG patients, the heterogeneity of MuSK antibodies in their binding to functional domains of MuSK suggests a diversity to MuSK-implicated pathophysiology in MG.

The inhibited MuSK-Dvl interaction decreases the frequency of spontaneous synaptic currents (SSCs) in association with the decreased SSC amplitude, suggesting a defect in ACh release upregulation, which may reflect retrograde Wnt-MuSK (CRD)-Dvl signaling at the nerve terminal[40,46]

(Fig. 2). The antibody-induced disturbance in bidirectional Wnt signaling via MuSK CRD may, at least in part, be compatible with presynaptic abnormalities including the absence of ACh release upregulation to compensate for postsynaptic failure found in anti-MuSK-positive MG patients[53] and animal models.[54–58] Also, the muscle Lrp4 (independent of MuSK and agrin) regulates presynaptic differentiation, including synaptic vesicles and active zones in addition to its pivotal role in postsynaptic AChR clustering via MuSK; Lrp4 in motoneurons is dispensable for NMJ formation when Lrp4 is available from muscles.[59,60] This evidence may also be worth investigating if Lrp4 antibodies reported in MG[37–39] could cause both post- and presynaptic dysfunctions contributing to disease severity.

Reportedly, biglycan, an extracellular matrix protein that is selectively enriched in postsynaptic membranes, interacts with the two domains of MuSK (Lrp4-reactive Ig1 domain and Wnt-reactive CRD) at the junctional region and participates in synapse stabilization, including MuSK, AChR clusters, and acetylcholinesetase.[61] Biglycan stabilization appears similar to provided by Collagen Q,[62] whose interaction with MuSK is interfered with at the C terminus by MuSK antibodies[63] (Fig. 2). Erbin also interacts with MuSK and is essential for the crosstalk between agrin-MuSK and neuregulin1-ErbB receptor kinases signaling pathways that both contribute to AChR clustering[64,65] (Fig. 2). The transmembrane dystroglycan complex participates in the agrin-laminin (α4, α5, and β2)-rapsyn signaling cascade, which helps stabilize AChR clusterings in collaboration with MuSK-mediated signals.[66] Adenomatous polyposis coli (APC), a component of the β-catenin degradation complex, acts as a Wnt downstream effector and participates in agrin-induced AChR clustering, thereby contributing to agrin- and Wnt-mediated signaling pathways.[40,67]

Calcium-release and calcium-influx channels involved in muscle contractile machinery: ryanodine receptor-1 and TRPC

MG-associated thymoma expresses antigens that trigger antibody responses, which play a part in disease generation and modification. Antibodies against the ryanodine receptor-1 (RyR1), which physically interacts with the dihydropyridine

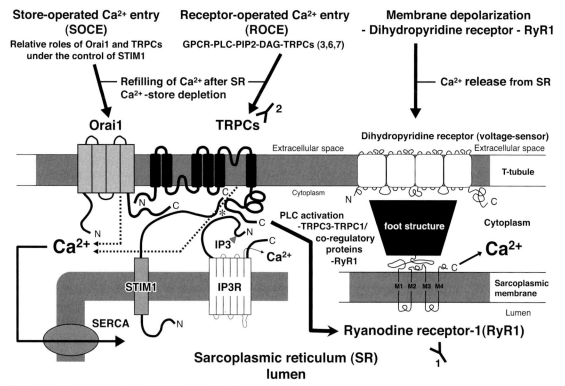

* Homer 1 (forms a complex with TRPCs and IP3R)

Figure 3. Pivotal organization for Ca^{2+}-mediated muscle contraction and targets of antibodies in thymoma-associated MG. RyR1 interacts voltage dependently with dihydropyridine receptor (DHPR) in the T-tubular membrane, thereby triggering sarcoplasmic Ca^{2+} release for the excitation–contraction coupling (right). Non–voltage gated Ca^{2+} influx channels are termed TRPCs. TRPC3 is activated by phospholipase C (PLC)–mediated signaling and engages with RyR1 via the triadic bridging complex (TRPC1 and possibly coregulatory proteins) to cause Ca^{2+} release from the sarcoplasmic reticulum (SR) (bold and crooked arrow from middle to lower right) in collaboration with the voltage-dependent, DHPR-mediated signaling. Three mechanisms act on refilling Ca^{2+} after depletion of sarcoplasmic Ca^{2+}: (1) receptor-operated Ca^{2+} entry (ROCE) via the PLC-phosphatidylinositol 4,5-bisphosphate (PIP2)-diacylglycerol (DAG) signaling pathway acting on the TRPCs 3, 6, 7 (middle); (2) store-operated Ca^{2+} entry (SOCE) regulated by relative roles of Orai1 and TRPCs under the control of STIM1 (Ca^{2+} sensor) (left) (dotted lines with arrows); (3) SOCE through TRPCs after the inositol triphosphate (IP3)–IP3 receptor (IP3R) interaction triggered by PLC-generated IP3-binding, followed by dissociation of the TRPCs-Hormer1 (* in figure)–IP3R complex, which allows STIM1 access to gate open TRPCs (lower middle). GPCR, G protein–coupled receptors; Orai1, Ca^{2+} release–activated Ca^{2+} messenger-1; STIM1, stromal interaction molecule-1 (Ca^{2+} sensor); SERCA, sarcoplasmic/endoplasmic reticulum Ca^{2+}ATPase. Y marks indicate the targets of antibodies detected in thymoma-associated MG: (Y1) RyR1; (Y2) TRPC3.

receptor (DHPR: voltage sensor) in the T-tubular membrane, impair sarcoplasmic Ca^{2+} release, and thereby cause muscle contractile weakness[68] (Fig. 3). Our search for RyR1 epitopes in 25 MG patients[68] showed that residues 4997–5017 (C-terminal transmembrane segment, which is expressed in thymoma epithelial cells and is suspected of inducing breakdown in tolerance to RyR1[69]) and residues 5019–5038 (C-terminal tail which protrudes into cytoplasm outside the sarcoplasmic reticulum and can form a functional Ca^{2+} release channel[70]) were pre-dominantly recognized by antibodies (64% antibody positivity for both segments, mostly associated with thymoma), while residues 1191–1216 (a region toward the N-terminus that faces the loop between domains II and III of DHPR and is within the reported main immunogenic region, MIR[71]) were antigenic in only a few patients (12% antibody positivity). The rarity of antibodies against the N-terminal sequence in our study may reflect the possibility that our synthetic peptides used as antigens did not detect conformation-specific antibodies that recognize MIR and allosterically inhibit RyR1 function.[71] However, our frequent detection of antibodies against the C-terminal tail is compatible with a direct inhibition of sarcoplasmic Ca^{2+} release.[68,70] The access of anti-RyR1 antibodies across the cell membrane to their intracellular targets is controversial and may follow complement-mediated skeletal muscle membrane damage arising from anti-AChR antibodies.

The membrane depolarization-induced, DHPR-mediated signal collaborates with the non–voltage gated Ca^{2+} influx channel, TRPC, for sarcoplasmic Ca^{2+} release.[72,73] Of seven types of TRPC, TRPC3 is activated via a PLC-PIP2-DAG signaling pathway and thereby regulates the sarcoplasmic Ca^{2+} release by functional linking to RyR1 via triadic bridging proteins, including TRPC1 and possibly coregulatory proteins (junctophylins 1 and 2, homer, mitsugumin29, calreticulin, and calmodulin)[74,75] (Fig. 3). The TRPC3-knockdown mouse skeletal muscle in which expression of RyR1 was not significantly changed demonstrated an amplitude reduction of 40% in the depolarization-induced sarcoplasmic Ca^{2+} release compared with the wild type.[74] This finding suggests that sarcoplasmic Ca^{2+} release depends partly on the TRPC3-mediated signal; the TRPC3-knockdown increased TRPC1 expression almost twofold, possibly as a compensatory mechanism for missing TRPC3.[74,75]

TRPCs, including TRPC3, also refill Ca^{2+} after depletion of sarcoplasmic Ca^{2+} stores due to the activation of internal Ca^{2+} channels such as RyR1 and IP3R[12] through two Ca^{2+} entry pathways: the receptor-operated Ca^{2+} entry (ROCE) and the store-operated Ca^{2+} entry (SOCE). These two pathways are separated but exhibit overlapping phenomena.[73] ROCE is triggered by the activation of G protein–coupled receptors, followed by PLC activation and the production of DAG from PIP2; DAG binds to TRPC3 allowing Ca^{2+} entry[11,76,77] (Fig. 3). The intracellular Ca^{2+} machinery based on SOCE was clarified following the discovery of the stromal interaction molecule-1 (Ca^{2+} sensor: STIM1)[78] and the Ca^{2+} release-activated Ca^{2+} messenger-1 (Ca^{2+} permeable channel: Orai1).[79] SOCE operates via Ca^{2+} influx channels which are assembled as TRPCs-STIM1, Orai1-STIM1, or TRPCs-Orai1-STIM1 complexes,[80–88] in which STIM1 acts as a Ca^{2+} sensor (Fig. 3). In the skeletal muscle, STIM1[89] and Orai1[90] are expressed at high levels and con-

tribute to Ca^{2+} refilling after the depletion of sarcoplasmic Ca^{2+} stores.[91–97] In addition, TRPCs interacts with STIM1 and Homer1, the latter belonging to a family of scaffolding proteins that couples TRPCs to IP3R to keep TRPCs in the closed state.[12] Following the stored Ca^{2+} depletion caused by the IP3-IP3R interaction, the dissociation of the TRPCs-Homer1-IP3R complex allows STIM1 access to gate open TRPCs[12] (Fig. 3).

In view of the roles of TRPC3 in the release of sarcoplasmic Ca^{2+} by functional engagement with RyR1 and in the restocking of sarcoplasmic Ca^{2+} stores by ROCE and SOCE, we assessed for antibodies against TRPC3 using antigenic peptide corresponding to its extracellularly exposed segment (residues 611–640)[98] in 25 MG patients. Results showed that TRPC3 antibodies were detected in 9 patients (36%) who were also positive for RyR1 antibodies and had a Myasthenia Gravis Foundation of America clinical severity score of grade III or higher.[99] Positive predictive values for thymoma were 50% for TRPC3 antibodies and 94% for RyR1 antibodies, but the specificity was 89% for both types of antibodies.[99] It remains to be seen if the TRPC3 protein is expressed in thymoma-epithelial cells as is the RyR1 protein.[69,100]

Conflicts of interest

The author declares no conflicts of interest.

References

1. Pang, G. & T.C. Südhof. 2010. Cell biology of Ca^{2+}-triggered exocytosis. *Curr. Opin. Cell Biol.* **22:** 496–505.
2. Smith, S.M., R. Renden & H. von Gersdoff. 2008. Synaptic vesile endocytosis: fast and slow modes of membrane retrieval. *Trends Neurosci.* **31:** 559–568.
3. Yamashita, T. 2012. Ca^{2+}-dependent regulation of synaptic vesicle endocytosis. *Neurosci. Res.* **73:** 1–7.
4. Daly, C. & E.B. Ziff. 2002. Ca^{2+}-dependent formation of a dynamin-synaptophysin complex. Potential role in synaptic vesicle endocytosis. *J. Biol. Chem.* **277:** 9010–9015.
5. Deák, F. *et al.* 2004. Synaptobrevin is essential for fast synaptic-vesicle endocytosis. *Nat. Cell Biol.* **6:** 1102–1108.
6. Xue, L. *et al.* 2012. A membrane pool retrieved via endocytosis overshoot at nerve terminals: a study of its retrieval mechanism and role. *J. Neurosci* **32:** 3398–3404.
7. Zhang, Q., Y. Li & R.W. Tsien. 2009. The dynamic control of kiss-and-run and vesicular reuse probed with single nanoparticles. *Science* **323:** 1488–1453.
8. Meunier, F.A. *et al.* 2010. Sustained synaptic vesicle recycling by bulk endocytosis contributes to the maintenance of high-rate neurotransmitter release stimulated by glycerotoxin. *J. Cell Sci.* **123:** 1131–1140.

9. Santafé, M.M. *et al.* 2006. Muscarinic autoreceptors modulate transmitter release through protein kinase C and protein kinase A in the rat motor nerve terminal. *Eur. J. Neurosci.* **23:** 2048–2056.

10. Amaral, M.D. & L. Pozzo-Miller. 2012. Intracellular Ca^{2+} stores and Ca^{2+} influx are both required for BDNF to rapidly increase quantal vesicular transmitter release. *Neural Plast.* **2012:** 203536.

11. Lemonnier, L., M. Trebak & J.W. Putney, Jr. 2008. Complex regulation of the TRPC3, 6 and 7 channel subfamily by diacylglycerol and phosphatidylinositol- 4,5-bisphosphate. *Cell Calcium* **43:** 506–514.

12. Yuan, J.P. *et al.* 2012. The closing and opening of TRPC channels by Homer1 and STIM1. *Acta Physiol. (Oxf.)* **204:** 238–247.

13. Bauer, C.S. *et al.* 2007. Potentiation of exocytosis by phospholipase C-coupled G- protein-coupled receptors requires the priming Munc13-1. *J. Neurosci.* **27:** 212–219.

14. Oliveria, L., M.A. Timóteo & P. Correia-de-Sá. 2009. Negative crosstalk between M1 and M2 muscarinic autoreceptors involves endogenous adenosine activating A1 receptors at the rat motor endplate. *Neurosci. Lett.* **459:** 127–131.

15. Garcia, N. *et al.* 2010. The interaction between topomyosin-related kinase B receptors and presynaptic muscarinic receptors modulates transmitter release in adult rodent motor nerve terminals. *J. Neurosci.* **30:** 16514–16522.

16. Minic, J. *et al.* 2002. Regulation of acetylcholine release by muscarinic receptor at the mouse neuromuscular junction depends on the activity of acetylcholinesterase. *Eur. J. Neursci.* **148:** 432–440.

17. Santafé, M.M. *et al.* 2007. Coupling of presynaptic muscarinic autoreceptors to serine kinases in low and high release conditions on the rat motor nerve terminal. *Neuroscience* **148:** 432–440.

18. Garcia, N. *et al.* 2005. Expression of muscarinic acetylcholine receptors (M1-, M2-, M3- and M4-type) in the neuromuscular junction of the newborn and adult rat. *Histol Histopathol.* **20:** 733–743.

19. Hulme, E.C., N.J.M. Birdsall & N.J. Buckley. 1990. Muscarinic receptor subtypes. *Annu. Rev. Pharmacol. Toxicol.* **30:** 633–673.

20. Kim, J.Y. & D. Saffen. 2005. Activation of M1 muscarinic acetylcholine receptors stimulates the formation of a multiprotein complex centered on TRPC6 channels. *J. Biol. Chem.* **280:** 32035–32047.

21. Takamori, M. *et al.* 2007. Autoantibodies against M1 muscarinic acetylcholine receptor in myasthenic disorders. *Eur. J. Neurol.* **14:** 1230–1235.

22. Takamori, M. 2008. Lambert-Eaton myasthenic syndrome: search for alternative autoimmune targets and possible compensatory mechanisms based on presynaptic calcium homeostasis. *J. Neuroimmunol.* **200–201:** 145–152.

23. Lang, B. *et al.* 2003. Pathogenic autoantibodies in the Lambert-Eaton myasthenic syndrome. *Ann. N.Y. Acad. Sci.* **998:** 187–195.

24. Nishimune, H. 2012. Molecular mechanism of active zone organization at vertebrate neuromuscular junctions. *Mol. Neurobiol.* **45:** 1–16.

25. Carlson, S.S., G. Valdez & J.R. Sanes. 2010. Presynaptic calcium channels and α3-integrins are complexed with synaptic cleft laminins, cytoskeletal elements and active zone components. *J. Neurochem.* **115:** 654–666.

26. Kaeser, P.S. *et al.* 2012. RIM genes differentially contribute to organizing presynaptic release sites. *Proc. Natl. Acad. Sci. USA* **109:** 11830–11835.

27. Wu, H., W.C. Xiong & L. Mei. 2010. To build a synapse: signaling pathways in neuromuscular junction assembly. *Development* **137:** 1017–1033.

28. Linnoila, J. *et al.* 2008. A mammalian homolog of Drosophila tumorous imaginal discs, Tid1, mediates agrin signaling at the neuromuscular junction. *Neuron* **60:** 625–641.

29. Luo, S. *et al.* 2008. Hsp90 beta regulates rapsyn turnover and subsequent AChR cluster formation and maintenance. *Neuron* **60:** 97–110.

30. Lee, Y., J. Rudell & M. Ferns. 2009. Rapsyn interacts with the muscle acetylcholine receptor via alpha-helical domains in the alpha, beta, and epsilon subunit intracellular loops. *Neuroscience* **163:** 222–232.

31. Yamanashi Y., T. Tezuka & K. Yokoyama. 2012. Activation of receptor protein- tyrosine kinases from the cytoplasmic component. *J. Biochem.* **151:** 353–359.

32. Hallock, P.T. *et al.* 2010. Dok-7 regulates neuromuscular synapse formation by recruiting Crk and Crk-L. *Genes Dev.* **24:** 2451–2461.

33. Weatherbee, S.D., K.V. Anderson & L.A. Niswander. 2006. LDL-receptor-related protein 4 is crucial for formation of the neuromuscular junction. *Development* **133:** 4993–5000.

34. Zhang, B. *et al.* 2008. Lrp4 serves as a coreceptor of agrin. *Neuron* **60:** 285–297.

35. Kim, N. *et al.* 2008. Lrp4 is a receptor for agrin and forms a complex with MuSK. *Cell* **135:** 334–342.

36. McConville, J. *et al.* 2004. Detection and characterization of MuSK antibodies in seronegative myasthenia gravis. *Ann. Neurol.* **55:** 580–584.

37. Higuchi, O. *et al.* 2011. Autoantibodies to low-density lipoprotein receptor-related protein 4 in myasthenia gravis. *Ann. Neurol.* **69:** 418–422.

38. Pevzner, A. *et al.* 2011. Anti-Lrp4 autoantibodies in AChR- and MuSK-antibody-negative myasthenia gravis. *J. Neurol.* **259:** 427–435.

39. Zhang, B. *et al.* 2012. Autoantibodies to lipoprotein-related protein 4 in patients with double-seronegative myasthenia gravis. *Arch. Neurol.* **69:** 445–451.

40. Koles, K. & V. Budnik. 2012. Wnt signaling in neuromuscular junction development. *Cold Spring Harb. Perspect. Biol.* **4:** a008045.

41. Koles, J. *et al.* 2012. Mechanism of evenness interrupted (Evi)-exosome release at synaptic boutons. *J. Biol. Chem.* **287:** 16820–16834.

42. Zhang, B. *et al.* 2012. Wnt proteins regulate acetylcholine receptor clustering in muscle cells. *Mol. Brain* **5:** 7.

43. Strochlic, L. *et al.* 2012. Wnt4 participates in the formation of vertebrate neuromuscular junction. *PLoS ONE* **7:** e29976.

44. Jing, L. *et al.* 2009. Wnt signals organize synaptic prepattern and axon guidance through the zebrafish unplugged/MuSK receptor. *Neuron* **61:** 721–733.

45. Henriquez, J.P. *et al.* 2008. Wnt signaling promotes AChR aggregation at the neuromuscular synapse in collaboration with agrin. *Proc. Natl. Acad. Sci. USA* **105:** 18812–18817.

46. Luo, Z.G. *et al.* 2002. Regulation of AChR clustering by Dishevelled interacting with MuSK and PAK1. *Neuron* **35:** 489–505.

47. Wang, J. *et al.* 2008. Wnt/beta-catenin signaling suppresses Rapsyn expression and inhibits acetylcholine receptor clustering at the neuromuscular junction. *J. Biol. Chem.* **283:** 21668–21675.

48. Henriquez, J.P. & P.C. Salinas. 2011. Dual roles for Wnt signaling during the formation of the vertebrate neuromuscular junction. *Acta Physiol. (Oxf.)* **204:** 128–136.

49. Stiegler, A.L., S.J. Burden & S.R. Hubbard. 2006. Crystal structure of the agrin-responsive immunoglobulin-like domains 1 and 2 of the receptor tyrosine kinase MuSK. *J. Mol. Biol.* **364:** 424–433.

50. Zhang, W. *et al.* 2011. Agrin binds to the N-terminal region of Lrp4 protein and stimulates association between Lrp4 and the first immunoblobul-like domain in muscle-specific kinase (MuSK). *J. Biol. Chem.* **286:** 40624–40630.

51. Zong, Y. *et al.* 2012. Structural basis of agrin-Lrp4-MuSK signaling. *Genes Dev.* **26:** 247–258.

52. Stiegler, A.L., S.J. Burden & S.R. Hubbard. 2009. Crystal structure of the Frizzled-like cysteine-rich domain of the receptor tyrosine kinase MuSK. *J. Mol. Biol.* **393:** 1–9.

53. Niks, E.H. *et al.* 2010. Pre- and postsynaptic neuromuscular junction abnormalities in musk myasthenia. *Muscle Nerve* **42:** 283–288.

54. Cole, R.N. *et al.* 2008. Anti-MuSK patient antibodies disrupt the mouse neuromuscular junction. *Ann. Neurol.* **63:** 782–789.

55. Richman, D.P. *et al.* 2011. Acute severe animal model of anti-muscle-specific kinase myasthenia. *Arch. Neurol.* **69:** 453–460.

56. Klooster, R. *et al.* 2012. Muscle-specific kinase myasthenia gravis IgG4 autoantibodies cause severe neuromuscular junction dysfunction in mice. *Brain* **135:** 1081–1101.

57. Mori, S. *et al.* 2012. Antibodies against muscle-specific kinase impair both presynaptic and postsynaptic functions in a murine model of myasthenia gravis. *Am. J. Pathol.* **180:** 798–810.

58. Viegas, S. *et al.* 2012. Passive and active immunization models of MuSK-ab positive myasthenia: electrophysiological evidence for pre and postsynaptic defects. *Exp. Neurol.* **234:** 506–512.

59. Wu, H. *et al.* 2012. Distinct roles of muscle and motoneuron Lrp4 in neuromuscular junction formation. *Neuron* **75:** 94–107.

60. Yumoto, N., N. Kim & S.J. Burden. 2012. Lrp4 is a retrograde signal for presynaptic differentiation at neuromuscular synapses. *Nature* **489:** 438–442.

61. Amenta, A.R. *et al.* 2012. Biglycan is an extracellular MuSK binding protein important for synaptic stability. *J. Neurosci.* **32:** 2324–2334.

62. Sigoillot, S.M. *et al.* 2010. ColQ controls postsynaptic differentiation at the neuromuscular junction. *J. Neurosci.* **30:** 13–23.

63. Kawakami, Y. *et al.* 2011. Anti-MuSK autoantibodies block binding of collagen Q to MuSK. *Neurology* **77:** 1819–1826.

64. Simeone, L. 2010. Identification of Erbin interlinking MuSK and ErbB2 and its impact on acetylcholine receptor aggregation at the neuromuscular junction. *J. Neurosci.* **30:** 6620–6634.

65. Ngo, S.T. *et al.* 2012. Neuregulin-1 potentiates agrin-induced acetylcholine receptor clustering through muscle-specific kinase phosphorylation. *J. Cell Biol.* **125:** 1531–1543.

66. Pilgram, G.S.K. *et al.* 2010. The roles of the dystrophin-associated glycoprotein complex at the synapse. *Mol. Neurobiol.* **41:** 1–21.

67. Wang, J. *et al.* 2003. Regulation of acetylcholine receptor clustering by the tumor suppressor APC. *Nat. Neurosci.* **6:** 1017–1018.

68. Takamori, M. *et al.* 2004. Anti-ryanodine receptor antibodies and FK506 in myasthenia gravis. *Neurology* **62:** 1894–1896.

69. Kusner, L.L., Å. Mygland & H.J. Kaminski. 1998. Ryanodine receptor gene expression thymomas. *Muscle Nerve* **21:** 1299–1303.

70. Bhat, M.B. *et al.* 1997. Functional release channel formed by the carboxyl-terminal protein of ryanodine receptor. *Biophys. J.* **73:** 1329–1336.

71. Skeie, G.O. *et al.* 2003. Ryanodine receptor antibodies in myasthenia gravis: epitope mapping and effect on calcium release in vitro. *Muscle Nerve* **27:** 81–89.

72. Gees, M., B. Colsoul & B. Nilius. 2010. The role of transient receptor potential cation channels in Ca^{2+} signaling. *Cold Spring Harb. Perspect. Biol.* **2:** a003962.

73. Birnbaumer, L. 2009. The TRPC class of ion channels: a critical review of their roles in slow, sustained increases in intracellular Ca^{2+} concentrations. *Annu. Rev. Pharmacol. Toxicol.* **49:** 395–426.

74. Lee, E.H. *et al.* 2006. Functional coupling between TRPC3 and RyR1 regulates the expressions of key triadic proteins. *J. Biol. Chem.* **281:** 10042–10048.

75. Woo, J.S. *et al.* 2008. TRPC3-interacting triadic proteins in skeletal muscle. *Biochem. J.* **411:** 399–405.

76. DeHaven, W.I. *et al.* 2009. TRPC channels function independently of STIM1 and Orai1. *J. Physiol.* **587:** 2275–2298.

77. Harteneck, C. & M. Gollasch. 2011. Pharmacological modulation of diacylglycerol-sensitive TRPC3/6/7 channesls. *Curr. Pharm. Biotechnol.* **12:** 35–41.

78. Roos, J. *et al.* 2005. STIM1, an essential and conserved component of store-operated Ca2+ channel function. *J. Cell Biol.* **169:** 435–445.

79. Vig, M. *et al.* 2006. CRACM1 is a plasma membrane protein essential for store-operated Ca^{2+} entry. *Science* **312:** 1220–1223.

80. Ong, H.L. *et al.* 2007. Dynamic assembly of TRPC1-STIM1-Orai1 ternary complex is involved in store-operated calcium influx. Evidence for similarities in stor-operated and calcium release-activated calcium channel components. *J. Biol. Chem.* **282:** 9105–9116.

81. Cheng, K.T. *et al.* 2011. Contribution of TRPC1 and Orai1 to Ca(2+) entry activated by store depletion. *Adv. Exp. Med. Biol.* **704:** 435–449.

82. Liao, Y. *et al.* 2009. A role for Orai1 in TRPC-mediated Ca^{2+} entry suggests that a TRPC:Orai1 complex may mediate store and receptor operated Ca^{2+} entry. *Proc. Natl. Acad. Sci. USA* **106:** 3202–3206.

83. Lee, K.P. *et al.* 2010. An endoplasmic reticulum/plasma membrane junction: STIM1/Orai1/TRPCs. *FEBS Lett.* **584:** 2022–2027.

84. Yuan, J.P. *et al.* 2007. STIM1 heteromultimerizes TRPC channels to determine their function as store-operated channels. *Nat. Cell Biol.* **9:** 636–645.

85. Yuan, J.P. *et al.* 2009. TRPC channels as STIM1-regulated SOCs. *Channels (Austin)* **3:** 221–225.

86. Kim, M.S. *et al.* 2009. Native store-operated Ca^{2+} influx requires the channel function of Orai1 and TRPC1. *J. Biol. Chem.* **284:** 9733–9741.

87. Shen, W.W., M. Frieden & N. Demaurex. 2011. Remodelling of the endoplasmic reticulum during store-operated calcium entry. *Biol. Cell* **103:** 365–380.

88. Berna-Erro, A., P.C. Redondo & J.A. Rosado. 2012. Store-operated Ca(2+) entry. *Adv. Exp. Med. Biol.* **740:** 349–382.

89. Stiber, J. *et al.* 2008. STIM1 signaling controls store operated calcium entry required for development and contractile function in skeletal muscle. *Nat. Cell Biol.* **10:** 688–697.

90. Vig, M. *et al.* 2008. Defective mast cell effector functions in mice lacking the CRACM1 pore subunit of store-operated calcium release-activated calcium channels. *Nat. Immunol.* **9:** 89–96.

91. Dirksen, R.T. 2009. Checking your SOCCs and feet: the molecular mechanisms of Ca2+ entry in skeletal muscle. *J. Physiol.* **587:** 3139–3147

92. Launikonis, B.S., R.M. Murphy & J.N. Edwards. 2010. Toward the roles of store-oeprated Ca(2+) entry in skeletal muscle. *Pflugers Arch.* **460:** 813–823.

93. Shin, D.M. & S. Maullem. 2008. Skeletal muscle dressed in SOCs. *Nat. Cell Biol.* **10:** 639–641.

94. Lee, E.H. 2010. Ca2+ channels and skeletal muscle diseases. *Prog. Biophys. Mol. Biol.* **103:** 35–43.

95. Kiviluoto, S. *et al.* 2011. STIM1 as a key regulator for Ca^{2+} homeostasis in skeletal-muscle development and function. *Skeletal Muscle* **1:** 16.

96. Stiber, J.A. & P.B. Rosenberg. 2011. The role of store-operated calcium influx in skeletal muscle signaling. *Cell Calcium* **49:** 341–349.

97. Seth, M. *et al.* 2012. Dynamic regulation of sarcoplasmic reticulum Ca(2+) stores by stromal interaction molecule 1 and sarcolipin during muscle differentiation. *Dev. Dyn.* **241:** 839–847.

98. Mori, Y. *et al.* 1998. Differential distribution of TRP Ca^{2+} channel isoforms in mouse brain. *NeuroReport* **9:** 507–515.

99. Takamori, M. 2008. Autoantibodies against TRPC3 and ryanodine receptor in myasthenia gravis. *J. Neuroimmunol.* **200:** 142–144.

100. Iwasa, K., K. Komai & M. Takamori. 1998. Spontaneous thymoma rat as a model for myasthenic weakness caused by anti-ryanodine receptor antibodies. *Muscle Nerve* **21:** 1655–1660.

Ann. N.Y. Acad. Sci. ISSN 0077-8923

ANNALS OF THE NEW YORK ACADEMY OF SCIENCES

Issue: *Myasthenia Gravis and Related Disorders*

Active zones of mammalian neuromuscular junctions: formation, density, and aging

Hiroshi Nishimune

Department of Anatomy and Cell Biology, University of Kansas Medical School, Kansas City, Kansas

Address for correspondence: Hiroshi Nishimune, Ph.D., University of Kansas Medical School, 3901 Rainbow Blvd., MS 3051, HLSIC 2073, Kansas City, KS, 66160. hnishimune@kumc.edu

Presynaptic active zones are synaptic vesicle release sites that play essential roles in the function and pathology of mammalian neuromuscular junctions (NMJs). The molecular mechanisms of active zone organization use presynaptic voltage-dependent calcium channels (VDCCs) in NMJs as scaffolding proteins. VDCCs interact extracellularly with the muscle-derived synapse organizer, laminin $\beta 2$ and interact intracellularly with active zone–specific proteins, such as Bassoon, CAST/Erc2/ELKS2alpha, ELKS, Piccolo, and RIMs. These molecular mechanisms are supported by studies in P/Q- and N-type VDCCs double-knockout mice, and they are consistent with the pathological conditions of Lambert–Eaton myasthenic syndrome and Pierson syndrome, which are caused by autoantibodies against VDCCs or by a laminin $\beta 2$ mutation. During normal postnatal maturation, NMJs maintain the density of active zones, while NMJs triple their size. However, active zones become impaired during aging. Propitiously, muscle exercise ameliorates the active zone impairment in aged NMJs, which suggests the potential for therapeutic strategies.

Keywords: Bassoon; calcium channel; exercise; laminin; motor neuron; synapse

Introduction

Synaptic vesicles at adult mammalian neuromuscular junctions (NMJs) accumulate near the electron-dense material of presynaptic active zones (Fig. 1). Synaptic transmission is initiated by Ca^{2+} influx through presynaptic P/Q-type VDCCs[1,2] and synaptic vesicle fusion at the active zones.[3] The cytosolic regions of these active zones form large protein complexes, which are detected as electron-dense material extending from the presynaptic membrane toward the cytosolic region on transmission electron micrographs.[4–6] The electron-dense materials align with postsynaptic junctional folds in adult NMJs.[7–9] These electron-dense materials of active zones distribute in a discrete pattern within one presynaptic terminal in mammalian NMJs,[10,6] similar to the salt crystals on a pretzel. The discrete distribution pattern of active zones is consistent with the distribution patterns of active zone–specific proteins that are detected using immunohistochemistry[11,12,9] and the distribution patterns of intramembranous particles on the P-face of presynaptic membranes

that are detected using freeze-fracture electron microscopy.[13,14] This discrete distribution pattern of active zones in mammalian NMJs is similar to *Drosophila* NMJs,[15–17] but different from frog NMJs that contain elongated continuous active zones.[18,5] Furthermore, the discrete distribution pattern of active zones within one mammalian NMJ is similar to large synapses of the central nervous system, the calyx of Held and large mossy fiber terminals in the hippocampus, that show discrete distribution patterns of active zone–specific proteins within a single presynaptic terminal.[19–21] The presynaptic active zone of central nervous system has been reviewed recently elsewhere.[22,23]

Impairments in active zone structure are known in two human neurological diseases, namely, Lambert–Eaton myasthenia syndrome (LEMS) and Pierson syndrome. LEMS patients exhibit a reduced number of NMJ active zones, reduced synaptic transmission, and weakened muscles because of autoantibodies against VDCCs and synaptic proteins.[24,14] Pierson syndrome patients exhibit a loss of NMJ active zones, impairments in synaptic

doi: 10.1111/j.1749-6632.2012.06836.x

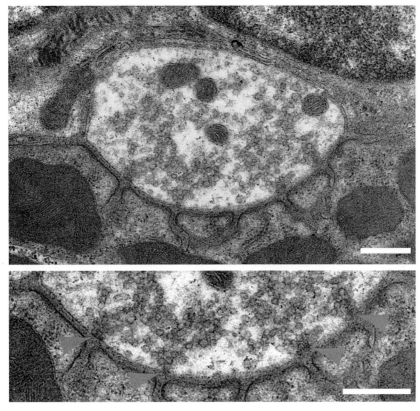

Figure 1. A transmission electron micrograph showing active zones in a mouse NMJ. The top micrograph shows an NMJ profile of a diaphragm from a wild-type mouse at postnatal day 85. The motor nerve terminal is colored in green and muscle in red. Synaptic vesicles are preferentially accumulating to four active zones. The bottom micrograph shows a high-magnification view of the presynaptic membrane area of the same NMJ. Orange arrowheads indicate electron-dense materials of the active zones that are accumulating synaptic vesicles and are aligned with postsynaptic junctional folds. Scale bars: 500 nm.

transmission, and denervation of NMJs because of the lack of laminin β2 caused by a genetic mutation.[25,26] These clinical phenotypes of Pierson syndrome are identical to phenotypes of laminin β2 knockout mice,[27] which suggest that the synapse organizer laminin β2 plays a role in active zone organization in humans. Furthermore, these studies suggest essential roles of active zones and their electron-dense materials in synaptic transmission at NMJs.

Molecular mechanisms of NMJ active zone organization

What is known about the molecular mechanism to organize NMJ active zones? The synapse organizer, laminin β2, is an extracellular matrix protein secreted by muscles that specifically concentrates in the synaptic cleft of NMJs.[28,29] Laminin β2 knockout mice demonstrate a loss of active zones, impairment of presynaptic differentiation, and an attenu-

ation of miniature endplate potential frequency and quantal content at NMJs.[27,30] These data suggest a role of laminin β2 in the organization of NMJ active zones. However, a specific receptor for this active zone organizer was previously unknown because the well-known laminin receptors, such as integrins and dystroglycans, do not distinguish between synaptic and nonsynaptic laminins (with or without laminin β2).[31–33] In a search for a specific receptor, laminin β2 was shown to bind directly and specifically to P/Q- and N-type VDCCs,[11] both of which are concentrated at presynaptic terminals in mammalian NMJs.[1,34] These VDCC pore-forming subunits bind to synaptic laminins containing laminin β2 but not to nonsynaptic laminins, which contain laminin β1.[11] Furthermore, synaptic laminins bind to VDCCs that are highly concentrated at presynaptic terminals in NMJs (e.g., P/Q- and N-types) but not to other VDCCs (e.g., R- and L-type VDCCs

[Cav1.2]).[11] Therefore, these VDCCs are the first receptors that specifically bind synaptic laminins. The interaction between laminin β2 and VDCC leads to the clustering of VDCCs and presynaptic components in cultured motor neurons,[11] which suggests presynaptic differentiation.

In vivo studies provide compelling support that extracellular interactions between laminins and VDCCs participate in the organization of NMJ active zones. The number of active zones decreases in P/Q-type VDCC knockout mice similar to laminin β2 knockout mice.[11] In addition, active zone number decreases in wild-type mice when the interaction between VDCC and laminin β2 is blocked by infusing an inhibitor of the interaction.[11] Moreover, P/Q- and N-type VDCC double knockout mice exhibit specific defects in the number of active zones, which is twice as severe as the defects in the single knockout mice of P/Q- or N-type VDCCs. However, the double knockout mouse displays normal axon projection, endplate recognition/innervation, and an accumulation of the synaptic vesicle-related proteins at presynaptic terminals without morphologically denervated endplates.[12] These results suggest that the termination of axonal outgrowth and the accumulation of synaptic vesicle proteins at NMJs are based on a cell adhesion-based signal or a retrograde signal from muscles to axons. However, active zone formation is based on a parallel or different signaling mechanisms utilizing VDCCs as a receptor for the active zone organizer.

The VDCCs that trigger synaptic vesicle release have been estimated to localize at or in close vicinity of active zones.[35–39,2] Adult mammalian NMJs rely on P/Q-type VDCCs for synaptic transmission.[34,40] However, the relative location of P/Q-type VDCCs and active zone proteins has not been analyzed in the immunohistochemistry studies of P/Q-type VDCCs in mammalian NMJs published by others.[41–44] Three-dimensional reconstruction of immunohistochemistry signals revealed that P/Q-type VDCCs distribute in a discrete punctate pattern within the NMJs and colocalize preferentially with the active zone protein Bassoon.[45] The punctate immunohistochemical-staining patterns of P/Q-type VDCCs and Bassoon were different from the diffuse distribution pattern of the synaptic vesicle-associated protein SV2, which suggests that these colocalization spots are discrete active zones within NMJs. This codistribution pattern of P/Q-type VD-

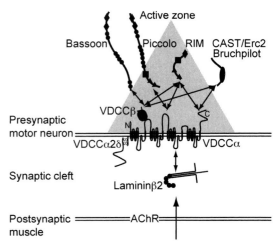

Figure 2. A diagram of the molecular mechanism of active zone organization in mammalian neuromuscular junctions. The diagram depicts interactions between the muscle-derived active zone organizer laminin β2, presynaptic voltage-dependent calcium channel (VDCC) subunits, and active zone proteins. The gray triangle depicts the electron-dense material of an active zone detected by electron microscopy. Horizontal double lines show pre- and postsynaptic membranes, and the space between these lines represents the synaptic cleft. The sizes of the proteins and the synaptic cleft are not in scale. Two-headed arrows represent some of the reported interactions.

CCs and Bassoon in NMJs is consistent with the direct binding of VDCCs and Bassoon (described below).[12]

Presynaptic VDCCs contribute to the tethering of the cytomatrix at the active zone (CAZ)[45] to the presynaptic membrane and organize the NMJ active zones by directly binding to active zone–specific proteins (Fig. 2). The active zone proteins, Bassoon, CAST/Erc2/ELKS2alpha, ELKS, and RIMs, interact with VDCC β subunits,[12,46–48] which form a tight complex with the pore-forming α subunits of P/Q- and N-type VDCCs.[49] The active zone proteins RIMs and Piccolo also interact with VDCC α subunits.[50–52] These CAZ proteins are likely to form a large protein complex[53–56] and become the electron-dense materials in the NMJ active zones. This view is further supported by the correlation between the loss of Bassoon immunohistochemical signals and the loss of active zone electron-dense materials in the NMJs of VDCC knockout mice.[11,12]

In summary, the muscle-derived active zone–organizer laminin β2 anchors the VDCC subunits and active zone–protein complex (Bassoon, CAST/ELKS/Erc family member, Piccolo, and

RIMs) from the extracellular side to organize NMJ active zones. P/Q-type VDCCs function as scaffolding proteins that link the extracellular interaction to cytosolic active zone proteins.[12,48] The three-dimensional alignment of P/Q-type VDCCs and Bassoon in NMJs strongly supports this molecular mechanism to organize the active zones.[57] The role of other NMJ organizers for active zone formation is less likely (Agrin, MuSK, and Lrp4) or not clear (collagens and amyloid precursor protein) at this point and awaits further study.[58]

Bassoon interaction modulates VDCC inactivation

P/Q-type VDCCs and Bassoon bind directly in a coimmunoprecipitation assay.[12,45] Consistently, these two proteins preferentially colocalize in NMJs.[57] Furthermore, VDCCs and other active zone–specific proteins form protein complexes *in vitro* and *in vivo*.[12,47,48,51,52,56,57,59,60] These data raise the possibility of modifying VDCC function by the interacting active zone proteins. Indeed, Bassoon suppresses the inactivation property of P/Q-type VDCCs when the two proteins are co-expressed and analyzed using patch-clamp electrophysiology.[45] A significant depolarizing shift in the voltage dependence of inactivation is observed, which is similar to the effect of active zone protein RIM1 on VDCCs.[46,47] These results suggested that Bassoon suppresses inactivation and prolongs channel opening of P/Q-type VDCCs that are opened by repetitive depolarization. Therefore, Ca^{2+} influx through P/Q-type VDCCs is augmented by Bassoon and may contribute to the efficiency of NMJ synaptic transmission. An alternative possibility is that Bassoon preferentially increases the open time of VDCCs positioned in active zones, whereas those VDCCs without Bassoon located outside the active zones would not. This might be a way to enhance calcium entry to the active zones, similar to the role of SNARE proteins.[59] These hypotheses are consistent with the Bassoon-dependent increase in Ca^{2+} influx through L-type VDCCs in the inner hair cells of the auditory system.[60] Other modifications of VDCC function by active zone–specific proteins have been reported by other groups.[46,60,47,61,52,62] The functional modification of VDCCs by Bassoon is likely to occur in addition to the previously reported role of Bassoon in synaptic vesicle tethering to the presynaptic membranes.[60,63,64] In summary,

active zone–specific proteins play a role in synaptic transmission by binding to presynaptic VDCC complexes, modifying channel function, and tethering synaptic vesicles.

The functional modification of VDCCs by active zone proteins does not seem to contribute to active zone formation. The synapse organizer laminin β2 induces presynaptic differentiation in cultured motor neurons despite P/Q- and N-type VDCC blockade by specific toxins, providing evidence for dispensability of Ca^{2+} influx into nerve terminals for active zone formation.[11] This finding suggests that ion channel activity or the modification of channel function may not be required for the formation of NMJ active zones.

Active zone density

NMJ active zones distribute in a discrete pattern (like the salt crystals on a pretzel) within one presynaptic terminal of mammalian NMJs. Freeze-fracture electron microscopy has revealed active zones based on the intramembranous particles[13,14] at a density of 2.4–2.7 active zones per square micometers in mouse and human adult NMJs.[14,65,66] The density of active zones that are labeled by Bassoon immunohistochemistry is 2.3 active zones per square micometers in mouse NMJs.[9] Importantly, the active zone densities match in two species using two different techniques, which suggests that the active zones of mammalian NMJs are maintained at 2.3–2.7 active zones per square micometers.

The density of NMJ active zones is maintained at a constant level during postnatal maturation in mice. The density of active zones that are labeled by Bassoon immunohistochemistry remains constant at 2.3 active zones per square micometer, whereas the synapse size and active zone numbers increase more than threefold during the first two months of postnatal maturation in mouse NMJs (Fig. 3).[9] What is the significance of maintaining a constant density of active zones while NMJs enlarge and change its morphology? A regulated distance between active zones ensures access to synaptic vesicles and Ca^{2+}-buffering systems in the presynaptic terminal,[37,39] which may isolate active zones as independent units and limit calcium-dependent short-term plasticity.[59] It also aids the effective clearance of neurotransmitters in the synaptic cleft by maintaining the local neurotransmitter concentrations under a certain level.[67] In addition, a constant active zone

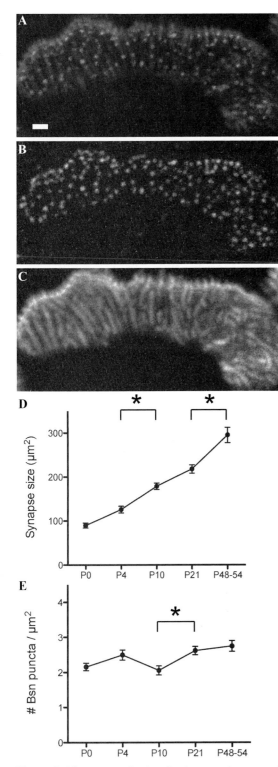

density allows postsynaptic membranes to maintain a constant density of neurotransmitter receptors during maturation, which secures the safety factor of NMJ neurotransmission.[68] These points support the advantages of maintaining the active zone density for the efficacy of synaptic transmission at NMJs.

How do active zones maintain regulated distance between themselves in presynaptic terminals? Laminin α4 is an extracellular matrix molecule concentrated in the synaptic cleft of mouse NMJs, but it is excluded under the active zones and from junctional folds.[8] Interestingly, laminin α4 knockout mice display normal numbers of NMJ active zones, but the active zones are not placed at the normal position facing the junctional folds.[8] Therefore, laminin α4 plays a role in the specification of the active zone location in mouse NMJs. In the cytosolic side, cytoskeletal structures like presynaptic particle web, or cytoskeletal protein complexes that bind to VDCCs and active zone proteins may regulate the distance between the active zones.[69,55,56] However, the molecular mechanism that control the number and spacing of active zones is further studied in *Drosophila* NMJs.[70–74,58]

Impairment of active zones in aged NMJs and recovery by exercise

Active zone density is maintained during the NMJ maturation; however, active zones are impaired in aged animals. Decreased Bassoon protein levels have been detected in the NMJs of aged mice and rats.[9,57] Would the reduced Bassoon protein level in aged NMJs affect NMJ function? Lack of Bassoon is known to cause an impairment of synaptic vesicle trafficking to presynaptic membranes in central nervous system and sensory neurons.[60,63,64] As mentioned in the electrophysiological analyses

in adult NMJs. A fluorescent immunohistochemical staining showing Bassoon (green in A, B) and acetylcholine receptors (red in A, C) in sternomastoid muscle of an adult mouse. Many Bassoon puncta are localized on top of the postsynaptic folds, which were visualized as bright lines of α-bungarotoxin staining. (D) The synapse size (measured by the α-bungarotoxin stained area) shows about threefold enlargement during the perinatal to adult stages. (E) The density of the Bassoon puncta stays at a relatively constant level (2.3 puncta/μm^2) during the postnatal development of NMJs. Asterisks indicate significant differences by one-way ANOVA analysis ($P < 0.05$). Modified from Ref. 9, ©Wiley-Blackwell.

Figure 3. The constant density of active zones in postnatal mouse NMJs. (A–C) The active zone–specific protein Bassoon forms puncta that are aligned with postsynaptic junctional folds

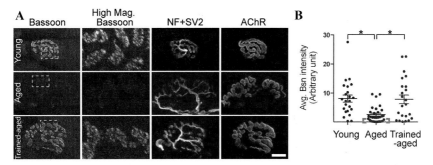

Figure 4. Exercise ameliorates the decrease in active zone protein level observed in aged NMJs. (A) NMJs of aged rats (aged, two-year-old rats) exhibit lower Bassoon signal intensity compared to young adult rats (young, postnatal day 56). Aged rats that underwent isometric strength training of muscles for two months (trained aged) show higher Bassoon immunohistochemical signal intensity compared to the NMJs of untrained aged rats (aged). Highly magnified Bassoon staining of the area marked by white dotted boxes are shown in the second column from the left (High Mag. Bassoon). Nerve and endplate morphology is shown using antineurofilament and anti-SV2 antibodies (NF + SV2) and α-bungarotoxin for acetylcholine receptors (AChR). Scale bar: 10 μm. (B) Average signal intensity of Bassoon is significantly higher in NMJs of young rats and trained-aged rats compared to those of untrained-aged rats (scatter plot shows each NMJ data, and whiskers show mean ± standard error in arbitrary intensity units). The red bracket indicates a subgroup of aged NMJs with a minuscule level of Bassoon signal. Young rats and trained-aged rats do not show a significant difference. Modified from Ref. 57.

of VDCC–Bassoon interaction, Ca^{2+} influx is decreased in VDCCs without Bassoon,[57] which may weaken synaptic transmission. Furthermore, impaired NMJ synaptic transmission is known in human diseases and knockout mice that have decreased numbers of active zones.[2,30,26] Taken together, the reduced Bassoon protein level in aged NMJs is likely to weaken synaptic transmission. This view is consistent with the attenuation of synaptic function in aged NMJs compared to young adult NMJs, including stronger synaptic depression during repeated stimulation,[75] reduced endplate potential amplitude (plateau level) after repetitive stimulation,[76] and the reduced frequency of miniature endplate potentials.[77,76] In summary, active zone protein loss may be a part of the molecular mechanism that causes impairment of aged NMJs.

This active zone impairment in aged NMJs is ameliorated by muscular exercise. Exercise intervention is beneficial for the nervous system because exercise upregulates neurotrophins[78–81] and improves recovery after nerve injury.[82] In addition, an effect of exercise on presynaptic active zones was demonstrated in our recent study.[57] Isometric strength exercise ameliorated the loss of Bassoon in the aged NMJs of two-year-old rats. The mean intensity of Bassoon immunohistochemical signal in the NMJs of exercised-aged rats was similar to young adult rats (Fig. 4). Importantly, the improvement in this active zone protein in aged NMJs after exercise is

consistent with improvements in NMJ function after endurance training in aged mice revealed using electrophysiology.[83] Furthermore, the beneficial effects of exercise in the attenuation or reversal of age-related changes in NMJs have been observed in human and rodents by several groups as well.[84,85] In summary, the exercise-induced preservation of active zone proteins in aged NMJs is likely to exert a positive effect on NMJ function.

Summary

Recent findings related to NMJ active zones are summarized in this review, including the molecular mechanisms of formation, density, impairments during aging, and recovery by exercise. The transsynaptic signaling between the active zone organizer laminin β2 secreted by muscle, its specific receptor presynaptic VDCCs, and active zone–specific proteins play an important role in active zone organization. The interactions of VDCCs and active zone proteins modulate VDCC function but may cause presynaptic impairment in aged NMJs because of the loss of active zone proteins. However, this loss of active zone proteins in aged NMJs is ameliorated by muscular exercise.

The impaired condition of aged NMJs and pathological conditions of Lambert–Eaton myasthenic and Pierson syndromes reiterate the importance of active zones in NMJ function. Furthermore, impairments in active zones may underlie the etiological mechanisms of other neuromuscular diseases. Propitious improvement of active zone protein levels in aged NMJs after muscle exercise creates a novel therapy for the maintenance and amelioration of NMJ functions under pathological conditions. However, the molecular mechanisms of these beneficial effects are not well known, which makes pharmacological intervention difficult. Patient conditions may not permit effective exercise interventions, because of restricted mobility. Therefore, further investigation to elucidate the organizational mechanisms in NMJ active zones is required for the development of novel therapeutic strategies.

Acknowledgments

The author thanks J. Chen, Y. Mori, J.A. Stanford, and T. Numata for their contributions to the findings described in this review, and R. Barohn for comments. The work in my laboratory is supported by Grants from the Whitehall Foundation, NIH-NCRR (RR024214), and NICHD (HD002528).

Conflict of interest

The author declares no conflicts of interest.

References

1. Rosato Siri, M.D. & O.D. Uchitel. 1999. Calcium channels coupled to neurotransmitter release at neonatal rat neuromuscular junctions. *J. Physiol.* **514**(Pt 2): 533–540.

2. Urbano, F.J. *et al.* 2003. Altered properties of quantal neurotransmitter release at endplates of mice lacking P/Q-type Ca^{2+} channels. *Proc. Natl. Acad. Sci. USA* **100**: 3491–3496.

3. Heuser, J.E. *et al.* 1979. Synaptic vesicle exocytosis captured by quick freezing and correlated with quantal transmitter release. *J. Cell Biol.* **81**: 275–300.

4. Couteaux, R. & M. Pecot-Dechavassine. 1970. Synaptic vesicles and pouches at the level of "active zones" of the neuromuscular junction. *C R Acad. Sci. Hebd. Seances. Acad. Sci. D.* **271**: 2346–2349.

5. Harlow, M.L. *et al.* 2001. The architecture of active zone material at the frog's neuromuscular junction. *Nature* **409**: 479–484.

6. Nagwaney, S. *et al.* 2009. Macromolecular connections of active zone material to docked synaptic vesicles and presynaptic membrane at neuromuscular junctions of mouse. *J. Comp. Neurol.* **513**: 457–468.

7. Hirokawa, N. & J.E. Heuser. 1982. Internal and external differentiations of the postsynaptic membrane at the neuromuscular junction. *J. Neurocytol.* **11**: 487–510.

8. Patton, B.L. *et al.* 2001. Properly formed but improperly localized synaptic specializations in the absence of laminin alpha4. *Nat. Neurosci.* **4**: 597–604.

9. Chen, J., T. Mizushige & H. Nishimune. 2012. Active zone density is conserved during synaptic growth but impaired in aged mice. *J. Comp. Neurol.* **520**: 434–452.

10. Rowley, K.L. *et al.* 2007. Synaptic vesicle distribution and release at rat diaphragm neuromuscular junctions. *J. Neurophysiol.* **98**: 478–487.

11. Nishimune, H., J.R. Sanes & S.S. Carlson. 2004. A synaptic laminin-calcium channel interaction organizes active zones in motor nerve terminals. *Nature* **432**: 580–587.

12. Chen, J., S.E. Billings & H. Nishimune. 2011. Calcium channels link the muscle-derived synapse organizer laminin beta2 to Bassoon and CAST/Erc2 to organize presynaptic active zones. *J. Neurosci.* **31**: 512–525.

13. Ellisman, M.H. *et al.* 1976. Studies of excitable membranes. II. A comparison of specializations at neuromuscular junctions and nonjunctional sarcolemmas of mammalian fast and slow twitch muscle fibers. *J. Cell Biol.* **68**: 752–774.

14. Fukunaga, H. *et al.* 1982. Paucity and disorganization of presynaptic membrane active zones in the lambert-eaton myasthenic syndrome. *Muscle Nerve* **5**: 686–697.

15. Jia, X.X., M. Gorczyca & V. Budnik. 1993. Ultrastructure of neuromuscular junctions in Drosophila: comparison of wild type and mutants with increased excitability. *J. Neurobiol.* **24**: 1025–1044.

16. Meinertzhagen, I.A. *et al.* 1998. Regulated spacing of synapses and presynaptic active zones at larval neuromuscular junctions in different genotypes of the flies Drosophila and Sarcophaga. *J. Comp. Neurol.* **393**: 482–492.

17. Liu, K.S. *et al.* 2011. RIM-binding protein, a central part of the active zone, is essential for neurotransmitter release. *Science* **334**: 1565–1569.

18. Ko, C.P. 1985. Formation of the active zone at developing neuromuscular junctions in larval and adult bullfrogs. *J. Neurocytol.* **14**: 487–512.

19. Satzler, K. *et al.* 2002. Three-dimensional reconstruction of a calyx of Held and its postsynaptic principal neuron in the medial nucleus of the trapezoid body. *J. Neurosci.* **22**: 10567–10579.

20. Dondzillo, A. *et al.* 2010. Targeted three-dimensional immunohistochemistry reveals localization of presynaptic proteins Bassoon and Piccolo in the rat calyx of Held before and after the onset of hearing. *J. Comp. Neurol.* **518**: 1008–1029.

21. Bednarek, E. & P. Caroni. 2011. Beta-adducin is required for stable assembly of new synapses and improved memory upon environmental enrichment. *Neuron* **69**: 1132–1146.

22. Schneggenburger, R., Y. Han & O. Kochubey. 2012. Ca(2+) channels and transmitter release at the active zone. *Cell Calcium* **52**: 199–207.

23. Sudhof, T.C. 2012. The presynaptic active zone. *Neuron* **75**: 11–25.

24. Lambert, E.H. & D. Elmqvist. 1971. Quantal components of end-plate potentials in the myasthenic syndrome. *Ann. N Y. Acad. Sci.* **183**: 183–199.

25. Zenker, M. *et al.* 2004. Human laminin beta2 deficiency causes congenital nephrosis with mesangial sclerosis and distinct eye abnormalities. *Hum. Mol. Genet.* **13**: 2625–2632.

26. Maselli, R.A. *et al.* 2009. Mutations in LAMB2 causing a severe form of synaptic congenital myasthenic syndrome. *J. Med. Genet.* **46**: 203–208.

27. Noakes, P.G. *et al.* 1995. Aberrant differentiation of neuromuscular junctions in mice lacking s-laminin/laminin beta 2. *Nature* **374**: 258–262.

28. Sanes, J.R. & Z.W. Hall. 1979. Antibodies that bind specifically to synaptic sites on muscle fiber basal lamina. *J. Cell Biol.* **83:** 357–370.

29. Hunter, D.D. *et al.* 1989. A laminin-like adhesive protein concentrated in the synaptic cleft of the neuromuscular junction. *Nature* **338:** 229–234.

30. Knight, D. *et al.* 2003. Functional analysis of neurotransmission at beta2-laminin deficient terminals. *J. Physiol.* **546:** 789–800.

31. Belkin, A.M. & M.A. Stepp. 2000. Integrins as receptors for laminins. *Microsc. Res. Tech.* **51:** 280–301.

32. Suzuki, N., F. Yokoyama & M. Nomizu. 2005. Functional sites in the laminin alpha chains. *Connect. Tissue Res.* **46:** 142–152.

33. Barresi, R. & K.P. Campbell. 2006. Dystroglycan: from biosynthesis to pathogenesis of human disease. *J. Cell Sci.* **119:** 199–207.

34. Uchitel, O.D. *et al.* 1992. P-type voltage-dependent calcium channel mediates presynaptic calcium influx and transmitter release in mammalian synapses. *Proc. Natl. Acad. Sci. USA* **89:** 3330–3333.

35. Pumplin, D.W., T.S. Reese & R. Llinas. 1981. Are the presynaptic membrane particles the calcium channels? *Proc. Natl. Acad. Sci. USA* **78:** 7210–7213.

36. Robitaille, R., E.M. Adler & M.P. Charlton. 1990. Strategic location of calcium channels at transmitter release sites of frog neuromuscular synapses. *Neuron* **5:** 773–779.

37. Llinas, R., M. Sugimori & R.B. Silver. 1992. Microdomains of high calcium concentration in a presynaptic terminal. *Science* **256:** 677–679.

38. Haydon, P.G., E. Henderson & E.F. Stanley. 1994. Localization of individual calcium channels at the release face of a presynaptic nerve terminal. *Neuron* **13:** 1275–1280.

39. Neher, E. 1998. Vesicle pools and Ca^{2+} microdomains: new tools for understanding their roles in neurotransmitter release. *Neuron* **20:** 389–399.

40. Protti, D.A. *et al.* 1996. Calcium channel blockers and transmitter release at the normal human neuromuscular junction. *Neurology* **46:** 1391–1396.

41. Day, N.C. *et al.* 1997. Differential localization of voltage-dependent calcium channel alpha1 subunits at the human and rat neuromuscular junction. *J. Neurosci.* **17:** 6226–6235.

42. Westenbroek, R.E., L. Hoskins & W.A. Catterall. 1998. Localization of Ca^{2+} channel subtypes on rat spinal motor neurons, interneurons, and nerve terminals. *J. Neurosci.* **18:** 6319–6330.

43. De Laet, A. *et al.* 2002. Immunohistochemical localization of voltage-activated calcium channels in the rat oesophagus. *Neurogastroenterol. Motil.* **14:** 173–181.

44. Santafé, M.M. *et al.* 2005. Changes in the neuromuscular synapse induced by an antibody against gangliosides. *Ann. Neurol.* **57:** 396–407.

45. Dresbach, T. *et al.* 2001. The presynaptic cytomatrix of brain synapses. *Cell Mol. Life Sci.* **58:** 94–116.

46. Kiyonaka, S. *et al.* 2007. RIM1 confers sustained activity and neurotransmitter vesicle anchoring to presynaptic Ca^{2+} channels. *Nat. Neurosci.* **10:** 691–701.

47. Uriu, Y. *et al.* 2010. Rab3-interacting molecule gamma isoforms lacking the Rab3-binding domain induce long lasting currents but block neurotransmitter vesicle anchoring in voltage-dependent P/Q-type Ca^{2+} channels. *J. Biol. Chem.* **285:** 21750–21767.

48. Billings, S.E., G.L. Clarke & H. Nishimune. 2012. ELKS1 and Ca^{2+} channel subunit beta4 interact and colocalize at cerebellar synapses. *Neuroreport* **23:** 49–54.

49. Catterall, W.A. 2000. Structure and regulation of voltage-gated Ca^{2+} channels. *Annu. Rev. Cell. Dev. Biol.* **16:** 521–555.

50. Shibasaki, T. *et al.* 2004. Interaction of ATP sensor, cAMP sensor, Ca^{2+} sensor, and voltage-dependent Ca^{2+} channel in insulin granule exocytosis. *J. Biol. Chem.* **279:** 7956–7961.

51. Shibasaki, T., Y. Sunaga & S. Seino. 2004. Integration of ATP, cAMP, and Ca^{2+} signals in insulin granule exocytosis. *Diabetes* **53:** S59–62.

52. Kaeser, P.S. *et al.* 2012. RIM genes differentially contribute to organizing presynaptic release sites. *Proc. Natl. Acad. Sci. USA* **109:** 11830–11835.

53. Takao-Rikitsu, E. *et al.* 2004. Physical and functional interaction of the active zone proteins, CAST, RIM1, and Bassoon, in neurotransmitter release. *J. Cell Biol.* **164:** 301–311.

54. Wang, X. *et al.* 2009. A protein interaction node at the neurotransmitter release site: domains of Aczonin/Piccolo, Bassoon, CAST, and Rim converge on the N-terminal domain of Munc13–1. *J. Neurosci.* **29:** 12584–12596.

55. Carlson, S.S., G. Valdez & J.R. Sanes. 2010. Presynaptic calcium channels and alpha3-integrins are complexed with synaptic cleft laminins, cytoskeletal elements and active zone components. *J. Neurochem.* **115:** 654–666.

56. Muller, C.S. *et al.* 2010. Quantitative proteomics of the Cav2 channel nano-environments in the mammalian brain. *Proc. Natl. Acad. Sci. USA* **107:** 14950–14957.

57. Nishimune, H. *et al.* 2012. Active zone protein Bassoon colocalizes with presynaptic calcium channel, modifies channel function, and recovers from aging related loss by exercise. *PLoS One* **7:** e38029.

58. Nishimune, H. 2012. Molecular mechanism of active zone organization at vertebrate neuromuscular junctions. *Mol. Neurobiol.* **45:** 1–16.

59. Catterall, W.A. & A.P. Few. 2008. Calcium channel regulation and presynaptic plasticity. *Neuron* **59:** 882–901.

60. Frank, T. *et al.* 2010. Bassoon and the synaptic ribbon organize Ca^{2+} channels and vesicles to add release sites and promote refilling. *Neuron* **68:** 724–738.

61. Han, Y. *et al.* 2011. RIM determines Ca(2) +channel density and vesicle docking at the presynaptic active zone. *Neuron* **69:** 304–316.

62. Kiyonaka, S. *et al.* 2012. Physical and functional interaction of the active zone protein CAST/ERC2 and the beta-subunit of the voltage-dependent Ca2+ channel. *J. Biochem.* **152:** 149–159.

63. Hallermann, S. *et al.* 2010. Bassoon speeds vesicle reloading at a central excitatory synapse. *Neuron* **68:** 710–723.

64. Mukherjee, K. *et al.* 2010. Piccolo and bassoon maintain synaptic vesicle clustering without directly participating in vesicle exocytosis. *Proc. Natl. Acad. Sci. USA* **107:** 6504–6509.

65. Fukunaga, H. *et al.* 1983. Passive transfer of Lambert-Eaton myasthenic syndrome with IgG from man to mouse depletes the presynaptic membrane active zones. *Proc. Natl. Acad. Sci. USA* **80:** 7636–7640.

66. Fukuoka, T. *et al.* 1987. Lambert-Eaton myasthenic syndrome: I. Early morphological effects of IgG on the presynaptic membrane active zones. *Ann. Neurol.* **22:** 193–199.

67. Massoulie, J. & S. Bon. 1982. The molecular forms of cholinesterase and acetylcholinesterase in vertebrates. *Annu. Rev. Neurosci.* **5:** 57–106.

68. Kelly, S.S. 1978. The effect of age on neuromuscular transmission. *J. Physiol.* **274:** 51–62.

69. Phillips, G.R. *et al.* 2001. The presynaptic particle web: ultrastructure, composition, dissolution, and reconstitution. *Neuron* **32:** 63–77.

70. Dickman, D.K. *et al.* 2006. Altered synaptic development and active zone spacing in endocytosis mutants. *Curr. Biol.* **16:** 591–598.

71. Pielage, J., R.D. Fetter & G.W. Davis. 2006. A postsynaptic Spectrin scaffold defines active zone size, spacing, and efficacy at the *Drosophila* neuromuscular junction. *J. Cell Biol.* **175:** 491–503.

72. Graf, E.R. *et al.* 2009. Rab3 dynamically controls protein composition at active zones. *Neuron* **64:** 663–677.

73. Wairkar, Y.P. *et al.* 2009. Unc-51 controls active zone density and protein composition by downregulating ERK signaling. *J. Neurosci.* **29:** 517–528.

74. Pielage, J. *et al.* 2011. Hts/Adducin controls synaptic elaboration and elimination. *Neuron* **69:** 1114–1131.

75. Smith, D.O. 1984. Acetylcholine storage, release and leakage at the neuromuscular junction of mature adult and aged rats. *J. Physiol.* **347:** 161–176.

76. Banker, B.Q., S.S. Kelly & N. Robbins. 1983. Neuromuscular transmission and correlative morphology in young and old mice. *J. Physiol.* **339:** 355–377.

77. Gutmann, E., V. Hanzlikova & F. Vysokocil. 1971. Age changes in cross striated muscle of the rat. *J. Physiol.* **216:** 331–343.

78. Dupont-Versteegden, E.E. *et al.* 2004. Exercise-induced gene expression in soleus muscle is dependent on time after spinal cord injury in rats. *Muscle Nerve* **29:** 73–81.

79. Cote, M.P. *et al.* 2011. Activity-dependent increase in neurotrophic factors is associated with an enhanced modulation of spinal reflexes after spinal cord injury. *J. Neurotrauma.* **28:** 299–309.

80. McCullough, M.J. *et al.* 2011. Glial cell line-derived neurotrophic factor protein content in rat skeletal muscle is altered by increased physical activity in vivo and in vitro. *Neuroscience* **174:** 234–244.

81. Schaser, A.J. *et al.* 2012. The effect of age and tongue exercise on BDNF and TrkB in the hypoglossal nucleus of rats. *Behav. Brain Res.* **226:** 235–241.

82. Udina, E., A. Puigdemasa & X. Navarro. 2011. Passive and active exercise improve regeneration and muscle reinnervation after peripheral nerve injury in the rat. *Muscle Nerve* **43:** 500–509.

83. Fahim, M.A. 1997. Endurance exercise modulates neuromuscular junction of C57BL/6NNia aging mice. *J. Appl. Physiol.* **83:** 59–66.

84. Vandervoort, A.A. 2002. Aging of the human neuromuscular system. *Muscle Nerve* **25:** 17–25.

85. Valdez, G. *et al.* 2010. Attenuation of age-related changes in mouse neuromuscular synapses by caloric restriction and exercise. *Proc. Natl. Acad. Sci. USA* **107:** 14863–14868.

Ann. N.Y. Acad. Sci. ISSN 0077-8923

ANNALS OF THE NEW YORK ACADEMY OF SCIENCES
Issue: *Myasthenia Gravis and Related Disorders*

The etiology of autoimmune diseases: the case of myasthenia gravis

Jean-François Bach

Académie des sciences, Paris, France

Address for correspondence: Jean-François Bach, Secrétaire Perpétuel, Académie des sciences—2eme division, 23 quai de conti, Paris 75006, France. jean-francois.bach@academie-sciences.fr

Autoimmune diseases comprise a wide variety of disorders, from those that are acute and spontaneously regressive to chronic diseases. Their occurrence is the sign of a loss of tolerance to self-antigens. With few exceptions, the etiology of autoimmune diseases has not been clearly established. In all cases, it is complex, involving genetic, epigenetic, and environmental factors. In this article I will attempt to analyze the various factors that have a triggering or protecting role, with particular reference to myasthenia gravis.

Keywords: myasthenia gravis; autoimmunity; genetics; epigenetics

Immunological factors involved in the loss of self-tolerance

All individuals normally carry identifiable autoreactive B and T cells. Intrathymic negative selection eliminates a great number of autoreactive T cells, in particular those that display high affinity receptors for self-antigens; however, this negative selection is not infallible. Many T cells with weak-to-moderate affinity for self-antigens survive the selection process and undergo peripheral stimulation, which can lead to the development of an autoimmune disease. The *AIRE* gene regulates this negative selection, which only leads to partial modulation of the efficiency of this process.[1]

Three main mechanisms contribute to autoreactive B and T cell activation: molecular mimicry, local inflammation of the target organ leading to increased immunogenicity of self-antigens, and polyclonal activation of B and T lymphocytes.

Molecular mimicry

Molecular mimicry is an old concept. Infectious agents are known to contain structural motifs that are also found in organ-specific self-antigens, such as sequential epitopes recognized by T cells and conformational epitopes recognized by antibodies. The two classic examples of this mechanism are rheumatic fever (cross-reaction between Streptococci and cardiac tissue) and Guillain–Barré syndrome (cross-reaction between *Campilobacter jejuni* bacteria and peripheral nerve gangliosides).[2] The concept can be extended to other autoimmune diseases, but there are still only few well-documented examples.

Local inflammation

The inflammation of an organ is known to increase the expression of molecules involved in antigen recognition. This is especially true in the case of viral infections. Theiler's virus at first induces a viral encephalitis rapidly followed by an autoimmune encephalitis because of the autoimmune T cell response triggered by the inflammation.[3] In addition to Theiler disease, this mechanism has been well established in experimental models, in particular for secondary cardiomyositis due to viral infection.[4] It is thought to be involved in many autoimmune diseases, such as multiple sclerosis and type 1 diabetes, but there is a lack of well-documented data supporting this etiology.[5] The chemical modification of some self-antigens is a related mechanism that leads to their recognition as being foreign and increases their immunogenicity. This is how the effects of penicillamin D on myasthenia gravis[6] and iodine on thyroiditis[7] are thought to be mediated.

doi: 10.1111/j.1749-6632.2012.06774.x

Polyclonal activation

A third mechanism is the polyclonal activation of autoreactive B or T cells. Activation can involve Th1 cells as is the case with interferon α[8] leading to the onset of various autoimmune diseases including myasthenia gravis.[9] Activation can lead to diminished immunoregulatory mechanisms. Treatment with anti-CD52 antibodies has been observed to lead to a significant depletion of circulating cells and to the onset of hyperthyroidism.[10] B cells undergo polyclonal activation in systemic lupus erythematosus with production of autoantibodies encoded by genes in germ-line configuration. What causes polyclonal activation is unclear and could be specific to the B lymphocytes of patients suffering from this disease.[11]

The search for etiologic agents

Two of the mechanisms mentioned above involve infectious agents. Very few autoimmune diseases have, however, been clearly linked to a specific pathogen. The explanation to the difficulty in identifying a link could be trivial. The infectious etiologic agent could be relatively common, and its effect on the onset of an autoimmune disease could be due to a genetic predisposition toward developing an immune response causing the disease. The infection might have occurred a long time before the clinical onset of the autoimmune disease making the identification of the pathogen difficult after many years.

There are numerous cases of homology between infectious agent proteins and autoantigens that can give rise to molecular mimicry.[12] Some authors have mentioned the possible involvement of a pathogen resembling the acetylcholine receptor in the onset of myasthenia gravis.[13] The search for mimetic structures is made difficult by the fact that the homology must involve a relatively large number of amino acids and that the search for conformational mimicry is very difficult. Furthermore, in the case of myasthenia gravis, the production of anti-RACh antibodies involves multiple receptor epitopes located on different chains as well as antibodies against other muscular antigens.[11] To date, it is unclear whether such autoantibodies are produced in parallel or whether there is a primary autoimmune reaction against a given antigen (RACh or another) followed by a secondary reaction against other epitopes (antigen spreading).

In spite of an intensive search for viruses, efforts yielded negative results for most of the autoimmune diseases examined. Recently, interesting studies investigated the possible role of the Epstein–Barr (EBV) virus, where different forms of the virus were found first in the brain of patients with multiple sclerosis and then in the thymus of patients suffering from myasthenia gravis.[14,15] Does this finding have an etiological implication or is the presence of EBV simply a bystander phenomenon? One hypothesis is that the activation and replication of EBV in memory B lymphocytes is a consequence of T cell activation of (through a bystander mechanism) or of autoreactive B cells. The possibility of a bystander effect linked to T cells is illustrated by the EBV reactivation observed in diabetic patients treated with a mitogenic anti-CD3 moncoclonal antibody.[16] In this case, one possibility is that the strong activation of T cells activates memory B cells. In fact, we have shown directly that the *in vitro* activation of T cells by an anti-CD3 antibody promotes replication and the activation of the EBV lytic cycle in B cells.[16] Before this hypothesis can be expanded, the results published for multiple sclerosis and myasthenia gravis need to be confirmed.[17]

In the case of drug-induced autoimmune diseases, which share the common characteristic of being regressive when treatment is interrupted, the situation is more complex because of the multiplicity of involved mechanisms. We have mentioned above penicillamin D[6] and interferon α[9] in the case of myasthenia gravis. There are many other examples, but they could represent specific situations and have limited importance in the context of spontaneous autoimmune diseases in which susceptibility genes may differ from those involved in the corresponding drug-induced autoimmune disease.

The role of genetic susceptibility

The role of genetic factors in the development of autoimmune diseases is well recognized. This is evident from the correlation rate for these diseases in monozygote twin pairs and even siblings. Two approaches have been used to identify the relevant genes.

The first approach is to look for an association between candidate genes and the disease in question. The most striking result has been the observation of a strong association between many autoimmune diseases and HLA genes. However, it should be noted that in most cases, the mechanism underlying this relationship is not as clear as initially thought. The central hypothesis of immune response genes (IR genes) is that a given HLA molecule presents a defined epitope causing the disease. However, other mechanisms need to be considered, in particular in the cases of rheumatoid arthritis,[18] myasthenia gravis,[19] and type 1 diabetes. For these two latter diseases, an important but yet unexplained role has been assigned to a locus located between HLA-B and TNF-α. Among other candidate genes, an important role in various autoimmune diseases has been recently given to the *PTPN22* gene, which is involved in the activation of T cells, in particular at the level of various cytokine signaling receptors.[20] Genes encoding the CTLA-4 molecule and the FCGR2 receptor are strongly suspected of a role in the predisposition to several autoimmune diseases, in particular, type 1 diabetes, myasthenia gravis, and systemic lupus erythematosus.[19,21] The data concerning other candidate genes, in particular the Toll-like receptor (TLR) genes, need to be confirmed.

In the case of myasthenia gravis, there is an association between the disease and RACh polymorphism.[21] This observation is all the more interesting because this association has been shown to be correlated with the regulation in the thymus of the negative selection mediated by RACh.[22]

One of the problems in understanding the role of candidate genes in autoimmune disease susceptibility is, with a few exceptions, the low relative risk for a given autoimmune disease carried by each of the genes, with the exception of the HLA genes that present a strong association with certain diseases such as type 1 diabetes, and an even stronger one with ankylosing spondylitis and narcolepsy[23] (but not with myasthenia gravis).[19] One can pose the question of whether these genes should really be considered as susceptibility genes or whether they are simply evidence of the involvement of the protein they encode in the pathophysiology of the disease. Another possibility is that the expression of these genes is highly reduced by epigenetic factors the existence and origin (role of the environment?) of which remain to be proven. Finally, systematic genomic screening has yielded surprising results with a large number of genes,[24] in fact, genetic regions that present a relative risk lower than that of candidate genes, raising the question of their relevance to disease etiology.

Additionally, because autoimmune diseases show a high level of concordance in twins and siblings, it is unlikely that the number of susceptibility genes would be high. This raises the question of the existence and definition of major susceptibility genes. Some models put the number of such major genes between two and four.

Extremely rare mutations that directly induce an autoimmune disease should of course be excluded from this discussion, such as, for example, mutations of the *FoxP3* gene (IPEX syndrome),[25] of the *AIRE* gene (APECED), and of the *NOD2* gene (Crohn's disease).[26]

The hygiene theory (revised by metagenomic studies of the intestinal flora)

Epidemiological data

The large increase in the frequency of most autoimmune (and allergic) diseases in developed countries over the last three decades is now a well-documented phenomenon.[27] It has been recently shown to be true for myasthenia gravis, at least for the forms occurring after the age of 30.[28,29] Not only has the number of cases increased, but for many diseases increasingly younger or older subjects are being affected. In parallel during the same period of time, a considerable decrease in the frequency of major infectious diseases has been observed, the main ones being tuberculosis and infantile diarrhea, which caused a large number of deaths until the 1960s.[29] The decrease in infections, although not general since many benign and severe infections are still observed, is explained by several factors including better hygiene, housing, water and food quality, improved nutrition, and the use of vaccines and antibiotics. The existence of a cause and effect relationship between the decline of infections and the increase of autoimmune and allergic diseases is currently being investigated.[30]

This hypothesis is corroborated by other epidemiological data. There is a north–south gradient in the prevalence of autoimmune diseases in both Europe and North America correlated with socioeconomic conditions.[27,30] Although epidemiological data from Africa are unreliable, there is every indication that the high frequency of infections observed is associated with very low frequencies of autoimmune and allergic diseases. These geographical variations are not due to genetic factors. When people migrate from countries of low incidence of certain autoimmune diseases, such as type 1 diabetes, to countries of high incidence, the frequency of the diseases increases as early as the first generation.[31]

Other epidemiological studies, mainly concerning allergic diseases and a few autoimmune diseases, have provided significant arguments in favor of the hygiene hypothesis, such as a higher frequency of hyperimmune diseases in first-born siblings and in children who were sent to nursery school at a late age[32] and a direct correlation between the onset of these diseases and the sanitary condition of the environment.

Cause and effect relationship

The causal relationship between the decline of infections and the increase in autoimmune diseases needs to be proven. Data are still lacking concerning human autoimmune diseases with the one exception concerning the improvement of some autoimmune pathologies after parasitic infestations.[33] By contrast, there is much more data concerning experimental models. Nonobese diabetic (NOD) mice housed in specific pathogen free (SPF) animal facilities of high sanitary quality present a very high frequency of diabetes unlike mice kept in conventional (less clean) facilities.[27] Interestingly, the infection of SFP mice with different infectious agents (bacteria, viruses, or parasites) completely prevents the onset of diabetes when the infection occurs at an early age.[27]

Germ-free mice present a complex problem. Results vary from one experimental model to another and even, depending on the publication, for the same given model. This is the case for NOD mice, where some authors observe an increase in diabetes in germ-free populations, while others do not.[34,35] For experimental allergic encephalomyelitis in transgenic mice that express a myelin basic protein-specific T cell receptor, the frequency of the disease is much lower in germ-free mice.[36] The same is observed in NZB mice.[37] The complexity of the problem lies in the fact that autoimmunity mechanisms are very different in these various models. Furthermore, the fact that germ-free mice suffer from immune deficiencies linked to an absence of exposure to infectious agents in their first days of life probably interferes in the development of au-

toimmune responses, while this is not the case in SPF mice.

The microbiome and autoimmune diseases

The human gut contains a very large quantity of bacteria belonging to over 200 species. These so-called commensal bacteria do not produce a specific pathogenic effect, but the composition of the microbiome, that is, the population of intestinal bacteria, could have an effect on the onset of some diseases. This idea was first evoked in the case of obesity when it was found that obese mice and humans present a reduced diversity of intestinal bacteria.[38] Similar observations were made for ulcerative colitis and Crohn's disease,[39] thus bringing us closer to autoimmune diseases. However, the two latter diseases are not strictly speaking autoimmune because the immune reactions are specifically directed against the intestinal commensal bacteria, making the interpretation of the data observed for these two diseases more complicated. A few recently published articles concerning experimental models and human diseases indicate that a decreased diversity in commensal bacteria is also observed in the case of various autoimmune diseases, in particular this has been reported for type 1 diabetes,[40,41] multiple sclerosis,[42] and rheumatoid arthritis.[43]

The possible link between microbiome composition and the development of some autoimmune diseases is supported by the demonstration that some commensal bacteria can slow the progression of several autoimmune diseases in experimental models. Segmented filamentous bacterium (SFB), which has been shown to induce the production of IL-17,[44] prevents the onset of type 1 diabetes in NOD mice.[45] These results have attracted great interest by the scientific community. However, they do not prove that the absence of some species of commensal bacteria has a role in the etiology of the disease because an essential control is lacking concerning the effect of other commensal bacteria in the development of these diseases. Of further interest is the fact that probiotic preparations, which are mixtures of commensal bacteria, can have a protective effect in the case of type 1 diabetes[46] in NOD mice as well as experimental colitis.[47]

All these considerations are interesting and deserve further studies. If the role of the microbiome in the predisposition to autoimmune diseases is confirmed, one can speculate a link to the hygiene hypothesis mentioned above. Both in mice and humans, reducing the exposure of newborns to an environment rich in pathogenic or nonpathogenic bacteria permanently modifies the intestinal microbiome. The major differences in the composition of the microbiomes of European and African children is a sufficiently convincing argument.[48] All of the factors mentioned above that participate in hygiene may affect the microbiome composition, whether they act on newborns directly or on mothers during pregnancy.

It should be noted, however, that if this hypothesis is confirmed, hygiene should not be considered as acting exclusively by means of the intestinal microbiome since, as mentioned above, several infections in young adults not linked to the gastrointestinal tract can prevent the onset of autoimmune diseases.

Molecular and cellular mechanisms underlying the protective effect of infections on autoimmune diseases

How commensal bacteria and pathogens prevent the onset of autoimmune diseases has yet to be clarified. Three types of mechanisms are currently being studied.[27]

The alteration of lymphocyte homeostasis by antigenic competition: immune responses developed against the "strong" antigens carried by infectious agents compete with the immune responses directed against autoantigens and allergens, which constitute "weak" antigens. At first, it was thought that this competition occurred during the antigen recognition phase at the level of dendritic cells. Now, it is thought to occur at the level of homeostatic factor consumption, in particular a number of cytokines such as IL-2, IL-15, and especially IL-7.

According to the bystander suppression hypothesis, antibacterial and anti-infectious responses in general induce regulatory T cells that display a suppressor effect that is not limited to infectious agents but that can also affect autoimmune responses.

The third hypothesis, regarding the stimulation of TLRs, involves bacterial ligands that act not as antigens but as stimulators of innate immunity receptors. TLR agonists are particularly interesting candidates for such a mechanism. The fact that many TLR agonists protect against the onset of type 1 diabetes in NOD mice[46] and experimental allergic encephalomyelitis[49] is a strong argument in favor of such a mechanism, which

may, however, seem paradoxical in the light of the potential role of TLRs in inducing autoimmune responses. The mechanism of action underlying stimulation of TLRs is complex and may even be different for each TLR. We have demonstrated in the NOD mouse model that TLR3 agonists involved iNKT cells while TLR4 agonists involved CD4+ FoxP3+ regulatory cells.[46]

General conclusions

The etiology of autoimmune diseases is clearly complex and involves multiple factors. There are a few cases where an external etiological agent can be found (rheumatic fever, Guillain–Barré syndrome, drug-induced autoimmune diseases). There are also very rare cases where autoimmune diseases have been linked to a point mutation in a gene involved in immunity (FoxP3, AIRE, and NOD2). In all the other cases, the importance of the genetic and environmental factors that either predispose or on the contrary oppose the onset of a particular disease needs to be assessed. Such an investigation is made complex by the fact that this situation will not only likely depend on the disease but also on factors intrinsic to the individuals.

Conflicts of interest

The author declares no conflicts of interest.

References

1. Mathis, D. & C. Benoist. 2009. AIRE. Annu. Rev. Immunol. 27: 287–312.
2. Yuki, N., K. Susuki, M. Koga, et al. 2004. Carbohydrate mimicry between human ganglioside GM1 and Campylobacter jejuni lipooligosaccharide causes Guillain–Barre syndrome. Proc. Natl. Acad. Sci. USA 101: 11404–11409.
3. Fuller, K.G., J.K. Olson, L.M. Howard, et al. 2004. Mouse models of multiple sclerosis: experimental autoimmune encephalomyelitis and Theiler's virus-induced demyelinating disease. Methods Mol. Med. 102: 339–361.
4. Rose, N.R. 2008. Autoimmunity in coxsackievirus infection. Curr. Top. Microbiol. Immunol. 323: 293–314.
5. Christen, U., C. Bender & M.G. von Herrath. 2012. Infection as a cause of type 1 diabetes? Curr. Opin. Rheumatol. 24: 417–423.
6. Penn, A.S., B.W. Low, I.A. Jaffe, et al. 1998. Drug-induced autoimmune myasthenia gravis. Ann. N.Y. Acad. Sci. 841: 433–449.
7. Barin, J.G., M.V. Taylor, R.B. Sharma, et al. 2005. Iodination of murine thyroglobulin enhances autoimmune reactivity in the NOD.H2 mouse. Clin. Exp. Immunol. 142: 251–259.
8. Batocchi, A.P., A. Evoli, S. Servidei, et al. 1995. Myasthenia gravis during interferon α therapy. Neurology 45: 382–383.

9. Borgia, G., L. Reynaud, I. Gentile, *et al.* 2001. Myasthenia gravis during low-dose IFN-α therapy for chronic hepatitis C. *J. Interferon Cytokine Res.* **21:** 469–470.

10. Coles, A.J., M. Wing, S. Smith, *et al.* 1999. Pulsed monoclonal antibody treatment and autoimmune thyroid disease in multiple sclerosis. *Lancet* **354:** 1691–1695.

11. Bach, J.F., S. Koutouzov & P.M. van Endert. 1998. Are there unique autoantigens triggering autoimmune diseases? *Immunol. Rev.* **164:** 139–155.

12. Oldstone, M.B. 2005. Molecular mimicry, microbial infection, and autoimmune disease: evolution of the concept. *Curr. Top. Microbiol. Immunol.* **296:** 1–17.

13. Im, S.H., D. Barchan, T. Feferman, *et al.* 2002. Protective molecular mimicry in experimental myasthenia gravis. *J. Neuroimmunol.* **126:** 99–106.

14. Cavalcante, P., L. Maggi, L. Colleoni, *et al.* 2011. Inflammation and Epstein–Barr virus infection are common features of myasthenia gravis thymus: possible roles in pathogenesis. *Autoimmune Dis.* 213092. Epub 2011 Sep 26.

15. Aloisi, F., B. Serafini, R. Magliozzi, *et al.* 2010. Detection of Epstein-Barr virus and B-cell follicles in the multiple sclerosis brain : what you find depends on how and where you look. *Brain* **133:** e157.

16. Keymeulen, B., S. Candon, S. Fafi-Kremer, *et al.* 2010. Transient Epstein–Barr virus reactivation in CD3 monoclonal antibody-treated patients. *Blood* **115:** 1145–1155.

17. Lassmann, H., G. Niedobitek, F. Aloisi, J.M. Middeldorp &NeuroProMiSe EBV Working Group. 2011. Epstein–Barr virus in the multiple sclerosis brain: a controversial issue—report on a focused workshop held in the Centre for Brain Research of the Medical University of Vienna, Austria. *Brain* **134**(Pt 9): 2772–2786.

18. Ronninger, M., M. Seddighzadeh, M.C. Eike, *et al.* 2012. Interaction analysis between HLA-DRB1 shared epitope alleles and MHC class II transactivator CIITA gene with regard to risk of rheumatoid arthritis. *PLoS One* **7:** e32861.

19. Giraud, M., C. Vandiedonck & H.J. Garchon. 2008. Genetic factors in autoimmune myasthenia gravis. *Ann. N.Y. Acad. Sci.* **1132:** 180–192.

20. Provenzano, C., R. Ricciardi, F. Scuderi, *et al.* 2012. PTPN22 and myasthenia gravis : replication in an Italian population and meta-analysis of literature data. *Neuromuscular Disorders* **22:** 131–138.

21. Garchon, H.J., F. Djabiri, J.P. Viard, *et al.* 1994. Involvement of human muscle acetylcholine receptor alpha-subunit gene (CHRNA) in susceptibility to myasthenia gravis. *Proc. Natl. Acad. Sci. USA* **91:** 4668–4672.

22. Giraud, M., R. Taubert, C. Vandiedonck, *et al.* 2007. An IRF8-binding promoter variant and AIRE control CHRNA1 promiscuous expression in thymus. *Nature* **448:** 934–937.

23. Dauvilliers, Y. & M. Tafti. 2006. Molecular genetics and treatment of narcolepsy. *Ann. Med.* **38:** 252–262.

24. Cho, J.H. & P.K. Gregersen. 2011. Genomics and the multifactorial nature of human autoimmune disease. *N. Engl. J. Med.* **365:** 1612–1623.

25. d'Hennezel, E., K. Bin Dhuban, T. Torgerson & C. Piccirillo. 2012. The immunogenetics of immune dysregulation, polyendocrinopathy, enteropathy, X linked (IPEX) syndrome. *J. Med. Genet.* **49:** 291–302.

26. Hugot, J.P., M. Chamaillard, H. Zouali, *et al.* 2001. Association of NOD2 leucine-rich repeat variants with susceptibility to Crohn's disease. *Nature* **411:** 599–603.

27. Bach, J.B. 2002. The effect of infections on susceptibility to autoimmune and allergic diseases. *N. Engl. J. Med.* **347:** 911–920.

28. Matsui, N., S. Nakane, Y. Nakagawa, *et al.* 2009. Increasing incidence of elderly onset patients with myasthenia gravis in a local area of Japan. *J. Neurol. Neurosurg. Psychiatr.* **80:** 1168–1171.

29. Casetta, I., E. Groppo, R. De Gennaro, *et al.* 2010. Myasthenia gravis: a changing pattern of incidence. *J. Neurol.* **257:** 2015–2019.

30. Okada, H., C. Kuhn, H. Feillet & J.F. Bach. 2010. The "hygiene hypothesis" for autoimmune and allergic diseases: an update. *Clin. Exp. Immunol.* **160:** 1–9.

31. Bodansky, H.J., A. Staines, C. Stephenson, *et al.* 1992. Evidence for an environmental effect in the aetiology of insulin dependent diabetes in a transmigratory population. *Br. Med. J.* **304:** 1020–1022.

32. Celedon, J.C., R.J. Wright, A.A. Litonjua, *et al.* 2003. Day care attendance in early life, maternal history of asthma, and asthma at the age of 6 years. *Am. J. Respir. Crit. Care Med.* **167:** 1239–1243.

33. Correale, J. & M.F. Farez. 2011. The impact of parasite infections on the course of multiple sclerosis. *J. Neuroimmunol.* **233:** 6–11.

34. Alam, C., E. Bittoun, D. Bhagwat, *et al.* 2011. Effects of a germ-free environment on gut immune regulation and diabetes progression in non-obese diabetic (NOD) mice. *Diabetologia.* **54:** 1398–1406.

35. Suzuki, T., T. Yamado, T. Takao, *et al.* 1987. Diabetogenic Effects of Lymphocyte Transfusion on the NOD or NOD Nude Mouse. Karger. Basel.

36. Berer, K., M. Mues, M. Koutrolos, *et al.* 2011. Commensal microbiota and myelin autoantigen cooperate to trigger autoimmune demyelination. *Nature* **479:** 538–541.

37. Unni, K.K., K.E. Holley, F.C. McDuffie & J.L. Titus. 1975. Comparative study of NZB mice under germfree and conventional conditions. *J. Rheumatol.* **2:** 36–44.

38. Ley, R.E. 2010. Obesity and the human microbiome. *Curr. Opin. Gastroenterol.* **26:** 5–11.

39. Hammer, H.F. 2011. Gut microbiota and inflammatory bowel disease. *Dig. Dis.* **29:** 550–553.

40. Brown, C.T., A.G. Davis-Richardson, A. Giongo, *et al.* 2011. Gut microbiome metagenomics analysis suggests a functional model for the development of autoimmunity for type 1 diabetes. *PLoS One* **6:** e25792.

41. Giongo, A., K.A. Gano, D.B. Crabb, *et al.* 2011. Toward defining the autoimmune microbiome for type 1 diabetes. *ISME J.* **5:** 82–91.

42. Power, C., J.M. Antony, K.K. Ellestad, *et al.* 2010. The human microbiome in multiple sclerosis: pathogenic or protective constituents? *Can. J. Neurol. Sci.* **37:** S24–S33.

43. Vaahtovuo, J., E. Munukka, M. Korkeamäki, *et al.* 2008. Fecal microbiota in early rheumatoid arthritis. *J. Rheumatol.* **35:** 1500–1505.

44. Wu, H.J., I.I. Ivanov, J. Darce, *et al.* 2010. Gut-residing seg-mented filamentous bacteria drive autoimmune arthritis via T helper 17 cells. *Immunity* **32:** 815–827.

45. Kriegel, M.A., E. Sefik, J.A. Hill, *et al.* 2011. Naturally trans-mitted segmented filamentous bacteria segregate with dia-betes protection in nonobese diabetic mice. *Proc. Natl. Acad. Sci. USA* **108:** 11548–11553.

46. Aumeunier, A., F. Grela, A. Ramadan, *et al.* 2010. Systemic Toll-like receptor stimulation suppresses experimental aller-gic asthma and autoimmune diabetes in NOD mice. *PLoS One* **5:** e11484

47. Mazmanian, S.K., J.L. Round & D.L. Kasper. 2008. A mi-crobial symbiosis factor prevents intestinal inflammatory disease. *Nature* **453:** 620–625.

48. De Filippo, C., D. Cavalieri, M. Di Paola, *et al.* 2010. Impact of diet in shaping gut microbiota revealed by a comparative study in children from Europe and rural Africa. *Proc. Natl. Acad. Sci. USA* **107:** 14691–14696.

49. Marta, M., A. Andersson, M. Isaksson, *et al.* 2008. Unex-pected regulatory roles of TLR4 and TLR9 in experimental autoimmune encephalomyelitis. *Eur. J. Immunol.* **38:** 565–575.

Ann. N.Y. Acad. Sci. ISSN 0077-8923

ANNALS OF THE NEW YORK ACADEMY OF SCIENCES

Issue: *Myasthenia Gravis and Related Disorders*

Defects of immunoregulatory mechanisms in myasthenia gravis: role of IL-17

Angeline Gradolatto,[1] Dani Nazzal,[1] Maria Foti,[2] Jacky Bismuth,[1] Frederique Truffault,[1] Rozen Le Panse,[1] and Sonia Berrih-Aknin[1]

[1]Unité mixte de recherche, CNRS UMR7215/INSERM U974/UPMC UM76/AIM, Thérapie des maladies du muscle strié, Institut de Myologie, Paris, France. [2]Genopolis Consortium, University of Milano-Bicocca, Italy

Address for correspondence: Sonia Berrih-Aknin, Unité Mixte de Recherche, CNRS UMR7215/INSERM U974/UPMC UM76/AIM, Thérapie des maladies du muscle strié, Groupe hospitalier Pitié-Salpêtrière, 105, boulevard de l'Hôpital, 75651 PARIS Cedex 13, France. sonia.berrih-aknin@upmc.fr

Deficient immunoregulation is consistently observed in autoimmune diseases. Here, we summarize the abnormalities of the T cell response in autoimmune myasthenia gravis (MG) by focusing on activation markers, inflammatory features, and imbalance between the different T cell subsets, including Th17 and regulatory T cells (T_{reg} cells). In the thymus from MG patients, T_{reg} cell numbers are normal while their suppressive function is severely defective, and this defect could not be explained by contaminating effector $CD127^{low}$ T cells. A transcriptomic analysis of T_{reg} cell and conventional T cell (T_{conv}; $CD4^+CD25^-$ cells) subsets pointed out an upregulation of Th17-related genes in MG cells. Together with our previous findings of an inflammatory signature in the MG thymus and an overproduction of IL-1 and IL-6 by MG thymic epithelial cells (TEC), these data strongly suggest that T cell functions are profoundly altered in the thymic pathological environment. In this short review we discuss the mechanisms of chronic inflammation linked to the pathophysiology of MG disease.

Keywords: myasthenia gravis; thymus; T_{reg} cells; Th17; inflammation; thymic epithelial cells

In most patients with myasthenia gravis (MG), the autoimmune response is mediated by antibodies against the acetylcholine receptor (AChR). The muscle is the target of the autoimmune attack and expresses reduced level of AChR, although it is under active compensatory mechanisms to limit the AChR decrease.[1,2] In this form of the disease, the thymus frequently displays structural and functional abnormalities either characterized by the presence of a tumor (thymoma, 15% of MG patients) or the presence of germinal centers (GCs) defined as thymic hyperplasia (60% of MG patients).[3] The hyperplastic MG thymus contains all the components necessary for an anti-AChR immune response including activated autoreactive B and T cells, antigen-presenting cells (APCs) and the autoantigen itself.[4–7] The role of the thymus in the production of the anti-AChR response was definitely and convincingly demonstrated in the model of immunodeficient mice where human anti-AChR antibodies were detectable when mice were grafted with MG thymus fragments or cells.[8,9]

Production of anti-AChR antibodies is dependent upon $CD4^+$ T cells.[10] Naive $CD4^+$ T cells can differentiate into several Th subsets including Th1, Th2, Th17, and T follicular effector cells (Tfh). On the basis of their respective cytokine profiles, responses to chemokines, and interactions with other cells, these T cell subsets can promote different types of inflammatory responses. Th1 cells produce the cytokine IFN-γ, which promotes Th1 differentiation, cytotoxic activity and upregulation of MHC class I and II.[11] Effector Th2 cells produce interleukin (IL)-4, IL-5, IL-9, IL-10, and IL-13. The discovery of the Th17 cells has revealed another proinflammatory T cell subset involved in several inflammatory disorders such as rheumatoid arthritis, multiple sclerosis, and Crohn disease. Th17 cells are characterized by their production of IL-17A, IL-17F, IL-21, IL-22, IL-26, and TNF-α, and by their expression

doi: 10.1111/j.1749-6632.2012.06791.x

of ROR-γt, the Th17 lineage-specific transcription factor. Tfh provide helper functions to B cells; they are one of the largest and most important subsets of effector T cells in lymphoid tissues. Finally, subsets of regulatory T (T_{reg}) cells regulate and counter-balance the immune response; they have distinct phenotypes and mechanisms of action and include $CD4^+CD25^+Foxp3^+$ T_{reg} cells, which are selected in the thymus (reviewed in Ref. 11).

Th subsets and activation markers in MG immune cells

MG patients have elevated numbers of blood mononuclear cells (MNC) expressing IFN-γ and IL-4, indicating that both Th1 and Th2 cells are involved in MG pathogenic mechanisms. The expression of these cytokines increases further upon culture of MNC from MG patients in the presence of AChR.[12] The implication of Th1 cells has also been suggested by the increased number of cells expressing CXCR3 (chemokine receptor preferentially expressed on Th1 cells) in the thymus and in $CD4^+$ peripheral T cells from MG patients.[13] CXCR3 expression was also upregulated in the experimental mouse model of myasthenia gravis (EAMG), suggesting that CXCR3 increase results from the immunization and inflammation processes. Interestingly, molecules inhibiting the binding of the CXCR3 ligand, CXCL10, to its receptor limit the severity of MG, indicating that this could be a new therapeutic approach.[14] The implication of the Th2 associated cytokine IL-10, which suppresses production of cytokines released by Th1 cells, has also been evaluated in EAMG. IL-10 caused earlier onset, and aggravated AChR-specific B cell responses and clinical signs of EAMG, although Th1 responses were suppressed.[15]

Tfh cells are a subset distinguishable from Th1 and Th2 cells by several criteria, including chemokine receptor expression (CXCR5), location/migration (B cell follicles), and function (B cell help).[16] Tfh activity classically occurs in GCs located in B cell follicles of secondary lymphoid organs, a site of immunoglobulin affinity maturation and isotype switching.[17] It appears that Tfh cells are also involved in MG. Indeed, MG patients showed a significantly higher frequency of $CXCR5^+CD4^+$ T cells in blood compared with the control group. In addition, the frequency of $CXCR5^+CD4^+$ T cells correlated with disease severity. After thymectomy and glucocorticoid treatment, the percentage of

$CXCR5^+$ $CD4^+$ T cells decreased gradually to the control level with a significant inverse correlation between the $CXCR5^+CD4^+$ T cell frequency and duration of the therapy.[18] Interestingly, major expansions in diverse TCR $V_β$ among $CD4^+$ T cells were associated with the $CD57^+CXCR5^+$ subset. Furthermore, the expression of markers for activation on these cells, lymphocyte trafficking, and B cell-activating ability persisted for more than three years, strengthening the hypothesis of a chronic activation. Thus, these data provide evidence for persistent clonally expanded B helper $CD4^+$ T cell populations in the blood of MG patients.[19]

Together, these data strongly support that in MG disease Th1, Th2, and Tfh cells are involved. Accordingly, several markers of activation related to T cell function have been associated with MG. IL-2 is known to be produced by T cells and is essential for the development of T_{reg} cells; but IL-2 acts also as B cell growth factor and stimulates antibody synthesis.[11] We showed that thymic lymphocytes from MG patients have an enhanced sensitivity to recombinant IL-2[20] and that serum levels of soluble IL-2R (sIL-2R) were increased in about a third of patients before thymectomy, and even more so in severely affected patients. Sequential sampling after thymectomy indicated a significant and progressive decline of sIL-2R levels within two years after surgery, which correlated with clinical improvement or remission.[21] In addition, increased sIL-2R titers were significantly associated with generalized and bulbar MG disease, while ocular cases were not different from controls,[22] indicating that sIL-2R is a marker of MG severity. MG patients have also higher serum levels of soluble adhesion molecules such sICAM-1 and sVCAM-1 than healthy control individuals, and plasmapheresis can induce their substantial decrease together with a decrease in anti-AChR Ab titer.[23]

The higher levels of activation markers consistently observed in MG patients support the hypothesis of a systemic and chronic activation that involves the different $CD4^+$ cell subsets as well as B cells. Accordingly, the B cell response is highly activated. Isolated B cells from thymic hyperplasia spontaneously produce anti-AChR antibodies.[4] In the periphery, total Ig production is higher in MG patients than in age-matched healthy control individuals,[24] suggesting that the increase in Ig synthesis is not restricted to anti-AChR antibodies. In this context, antibodies against several autoantigens other than AChR have been detected in MG patients, in particular muscle-cell antigens, such as titin or ryanodine receptor.[25] In addition, our microarray analysis in thymic tissue revealed an overexpression of most Ig genes spotted on the array in MG thymus compared to healthy tissue,[26,27] even unrelated to anti-AChR response. Together, these findings suggest that the production of anti-AChR antibodies in MG is probably linked to an overall stimulation of Ig production.

In a normal immune infectious response, a triggering agent stimulates an early inflammatory response that starts to control the infection, and this step is followed by immune suppression. As the infection is cleared, inflammation decreases while immune suppression continues to increase, resulting in the resolution of inflammation. Chronic inflammation could be due to impaired resolution despite the absence of infectious agents, because of inefficient immune suppression. The high level of inflammation observed in MG patients raises the possibility of potential defects in immune suppression mechanisms required for the resolution of the immune response.

Thymic T_{reg} cells from MG patients are severely defective

$CD4^+CD25^+$ T_{reg} cells have a major role in the control of the autoimmune response, and more generally in the immune response.[28] Qualitative or quantitative defects of T_{reg} cells have been demonstrated in many autoimmune diseases. In MG patients, we could not detect any changes in the number of $CD4^+CD25^+$ or $CD4^+CD25^{hi}$ T cells in the thymus.[29] We then evaluated the expression of Foxp3, a specific marker for T_{reg} cells. The percentage of Foxp3+ cells among $CD4^+$ cells (Fig. 1A), as well as the fluorescence intensity of Foxp3+ T cells (Fig. 1B), were similar in MG patients and controls. A recent report confirmed these observations by an immunofluorescence analysis of thymic sections. $CD4^+CD8^-$ Foxp3+ cells were predominantly found in the thymic medulla and their number declined with age, but there was no significant difference in the number or the distribution of these cells in the thymus between MG patients and controls.[30] In contrast, another group observed a decrease in the number of peripheral $CD4^+CD25^+$ T cells in MG patients;[31] in another study, however, the same team reported that there was no difference in peripheral T_{reg} cell numbers between MG

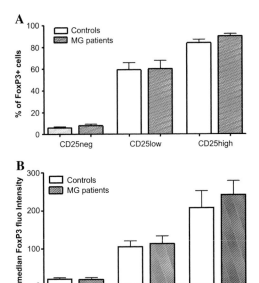

Figure 1. Foxp3 expression in $CD4^+$ thymic cells. The percentage of Foxp3+ cells (A) and the median fluorescence intensity of Foxp3 (B) were evaluated in $CD25^{neg}$, $CD25^{low}$, and $CD25^{high}$ gated cells by flow cytometry in MG patients ($n = 8$) compared to controls ($n = 8$). The results are expressed as mean value ± SEM.

patients and healthy individuals. Thus, if there are changes in the number of T_{reg} cells in MG patients, these changes must be subtle.[32] However, more recently, Zhang *et al.* showed that while the percentage of $CD4^+CD25^+$ T cells was not changed in MG patients Foxp3 was dramatically downregulated in peripheral $CD4^+CD25^+$ T cells at both mRNA and protein expression levels.[33] This discordance could be explained by technical differences, such as the use of anti-Foxp3 antibodies that recognize different epitopes, but it could also be due to biological differences related to different genetic backgrounds of the cohorts tested. Indeed, the study by Zhang *et al.* was carried out on Chinese patients, while patients included in the other studies were Caucasian.

If changes of T_{reg} markers are still a matter of debate in MG patients, their function appears to be clearly defective. We showed that T_{reg} cells from MG thymus have a severe defect in their suppressive function when co-cultured with autologous $CD4^+CD25^-$ T cells.[29] This result was confirmed by Zhang *et al.*,[33] and more recently by Luther *et al.* using peripheral blood cells.[34] To address the possibility that this defect may be attributable

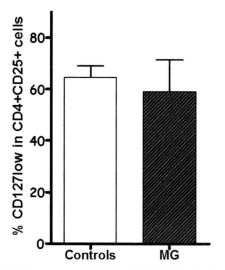

Figure 2. Expression of CD127 in CD4$^+$CD25$^+$ cells. The percentage of cells expressing low or negative level of CD127 was evaluated in CD4$^+$CD25$^+$ cells by flow cytometry in MG patients ($n = 4$) compared to controls ($n = 5$). The results are expressed as the mean value of the percentage of CD127$^{neg/low}$ in CD4$^+$CD25$^+$ cells ± SEM.

to the presence of a high number of activated effector cells in the isolated T$_{reg}$ population, we analyzed the expression of CD127, the IL-7 receptor, recently shown to discriminate between regulatory and effector function[35] in CD4$^+$CD25$^+$ T cells. MG and control CD4$^+$ thymocytes did not differ in CD127 expression by CD4$^+$CD25$^+$ T cells (Fig. 2). These results highly suggest that the defect in suppressive activity of thymic T$_{reg}$ cells in MG patients is not due to an excess of effector cells among the CD4$^+$CD25$^+$ T cell population. The defect of T$_{reg}$ cell function was further corroborated by data from EAMG rat models showing that administration of *ex vivo*-generated T$_{reg}$ cells to myasthenic rats inhibited the progression of experimental autoimmune MG and led to downregulation of humoral acetylcholine receptor-specific responses.[36] However, Nessi *et al.* showed that the action of T$_{reg}$ cells is more beneficial in preventing the events leading to EAMG development, rather than having an effect as a therapeutic approach.[37]

In our analysis of CD4$^+$CD25$^+$ thymic cells, we also observed that cells from MG patients express high levels of Fas and HLA-DR compared to controls. Interestingly, Fas (CD95) is overexpressed on autoreactive T cells from MG patients[7] and is upregulated by CD3-mediated activation.[38] Since the

CD4$^+$CD25$^+$ T cell population from MG thymi contains a large proportion of Fas^{hi} cells, we wondered whether the defect in suppressive activity of CD4$^+$CD25$^+$ T cells was due to this population, which was thought to include activated effector cells. After sorting CD4$^+$CD25$^+$Fas^{lo} and CD4$^+$CD25$^+$Fas^{hi} cells from MG thymi and testing their suppressive activity, we found that both subpopulations were unable to suppress the proliferation of CD4$^+$CD25$^-$ cells, while the same cell subsets from normal thymus suppressed the proliferation of their CD4$^+$CD25$^-$ counterparts.[29] Together, these results demonstrate that the defect of suppressive function in MG is severe whatever the subset of CD4$^+$CD25$^+$ T cells.

Relationship between defect of T$_{reg}$ cells and inflammatory events: role of IL-17

T$_{reg}$ cells are defective during MG pathogenesis. Since immunological investigations are carried out in MG patients when the disease is well established, it is not clear if the T$_{reg}$ dysfunction is a primary causal event or results from perturbations of the immune system during the disease development. It is possible that this defect is genetically or epigenetically predetermined, so that, in case of inflammation, the defective T$_{reg}$ cells would be unable to neutralize the inflammatory environment. It was indeed recently shown, in the model of type 1 diabetes, that the presence of a disease-associated IL-2RA haplotype led to diminished IL-2 responsiveness, resulting in lower levels of Foxp3 expression by T$_{reg}$ cells and a reduction in their ability to suppress proliferation of autologous T$_{conv}$ cells.[39] The potential involvement of IL-2RA polymorphism in MG has not yet been investigated.

However, it is also possible that the inflammatory environment reduces the functional activity of T$_{reg}$ cells. Indeed recent findings challenge the stability of T$_{reg}$ cells and demonstrate that T$_{reg}$ cells adapt to microenvironmental changes and, consequently, manifest functional plasticity by reprogramming into inflammatory T cells.[40] For example, it was shown that T$_{reg}$ cells stimulated with TGF-β exhibit sustained expression of Foxp3 while in the presence of TGF-β; on the other hand, IL-6 alone or in combination with IL-1 and IL-23 markedly downregulated Foxp3 expression and increased IL-17 production. Therefore, the T$_{reg}$ program appears to be turned off by IL-6, and T$_{reg}$ cells can be reprogrammed to the Th17 phenotype by TGF-β and IL-6.[41] A close relationship between CD4+Foxp3+ T_{reg} cells and proinflammatory IL-17–producing T cells was recently confirmed by the unexpected finding that human memory Foxp3+ T_{reg} cells secrete IL-17 *ex vivo* and constitutively express RORγt.[42] However, this finding is observed essentially in the periphery, as the normal human thymus does not contain IL-17–producing T_{reg} cells.[43] In the context described above in which MG TEC overproduce IL-6 and IL-1,[44,45] one might assume that such an environment could modify the balance between functional T_{reg} cells and inflammatory cells, namely Th17 cells, or, as suggested above, that T_{reg} cells themselves could be driven to secrete the proinflammatory IL-17.

Th17 cells and IL-17 pathway have been implicated in several autoimmune diseases such as experimental autoimmune encephalomyelitis, rheumatoid arthritis, psoriasis, and multiple sclerosis, in which levels of IL-17 mRNA were increased in both blood and cerebrospinal fluid.[46] Although Th17 cells appear to have a major role in inflammation and autoimmune responses, knowledge on the implication of this cell subset in human MG is very limited. A recent manuscript described high levels of IL-17 in the serum of generalized MG patients compared with controls.[47] Masuda *et al.* have evaluated the frequency of IL-17–producing CD4+ T cell subsets in peripheral blood mononuclear cells (PBMC) of patients with MG, but did not observe significant difference in RORγt mRNA expression between MG patients and healthy subjects.[48] Wang *et al.* showed an increase in Th17 cells and their associated cytokines in PBMC, but exclusively in MG patients with thymomas.[49] An imbalance of Th and T_{reg} cell subsets has also been demonstrated in EAMG rat model.[36,50] EAMG animals showed an upregulation of IL-17–related genes and down regulation of T_{reg} cell–regulated genes. Treatment with anti-IL-6 was sufficient to reverse gene expression and improve the disease at either the acute or chronic phase.[36]

The severe and consistent defects of immunoregulation in MG patients led us to analyze more deeply the T_{reg} and T_{conv} molecular contents by microarray technology. This experiment was performed by first sorting CD4+ cells, and then by isolating CD4+CD25+ and CD4+CD25− cells. Comparison of differentially expressed genes between T_{reg} and T_{conv}

cells from MG and controls separately confirmed the predominant expression of reference genes for the T_{reg} cell subset, such as Foxp3, CTLA4, GITR, and CD25. Interestingly, many genes of the IL-17 family (IL-17A, IL-17F, IL-21, IL-22, IL-26), together with Th1-specific genes such as IFN-γ and TNF-α, were upregulated in MG cells, compared to controls. These results were confirmed in our analysis on whole protein extracts from thymuses, in which a higher level of IL-17 was found in MG thymus compared to controls.

The increase in IFN-γ and IL-17–related genes indicated that both Th1 and Th17 cells are overrepresented in MG cells. Alternatively, it is possible that MG cell preparation included a high number of cells co-expressing IL-17 and IFN-γ. Several reports have recently focused on cells co-expressing IL-17A and IFN-γ (a cytokine normally associated with Th1 cells) adding to the complexity of Th17 cell heterogeneity. These IFN-γ/IL-17 double-producing cells are found in both mice and humans, often associated with infections. These findings indicate that cells of the Th17 lineage are plastic and fail to maintain a stable phenotype when cultured *in vitro* or when transferred *in vivo* to recipient mice in certain situations acquiring the ability to secrete additional cytokines (reviewed in Ref. 51).

Consequences of immune cell defects on chronic inflammation and pathophysiology of myasthenia gravis

The data described herein summarize the dysregulation of the immune system observed in MG patients. We propose that a primary event of yet unknown origin could cause inflammation in the thymus that would induce critical changes and lead to MG. The presence of the autoantigen AChR in the thymus, its high immunogenicity, and the possible regulation of its expression by pro-inflammatory cytokines make this molecule a potential autoimmune target in this highly activated site, which would perpetuate the autoimmune and inflammatory response.[52] Why AChR expressed in the thymus is not properly tolerated in MG patients is not clear. Both IFN-γ and AIRE are able to regulate AChR-alpha, and a defect of tolerance mechanisms would suggest a defect of AIRE in MG thymus before the onset of the disease. Because inflammation alters the expression of many genes including AIRE, this hypothesis will be very difficult to prove, since thymic tissues are only available after the onset of the disease.

The initial event(s) leading to an inflammatory response in the thymus could then trigger an overproduction *in situ* of various cytokines and chemokines,[53,54] which in turn would attract B and T cells from the periphery. Whether these cells are already activated when they reach the thymus is not clear. However, since the level of activation of these cells in the thymus is much higher than it is in the periphery,[7,20] we believe that the ongoing activation of the cells occurs in the thymus.

Once T cells are activated in the thymus, one could expect their activation status to be regulated by T_{reg} cells; but since MG T_{reg} cells are nonfunctional, the general level of activation and inflammation remains very high. The T_{reg} cell defect could be linked to the high IL-1 and IL-6 production by MG TEC, and these cytokines drive Foxp3$^+$ T cells to secrete IL-17.[43,44,55,] In this context, the question is: Why do TEC overproduce proinflammatory cytokines? The triggering event likely contributes to this overproduction, but it is possible that TECs from MG patients have the genetic background that allows a continuous and chronic activation status. Indeed, data showing that TECs kept a high activation status for at least two weeks *in vitro* away from the thymic environment support this hypothesis and deserve further investigation.

In conclusion, we propose that the primary triggering event induces inflammation of the thymus that remains chronic because of defective T_{reg} cells. Our continuing microarray experiments revealed the IL-17 pathway, and support a role for Th17 cells in chronic inflammation, a common feature in MG disease. Further functional analyses are ongoing to decipher more precisely the role of IL-17 in MG pathology.

Acknowledgments

The work presented here was supported by grants from The Association Francaise Contre les Myopathies (AFM) and The European Commission (MYASTAID, LSHM-CT-2006–037833) and (FIGHT-MG, Contract # FP7 HEALTH-2009-242-210).

Conflicts of interest

The authors declare no conflicts of interest.

References

1. Guyon, T. *et al.* 1994. Regulation of acetylcholine receptor alpha subunit variants in human myasthenia gravis. Quantification of steady-state levels of messenger RNA in muscle biopsy using the polymerase chain reaction. *J. Clin. Invest.* **94:** 16–24.
2. Guyon, T. *et al.* 1998. Regulation of acetylcholine receptor gene expression in human myasthenia gravis muscles. Evidences for a compensatory mechanism triggered by receptor loss. *J. Clin. Invest.* **102:** 249–263.
3. Berrih, S. *et al.* 1984. Anti-AChR antibodies, thymic histology, and T cell subsets in myasthenia gravis. *Neurology* **34:** 66–71.
4. Leprince, C. *et al.* 1990. Thymic B cells from myasthenia gravis patients are activated B cells. Phenotypic and functional analysis. *J. Immunol.* **145:** 2115–2122.
5. Melms, A. *et al.* 1988. Thymus in myasthenia gravis. Isolation of T-lymphocyte lines specific for the nicotinic acetylcholine receptor from thymuses of myasthenic patients. *J. Clin. Invest.* **81:** 902–908.
6. Wakkach, A. *et al.* 1996. Expression of acetylcholine receptor genes in human thymic epithelial cells: implications for myasthenia gravis. *J. Immunol.* **157:** 3752–3760.
7. Moulian, N. *et al.* 1997. Thymocyte Fas expression is dysregulated in myasthenia gravis patients with anti-acetylcholine receptor antibody. *Blood* **89:** 3287–3295.
8. Schonbeck, S. *et al.* 1992. Transplantation of thymic autoimmune microenvironment to severe combined immunodeficiency mice. A new model of myasthenia gravis. *J. Clin. Invest.* **90:** 245–250.
9. Aissaoui, A. *et al.* 1999. Prevention of autoimmune attack by targeting specific T-cell receptors in a severe combined immunodeficiency mouse model of myasthenia gravis [see comments]. *Ann. Neurol.* **46:** 559–567.
10. Christadoss, P. & M.J. Dauphinee. 1986. Immunotherapy for myasthenia gravis: a murine model. *J. Immunol.* **136:** 2437–2440.
11. Akdis, M. *et al.* 2011. Interleukins, from 1 to 37, and interferon-gamma: receptors, functions, and roles in diseases. *J. Allergy. Clin. Immunol.* **127:** 701–721 e701–e770.
12. Link, J. 1994. Interferon-gamma, interleukin-4 and transforming growth factor-beta mRNA expression in multiple sclerosis and myasthenia gravis. *Acta Neurol. Scand. Suppl.* **158:** 1–58.
13. Feferman, T. *et al.* 2005. Overexpression of IFN-induced protein 10 and its receptor CXCR3 in myasthenia gravis. *J. Immunol.* **174:** 5324–5331.
14. Feferman, T. *et al.* 2009. Suppression of experimental autoimmune myasthenia gravis by inhibiting the signaling between IFN-gamma inducible protein 10 (IP-10) and its receptor CXCR3. *J. Neuroimmunol.* **209:** 87–95.
15. Zhang, G.X. *et al.* 2001. Interleukin 10 aggravates experimental autoimmune myasthenia gravis through inducing Th2 and B cell responses to AChR. *J. Neuroimmunol.* **113:** 10–18.
16. Bauquet, A.T. *et al.* 2009. The costimulatory molecule ICOS regulates the expression of c-Maf and IL-21 in the development of follicular T helper cells and TH-17 cells. *Nat. Immunol.* **10:** 167–175.

17. Weinstein, J.S., S.G. Hernandez & J. Craft. 2012. T cells that promote B-cell maturation in systemic autoimmunity. *Immunol. Rev.* **247:** 160–171.

18. Saito, R. *et al.* 2005. Altered expression of chemokine receptor CXCR5 on T cells of myasthenia gravis patients. *J. Neuroimmunol.* **170:** 172–178.

19. Tackenberg, B. *et al.* 2007. Clonal expansions of CD4+ B helper T cells in autoimmune myasthenia gravis. *Eur. J. Immunol.* **37:** 849–863.

20. Cohen-Kaminsky, S. *et al.* 1989. Evidence of enhanced recombinant interleukin-2 sensitivity in thymic lymphocytes from patients with myasthenia gravis: possible role in autoimmune pathogenesis. *J. Neuroimmunol.* **24:** 75–85.

21. Cohen Kaminsky, S. *et al.* 1992. Follow-up of soluble interleukin-2 receptor levels after thymectomy in patients with myasthenia gravis. *Clin. Immunol. Immunopathol.* **62:** 190–198.

22. Confalonieri, P. *et al.* 1993. Immune activation in myasthenia gravis: soluble interleukin-2 receptor, interferon-gamma and tumor necrosis factor-alpha levels in patients' serum. *J. Neuroimmunol.* **48:** 33–36.

23. Tesar, V. *et al.* 2000. Soluble adhesion molecules and cytokines in patients with myasthenia gravis treated by plasma exchange. *Blood Purif.* **18:** 115–120.

24. Yoshikawa, H. *et al.* 2001. Analysis of immunoglobulin secretion by lymph organs with myasthenia gravis. *Acta Neurol. Scand.* **103:** 53–58.

25. Romi, F. *et al.* 2000. Muscle autoantibodies in subgroups of myasthenia gravis patients. *J. Neurol.* **247:** 369–375.

26. Cizeron-Clairac, G. *et al.* 2008. Thymus and Myasthenia Gravis: what can we learn from DNA microarrays? *J. Neuroimmunol.* **201–202:** 57–63.

27. Le Panse, R. *et al.* 2006. Microarrays reveal distinct gene signatures in the thymus of seropositive and seronegative myasthenia gravis patients and the role of CC chemokine ligand 21 in thymic hyperplasia. *J. Immunol.* **177:** 7868–7879.

28. Hori, S., T. Takahashi & S. Sakaguchi. 2003. Control of autoimmunity by naturally arising regulatory CD4+ T cells. *Adv. Immunol.* **81:** 331–371.

29. Balandina, A. *et al.* 2005. Functional defect of regulatory CD4(+)CD25+ T cells in the thymus of patients with autoimmune myasthenia gravis. *Blood* **105:** 735–741.

30. Matsui, N. *et al.* 2010. Undiminished regulatory T cells in the thymus of patients with myasthenia gravis. *Neurology* **74:** 816–820.

31. Fattorossi, A. *et al.* 2005. Circulating and thymic CD4 CD25 T regulatory cells in myasthenia gravis: effect of immunosuppressive treatment. *Immunology* **116:** 134–141.

32. Battaglia, A. *et al.* 2005. Circulating CD4+CD25+ T regulatory and natural killer T cells in patients with myasthenia gravis: a flow cytometry study. *J. Biol. Regul. Homeost. Agents* **19:** 54–62.

33. Zhang, Y. *et al.* 2009. The role of Foxp3+CD4+CD25hi Tregs in the pathogenesis of myasthenia gravis. *Immunol. Lett.* **122:** 52–57.

34. Luther, C. *et al.* 2009. Prednisolone treatment induces tolerogenic dendritic cells and a regulatory milieu in myasthenia gravis patients. *J. Immunol.* **183:** 841–848.

35. Liu, W. *et al.* 2006. CD127 expression inversely correlates with Foxp3 and suppressive function of human CD4+ T reg cells. *J. Exp. Med.* **203:** 1701–1711.

36. Aricha, R. *et al.* 2011. Blocking of IL-6 suppresses experimental autoimmune myasthenia gravis. *J. Autoimmunol.* **36:** 135–141.

37. Nessi, V. *et al.* 2010. Naturally occurring CD4+CD25+ regulatory T cells prevent but do not improve experimental myasthenia gravis. *J. Immunol.* **185:** 5656–5667

38. Moulian, N. *et al.* 1998. Two signaling pathways can increase fas expression in human thymocytes. *Blood* **92:** 1297–1307.

39. Garg, G. *et al.* 2012. Type 1 diabetes-associated IL2RA variation lowers IL-2 signaling and contributes to diminished CD4+CD25+ regulatory T cell function. *J. Immunol.* **188:** 4644–4697.

40. da Silva Martins, M. & C. Piccirillo. 2012. Functional stability of Foxp3(+) regulatory T cells. *Trend. Molecul. Medi.* **18:** 454–516.

41. Yang, X. O. *et al.* 2008. Molecular antagonism and plasticity of regulatory and inflammatory T cell programs. *Immunity* **29:** 44–56.

42. Ayyoub, M. *et al.* 2009. Human memory FOXP3+ Tregs secrete IL-17 ex vivo and constitutively express the T(H)17 lineage-specific transcription factor RORgamma t. *Proc. Natl. Acad. Sci. USA* **106:** 8635–8640.

43. Voo, K.S. *et al.* 2009. Identification of IL-17-producing FOXP3+ regulatory T cells in humans. *Proc. Natl. Acad. Sci. USA* **106:** 4793–4798.

44. Aime, C., S. Cohen-Kaminsky & S. Berrih-Aknin. 1991. In vitro interleukin-1 (IL-1) production in thymic hyperplasia and thymoma from patients with myasthenia gravis. *J. Clin. Immunol.* **11:** 268–278.

45. Cohen-Kaminsky, S. *et al.* 1993. Interleukin-6 overproduction by cultured thymic epithelial cells from patients with myasthenia gravis is potentially involved in thymic hyperplasia. *Eur. Cytokine Netw.* **4:** 121–132.

46. Marwaha, A.K. *et al.* 2012. TH17 cells in autoimmunity and immunodeficiency: protective or pathogenic? *Front. Immunol.* **3:** 1–8.

47. Roche, J.C. *et al.* 2011. Increased serum interleukin-17 levels in patients with myasthenia gravis. *Muscle Nerve* **44:** 278–280.

48. Masuda, M. *et al.* 2010. Clinical implication of peripheral CD4+CD25+ regulatory T cells and Th17 cells in myasthenia gravis patients. *J. Neuroimmunol.* **225:** 123–131.

49. Wang, Z. *et al.* 2012. T helper type 17 cells expand in patients with myasthenia-associated thymoma. *Scand. J. Immunol.* **76:** 54–61.

50. Mu, L. *et al.* 2010. Disequilibrium of T helper type 1, 2, and 17 cells and regulatory T cells during the development of experimental autoimmune myasthenia gravis. *Immunol.* **128**(1 supp): e826–e836.

51. Morrison, P. J., S.J. Ballantyne & M.C. Kullberg. 2011. Interleukin-23 and T helper 17-type responses in intestinal inflammation: from cytokines to T-cell plasticity. *Immunology* **133:** 397–408.

52. Poea-Guyon, S. *et al.* 2005. Effects of cytokines on acetylcholine receptor expression: implications for myasthenia gravis. *J. Immunol.* **174:** 5941–5949.

53. Meraouna, A. *et al.* 2006. The chemokine CXCL13 is a key molecule in autoimmune myasthenia gravis. *Blood* **108:** 432–440.

54. Berrih-Aknin, S. *et al.* 2009. CCL21 overexpressed on lymphatic vessels drives thymic hyperplasia in myasthenia. *Ann. Neurol.* **66:** 521–531.

55. Emilie, D. *et al.* 1991. In situ production of interleukins in hyperplastic thymus from myasthenia gravis patients. *Hum. Pathol.* **22:** 461–468.

Ann. N.Y. Acad. Sci. ISSN 0077-8923

ANNALS OF THE NEW YORK ACADEMY OF SCIENCES

Issue: *Myasthenia Gravis and Related Disorders*

Targeting plasma cells with proteasome inhibitors: possible roles in treating myasthenia gravis?

Alejandro M. Gomez,[1] Nick Willcox,[2] Peter C. Molenaar,[1] Wim Buurman,[1] Pilar Martinez-Martinez,[1] Marc H. De Baets,[1] and Mario Losen[1]

[1]School for Mental Health and Neuroscience, Maastricht University, Maastricht, the Netherlands. [2]Department of Clinical Neurology, University of Oxford, United Kingdom

Address for correspondence: Mario Losen, Department Neuroscience, Maastricht University, Universiteitssingel 50, 6229 ER, Maastricht, the Netherlands. m.losen@maastrichtuniversity.nl

Myasthenia gravis (MG) is treated primarily with broad-spectrum immuno-suppressants such as prednisone or azathioprine, which normally require several months to reduce autoantibody titers significantly. This delay may be caused by the resistance of the main antibody-producing cells, the plasma cells, to these drugs. In particular, long-lived plasma cells are resistant to immunosuppressive treatments and can produce (auto-) antibodies for months. Bortezomib is a proteasome inhibitor approved for treating patients with multiple myeloma, a plasma cell malignancy. Recent preclinical studies in cell cultures and animal models, and clinical studies in organ-transplant recipients, have demonstrated that bortezomib can kill non-neoplastic plasma cells within hours. This suggests that proteasome inhibitors could also be used for rapidly reducing autoantibody production in autoimmune diseases. We have begun to assess their potential in MG.

Keywords: bortezomib; plasma cell; myasthenia gravis; proteasome inhibition; autoimmunity

Introduction

Myasthenia gravis (MG) is an autoimmune disease characterized by muscle weakness caused by autoantibodies against postsynaptic proteins of the neuromuscular junction. In most MG-patients, they recognize the acetylcholine receptor (AChR)[1], but, in others, the muscle-specific kinase (MuSK)[2] or the low-density lipoprotein receptor-related protein (LRP4)[3] instead. Even though these antibodies cause similar clinical features (muscle weakness and fatigability), they are in fact the result of distinct autoimmune processes. For instance, in early-onset AChR-MG patients, the frequent thymic abnormalities include lymph node-type infiltrates with AChR-specific plasma cells,[4,5] whereas the MuSK-MG thymus hardly differs from that in age-matched controls.[6] Moreover, MuSK-MG is mediated by autoantibodies of the IgG4 subclass,[7] while those in AChR-MG are mainly complement-binding IgG1s and IgG3s.[8]

Many aspects of the underlying etiologies of these conditions remain to be defined, but different treatment responses to immunosuppressive drugs and monoclonal antibodies suggest that distinct antibody-producing cell populations are involved.[9] Plasma cells are the main antibody-producing cell type; they can be either short- or long-lived, and they do not divide. Importantly, they survive most immunosuppressive treatments, rendering them relevant targets for therapies aimed at reducing antibody production.

In this review, we focus on the importance of plasma cells as targets for therapy in autoimmune diseases, and on the potential applications of proteasome inhibitors for eliminating these high-rate antibody-producing cells, emphasizing the potential benefits of such therapies for treating MG patients.

Plasma cells in autoimmunity

Plasma cells are one vital end-product of B cell differentiation; unlike their immediate precursor plasmablasts, they do not proliferate or migrate into the circulation. Therefore, they are very rare in the blood and reside predominantly in the bone marrow and secondary lymphoid tissues such as spleen and

doi: 10.1111/j.1749-6632.2012.06824.x

Ann. N.Y. Acad. Sci. 1274 (2012) 48–59 © 2012 New York Academy of Sciences.

Control   EAMG

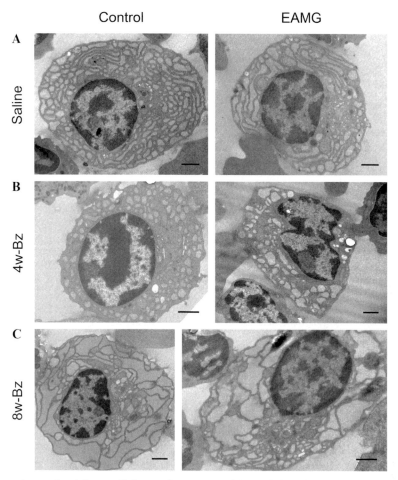

Figure 1. Electron micrographs of plasma cells from rat bone marrow. (A) Morphologically normal plasma cells after eight weeks of saline treatment. These cells are characterized by an elaborate endoplasmic reticulum (ER), which occupies most of the cytoplasm, and by an eccentric nucleus that contains patches of condensed chromatin (resembling a "cart-wheel" configuration). The Golgi apparatus is easy to distinguish. (B) Plasma cells from four-week bortezomib-treated animals. During bortezomib treatment, plasma cells frequently show morphological alterations, including distension of the ER cisternae, with disorganization of its normal structure and derangement of the Golgi complex. (C) Plasma cells from eight-week bortezomib-treated animals. Morphological alterations were similar to those in four-week treated animals, with more pronounced dilatation of the ER cisternae. Cells were stained with osmium tetroxide and contrasted with uranyl acetate and lead citrate. Scale bars, 1 μm. Reproduced, with permission, from Reference 39.

lymph nodes, where they are embedded in special niches. Their function is high-rate secretion of antibodies (3700 times more than by B lymphocytes;[10] i.e., >3,000 molecules/cell/second). Consequently, they are essential for maintaining antibody levels in serum and thus for humoral immune responses. Although antibody-producing cells were shown to survive for many months already in the 1960s,[11] long-lived plasma cells, and their contribution to humoral memory, have only been described accurately in the last decade.[12–14] Recent studies have demonstrated that their maintenance is largely independent of

continuous regeneration from memory B cells.[15,16] Moreover, the cellular and molecular components of the survival niches, where plasma cells must reside in the longer term, have been defined;[17] they include interactions via VCAM-1/VLA4, CXCL12/CXCR4, and IL-6/IL-6R.[18] While differentiating terminally, plasma cells almost completely downregulate most B cell markers (CD19, CD20, CD22, and MHC class II), though most do express CD38 and CD138. Crucial to their specialization is the upregulation of proteins related to endoplasmic reticulum (ER) stress and the unfolded protein response, including

Blimp-1 and XBP1.[19,20] The resulting intracellular differentiation is characterized by formation of extensive amounts of rough ER with densely arranged cisternae (Fig. 1) typical of professional secretory cells.

In recent years, long-lived plasma cells have proved to play a key role in antibody-mediated autoimmune diseases. For instance, in a mouse model of systemic lupus erythematosus (SLE), they produced substantial amounts of autoantibodies and were resistant to standard immunosuppression.[21] Furthermore, they appear to maintain the autoimmune response in Sjögren's syndrome[22] and in rheumatoid arthritis patients.[23]

Persisting long-lived plasma cells are probably also responsible for the typically slow time course of serum autoantibody decline seen in most MG patients during treatment with steroids and/or other immunosuppressive drugs. Convincing evidence implicating them in MG comes from retrospective studies of rituximab-treated MG-patients. In their long-term follow-up of a cohort of refractory MG-patients treated with the anti-CD20 antibody rituximab, Diaz-Manera *et al.* showed almost complete elimination of anti-MuSK autoantibodies, whereas anti-AChR levels did not change significantly.[9] Apparently therefore, autoantibodies against MuSK are made mainly by short-lived plasma cells that are continuously regenerated from autoreactive CD20 positive B cells. By contrast, those against the AChR most likely derive from long-lived plasma cells; so do total circulating IgGs and antitetanus toxoid antibodies, which also remained constant after CD20 depletion therapy, again implicating the long-lived plasma cell compartment that is expected to resist it.[9] Similarly, in a randomized phase II/III trial with rituximab in SLE patients,[24] autoantibody titers remained unchanged for at least one year, probably because they are maintained by long-lived plasma cells, even if circulating B cells are depleted completely.

Clearly, therefore, drugs targeting plasma cells may have a place in the therapy of autoimmune diseases.[25]

Bortezomib targets nonneoplastic plasma cells: *in vivo* studies

Most of the available immunosuppressive drugs are designed to halt proliferation of immune cells, but plasma cells are terminally differentiated and there are very few drugs that target them. Long-lived plasma cells are even resistant to whole-body irradiation.[26] Until recently, their neoplasms (in particular multiple myeloma) were notoriously hard to treat. Even benign plasma cells are typically resistant to most standard immunosuppressant treatments, including such novel drugs as mycophenolate mofetil (MMF),[15,27,28] and they express very few targets for therapeutic monoclonal antibodies. At present, one of the most effective FDA-approved drugs for plasma cell malignancies is the proteasome inhibitor bortezomib (also known as Velcade® or PS-341). It is currently used for treating patients with mantle cell lymphoma as well as multiple myeloma.[29,30] However, peripheral neuropathy (PN) is a major side effect of bortezomib-—when used repeatedly. PN can be very disabling in up to 30% of treated patients and has seriously discouraged off-label testing of bortezomib in clinical conditions other than cancers. Recent advances in its use (e.g., subcutaneous instead of intravenous administration[31] and lower but effective dose regimens[32]) are showing promise for reducing these risks and thus for broadening its future applicability in other diseases. Recently, a second proteasome inhibitor, carfilzomib (also known as Kyprolis™ or PR-171), has been approved for the treatment of multiple myeloma. By analogy, it is likely to be effective against autoimmune plasma cells as well. Since carfilzomib does not increase the risk of PN in multiple myeloma patients,[33] this particular side effect of bortezomib may not be proteasome specific.[34]

Proteasome inhibition is toxic for myeloma cells because it (a) causes accumulation of misfolded proteins in the ER, triggering the terminal unfolded protein response that ultimately leads to apoptosis;[35] (b) prevents the activation of the transcription factor NF-κB that is crucial for expression of cytokines, chemokines and their receptors, which ensure plasma cell survival.[36] In fact, it is now clear that it is mainly the high-rate production of proteins that sensitizes certain cell types toward proteasome inhibition.[37] That is why Neubert *et al.* predicted that bortezomib would be toxic to nonneoplastic plasma cells too, since they also secrete antibodies in large amounts.[38]

Initial studies in animal models demonstrated that proteasome inhibition could indeed kill nonneoplastic plasma cells (Table 1). In an SLE model, plasma cells (whether short- or long-lived) were

Table 1. Summary of *in vitro* and *in vivo* studies with bortezomib (Btz) in nonneoplastic models of disease

References	Disease model	Btz dose and schedule(s)	Effects on PC	Main findings
***In vitro* studies**				
Perry *et al.*[27]	PC from the BM of renal-transplant recipients	1 mg/L for 24 h or 72 hours	Btz induced apoptosis in more than 60% of PC already after 24 hours	Btz, but not Rtx or IVIg, blocked the production of allo-antibodies by PC after 72 hours. A dose-response curve showed that Btz is effective at concentrations ≥1 mg/L
Gomez et al., unpublished data	Thymic cells from MG patients	1 mg/L twice (days 7 and 11) in a 14-day culture schedule	No Btz-exposed PC survived to day 14. In cultures with Dx, Len or saline, significantly more PC survived until day 14	Autoantibody and IgG production were completely blocked by Btz, but not by Dx, Len, or saline. On dose-response testing, Btz eliminated PC at concentrations ≥4 μg/L
***In vivo* studies**				
Neubert *et al.*[38]	SLE-like mice (NZB/W F1; MRL/lpr)	0.75 mg/kg - Twice at 36 h interval (A) - Three times in one week (B) - Twice weekly for 40 weeks (C)	>60% reduction of both short- and long-lived PC in the BM, from 48 h after the first dose (A)	Significant reduction of anti-ds-DNA antibody titers only with Btz treatment (not Dx or Cy) (B). Long-term treatment with Btz improved the clinical condition of these mice (C)
Gomez *et al.*[39]	EAMG rats	0.2 mg/kg - For prevention: Twice weekly for eight weeks (8w-Btz) - For treatment: four weeks Btz, starting four weeks after induction of the model (4w-Btz)	Strong reduction of total PC in the BM, with both regimens	Significant reduction of anti-AChR antibody titers and total IgG levels in both the 8w-Btz and the 4w-Btz groups, i.e., also when autoantibodies were already present (4w-Btz)

Continued

Table 1. *Continued*

References	Disease model	Btz dose and schedule(s)	Effects on PC	Main findings
Vogelbacher *et al.*[40]	Chronic allograft nephropathy model in rats	0.2 mg/kg - Twice weekly for nine weeks	Significant depletion of PC in the BM and the spleen	Significant reduction of allo-antibody titers and IgG-producing cells. Some additive actions were suggested for Btz and the mTOR-inhibitor sirolimus
Meslier Y. *et al.*[41]	Experimental hemophilia-A mice that develop antifactor VIII antibodies	0.75 mg/kg - For prevention: Btz twice weekly for four weeks. - For treatment: Btz twice weekly for 10 weeks	Both short- and long-lived PC were strongly reduced by Btz in the spleen, but not in the BM, with the preventive schedule. The number of autoreactive PC in BM was not reduced by Btz treatment.	Btz was effective in preventing antifactor VIII antibody responses but hardly reduced them once they were established
Ichikawa *et al.*[42]	SLE-like mice (NZB/W F1, ONX 0914, NZB/NZW)	0.5 mg/kg - Twice weekly for 13 weeks	Btz decreased by >90% the number of PC in the spleen and the BM	Greater sensitivity of autoantibody- than total IgG- secreting PC to proteasome inhibition. New proteasome inhibitors (carfilzomib and ONX 0914) also gave positive results
Bontscho *et al.*[43]	Mouse model of vasculitis due to anti-neutrophil cytoplasmic antibodies (ANCA)	0.75 mg/kg twice weekly - Early treatment: five weeks of Btz, starting three weeks after induction of the model - Late treatment: three weeks of Btz, starting five weeks after induction of the model	Spleen and BM PC were significantly reduced by Btz. Autoreactive PCs were more susceptible to Btz treatment.	Btz significantly reduced autoantibody titers already one week into early treatment, and protected against development of clinical signs Late treatment reduced antibody titers at the endpoint but did not improve the clinical condition. Combined steroid/Cy significantly reduced PC numbers in the spleen, but not in BM

AMR, antibody-mediated transplant rejection; BM, bone marrow; Btz, bortezomib; Cy, cyclophosphamide; Dx, dexamethasone; EAMG, experimental autoimmune myasthenia gravis; IVIg, intravenous immunoglobulin; Len, lenalidomide; PC, plasma cell; Rtx, rituximab.

depleted as early as 48 hours after treatment by inducing apoptosis in them.[38] Moreover, long-term treatment (>30 weeks) decreased autoantibody titers almost to background levels, while approximately halving total IgG levels (possibly reflecting partial recovery of plasma cells after the treatment was stopped). Hence, proteasome inhibition ameliorated the lupus-like nephritis signs in these mice and prolonged their survival. Similarly, we have demonstrated that bortezomib significantly depletes bone marrow plasma cells in an animal model of MG (experimental autoimmune myasthenia gravis, EAMG).[39] In that study, we treated EAMG-rats with bortezomib twice weekly for four weeks, starting four weeks after immunization with *Torpedo* AChR (by when serum autoantibodies against rat AChR were present). At the end of the experiment, plasma cell numbers and autoantibody titers were significantly lower in bortezomib-treated rats than in saline-injected controls; titers were reduced by 60% after four weeks of treatment. Interestingly, in bone marrow plasma cells, bortezomib induced ultrastructural changes (swelling of the endoplasmic reticulum) characteristic of ER stress (Fig. 1B, C).

Bortezomib is toxic for nonneoplastic plasma cells: *in vitro* studies

Recent *in vitro* studies have focused on the sensitivity of nonmalignant plasma cells to proteasome inhibition (Table 1),[27,38–43] and especially—in antibody-mediated kidney transplant rejection—on its potential for depleting allo-reactive (anti-HLA) plasma cells. In one of the first such studies,[27] bortezomib, but not rituximab or IVIg, induced apoptosis within 72 hours in plasma cells cultured from the bone marrow of transplant recipients. In addition, it completely blocked allo-antibody production in these cultures, while rituximab had no significant effect. These results, along with pilot clinical studies *in vivo*,[44] prompted the off-label use of bortezomib for preventing transplant rejection in patients, as discussed later in this review.

To extend this approach to autoimmune disease, we took advantage of the very prevalent lymph node-like infiltration into the early-onset MG thymus,[4,6,45,46] where germinal centers form close to rare muscle-like myoid cells,[4] and plasma cells spontaneously secrete anti-AChR antibodies.[5,45,46] Since the thymus is removed surgically in many of these patients as part of treatment, it is an accessible

and valuable source of specific autoreactive plasma cells for research.[5] In culture, these continue spontaneously secreting substantial amounts of AChR autoantibodies for several weeks (at least)—even after irradiation, a feature unique to plasma cells.[5] They are apparently sustained by "feeder effects" from accessory thymic cell types (e.g., fibroblasts and macrophages).[5,45,46]

We therefore exploited this source of autoimmune plasma cells as a test-bed for evaluating their sensitivity to drugs used against myelomas. These included bortezomib, dexamethasone, and the thalidomide derivative lenalidomide (now also approved for antimyeloma therapy); we measured (auto-) antibody and total IgG production and plasma cell survival after two weeks in culture (unpublished results). Bortezomib proved to target plasma cells with surprising efficiency; they were already almost undetectable after 24 hours, and even at 60 times lower concentrations than those reached in patients' plasma.[31] Plasma cells appeared apoptotic as soon as eight hours after adding bortezomib to the cultures. Moreover, autoantibody and total IgG production were completely blocked upon addition of bortezomib, whereas dexamethasone caused a mild but statistically significant reduction and lenalidomide had no significant effect. Importantly, at the doses used, none of these drugs caused extra death of thymic cells by day 14 (i.e., above the rate of apoptosis expected of thymocytes). Thus, bortezomib's toxicity seems selective for plasma cells.

Experience with bortezomib in transplantation and autoimmune disorders

Since its introduction, there have been many clinical trials and case reports of bortezomib's benefits and side effects in multiple myeloma patients,[47] but few on its off-label use in nonneoplastic diseases (Table 2).[44,48–52] However, there are reports of positive outcomes in the treatment of autoimmune hemolytic anemia,[48,53] rheumatoid arthritis,[54] and SLE.[55] The most extensive studies have focused on the prevention of antibody-mediated rejection in renal transplant recipients.[56] Initially, bortezomib was only used as a last resort in patients who were refractory to several immunosuppressive drugs;[44] subsequently, in combination with plasma exchange, it also proved effective as primary treatment for rapidly reducing anti-HLA antibody levels in hyper acute transplant rejection.[57]

Table 2. Summary of clinical studies with bortezomib in transplantation and autoimmune disorders

Reference	Patients	Btz dose and schedule(s)	Main findings
Carson et al.[48]	Case report of refractory IgM-mediated autoimmune hemolytic anemia	1.3 mg/m^2 - Three doses of Btz	Improvement of symptoms and increase of hemoglobin levels after Btz treatment. IgM autoantibodies were significantly decreased
Hiepe et al.[59]	Four refractory SLE patients	1.3 mg/m^2 - Four cycles of Btz (days 1, 4, 8, 11) with 10-day treatment-free intervals. - 20 mg Dx was given in combination	Significant clinical improvement and reduction of lupus-associated antibodies. Total IgG levels and vaccine-specific antibodies were decreased, suggesting that the bone marrow PC were affected. The authors recommend a combination therapy of Btz with B cell depletion to ensure long-lasting improvement
Everly et al.[44]	Six renal transplant recipients with refractory AMR	1.3 mg/m^2 - One cycle of Btz (days 1, 4, 8, 11) - PE and Rtx were sometimes used as adjuvant therapy	Reversion of transplant rejection, amelioration of the clinical condition and reduction of allo-antibody titers. Effects were sustained for at least five months. No severe side effects reported
Walsh et al.[58]	30 renal transplant recipients with AMR. 13 had early onset AMR (< six months posttransplant) and 17 had late onset AMR (> six months posttransplant)	1.3 mg/m^2 - One cycle of Btz (days 1, 4, 8, 11) - PE and a single dose of Rtx were used as adjuvant therapies	Btz improved renal function and reduced allo-antibody titers in both early and late AMR, but more so in early than late AMR. Peripheral neuropathy was observed more frequently in late-onset AMR. There were no reports of severe cases (grades 3 or 4)
Sberro-Soussan et al.[51]	Four renal transplant recipients with AMR	1.3 mg/m^2 - One cycle of Btz (days 1, 4, 8, 11) plus maintenance immunosuppressive treatment	After five months' follow-up, no reductions in allo-antibody or IgG levels were observed. Bilateral conjunctivitis and prolonged fatigue were reported as severe side effects
Diwan et al.[49]	Eight sensitized renal-transplant candidates, with high anti-HLA antibody titers	1.3 mg/m^2 - One or four cycles of Btz (4 or 16 doses)	Monotherapy with Btz significantly reduced the number of both tetanus-specific and anti-HLA PC in the bone marrow of patients. Total PC numbers were also reduced by Btz, but not significantly

Continued

Table 2. *Continued*

Reference	Patients	Btz dose and schedule(s)	Main findings
			Treatment with Btz prolonged the reduction of anti-HLA antibodies by PE. No randomized paired-control group of bone marrow aspirates was included on this study
Everly *et al.*[50]	13 renal transplant recipients with refractory AMR	1.3 mg/m^2 - One or two cycles of Btz - PE and methylprednisone were used as adjuvant therapies	Anti-HLA antibody levels were reduced by ≥50% after one month of treatment; after one year, antibody titers were still low. Total IgG, antibodies against measles and tetanus toxoid remained unchanged, and at protective levels, at one year posttreatment. The authors suggest that the lower antibody production of protective PC makes them less susceptible to proteasome inhibition
Waiser *et al.*[52]	10 renal transplant recipients with AMR	1.3 mg/m^2 - One cycle of Btz (days 1, 4, 8, 11) - PE and IVIG were used as adjuvant therapies	Outcomes were compared to a historical group of patients treated with the same adjuvant therapy but with one single dose of Rtx instead of Btz. At 18 months posttreatment, graft survival was superior in Btz-treated patients Both Btz and Rtx significantly reduced peak anti-HLA antibody levels during the follow-up period, but neither eradicated existing allo-antibodies

AMR, antibody-mediated transplant rejection; Btz, bortezomib; Dx, dexamethasone; IVIg, intravenous immunoglobulin; PC, plasma cell; PE, plasma exchange; Rtx, rituximab; SLE, systemic lupus erythematosus.

Bortezomib reduced both numbers of allo-reactive plasma cells in the bone marrow and serum allo-antibody titers in strongly allo-sensitized renal patients prior to transplantation.[49] Moreover, it significantly increased graft survival in comparison to rituximab.[52] However, despite these positive findings, there is one other report that a single cycle of bortezomib as a monotherapy was not beneficial in subacute rejection when given after transplantation.[51] Moreover, it seems more effective in early than in late acute rejection.[58]

By contrast, there is much less published experience with proteasome inhibition in autoimmune diseases. To date, two reports have described a reduction of autoantibody titers and a clear increase of hemoglobin levels in cases of steroid/rituximab-refractory autoimmune hemolytic anemia.[48,53] In addition, in one multiple myeloma patient, the coincidental SLE improved substantially and anti-dsDNA titers declined significantly after just 3 cycles of bortezomib.[55] Similarly, Hiepe *et al.* recently reported significant clinical improvements and

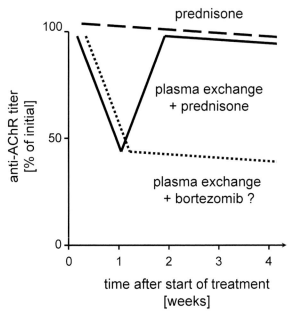

Figure 2. Schematic representation of predicted changes in anti-AChR antibody titers following different immunosuppressive treatments. Initial treatment with prednisone only (dashed line) normally requires several weeks to reduce autoantibody titers significantly. Plasma exchange (solid line) reduces them rapidly, but—even in patients also taking prednisone and other immunosuppressive drugs-—titers return almost to their initial levels within the next few weeks.[72] The combination of plasma exchange with bortezomib (dotted line) could induce a more lasting reduction in antibody titers, based on results of such a treatment in organ transplant recipients.[50]

autoantibody titer reductions in four patients with refractory SLE after treatment with bortezomib plus dexamethasone.[59] Protective vaccine-specific antibodies and total IgG levels were also decreased in these patients, suggesting that long-lived plasma cells were indeed depleted by proteasome inhibition. However, since repeated treatments were necessary to achieve sustained responses, combinations of bortezomib with agents that can also eliminate plasma cell precursors (i.e., rituximab) were recommended.

Proteasome inhibitors for myasthenia gravis patients?

Generally speaking, chronic autoimmune diseases such as MG can seriously affect quality of life because of persistence of clinical symptoms and/or side effects of long-term medication (e.g., diabetes, hypertension and osteoporosis caused by glucocorticoids[60]). Broad-spectrum immunosuppressive drugs, such as prednisone and azathioprine, ameliorate the symptoms in most MG patients. However, there is typically a long delay (six to eight weeks for steroids[60] and up to 18 months for aza-

thioprine[61]) before autoantibody titers decline and muscles strengthen significantly. That might well be because of treatment-resistant plasma cells. If so, their specific elimination could represent a novel and promising approach for treating MG. In time, we hope that there will be biomarkers to predict which MG patients will respond rapidly to standard immunosuppressants and which will need adjunctive plasma cell depletion to achieve earlier improvements, whether in acute severe or chronic refractory cases.

An important limitation in using bortezomib for nonmalignant diseases is the concern about development of PN, which is a serious but generally reversible side effect[62] that seems to depend on reaching a cumulative bortezomib-dose threshold during the first five cycles of treatment.[63] Whereas current regimens were designed for multiple myelomas (which are notoriously hard to treat), lower doses and short courses might be sufficient to deplete autoreactive plasma cells significantly, e.g., in MG. For instance, Diwan *et al.* showed that four cycles of bortezomib were already sufficient to significantly deplete bone marrow plasma cells in transplant recipients.[49] In a large clinical trial in myeloma patients, single weekly doses proved as effective as the established twice weekly schedule, with significantly lower risks of both any-grade PN (35% vs. 51%) and grade 3/4 PN (8% vs. 28%).[32] In addition, using the recently FDA-approved subcutaneous (instead of intravenous) route reduced the incidence and severity of PN (any grade PN 38% vs. 53%; grade 3/4 PN 6% vs. 16%).[31] Furthermore, second-generation proteasome inhibitors are now approved (carfilzomib) or being developed (some of them are already in use in clinical trials); they seem to be more selective than bortezomib and potentially less neurotoxic.[34,64] Another interesting possibility is to combine bortezomib with other drugs now being used for treating myelomas. These include the immunomodulatory drugs thalidomide and lenalidomide, drugs blocking the interactions that maintain plasma cells in their survival niches in the bone marrow (natalizumab[65] against VLA-4, tocilizumab[66] or siltuximab[67] against IL6, and plerixafor[68] against CXCR4), or drugs reactive with plasma cells directly (elotuzumab[69] against CS1, daratumumab[70] against CD38, or nBT062[71] against CD138).

Conclusions

In conclusion, proteasome inhibition has significant potential as an effective induction therapy, in combination with plasma exchange, for MG patients with high autoantibody titers and/or acute severe weakness. Removing autoreactive plasma cells should lead to more sustained reductions in autoantibody titers after plasma exchange (Fig. 2), a procedure, which, by itself, leads to only temporary reductions in autoantibodies in the plasma.[72] Additional immunosuppression with glucocorticoids (at lower than normal doses), azathioprine, MMF, or rituximab would probably be necessary to prevent generation of new autoreactive plasma cells—by when bortezomib will have served its purpose. Moreover, it might prove valuable in refractory MG.

To summarize, we consider that proteasome inhibition represents a promising new approach for MG treatment. Experience from animal models, from *in vitro* settings and from transplant recipients convincingly supports the potential of bortezomib for targeting plasma cells, the main antibody-producing cells. Naturally, future work is needed to confirm the potential of proteasome inhibition in antibody-mediated autoimmune diseases.

Acknowledgments

We thank Mr. H. Duimel and Dr. F. Verheyen for their help in preparing the electron micrographs, Mr. J. Hummel and Dr. K. Vrolix for their help with the thymic cell cultures, and Dr. M.E. Hill, Prof. H. Kaminski, Prof. A. Melms, and Prof. A.L. Goldberg for helpful discussions. A.M.G. was supported by a Marie-Curie fellowship from the European Union and a grant from the Prinses Beatrix Fonds (Project WAR08-12); P.M.-M. by grants from the Association Française contre les Myopathies and Genmab; N.W. by the UK Medical Research Council; M.L. by a Veni fellowship of The Netherlands Organization for Scientific Research and a fellowship of the Brain Foundation of the Netherlands.

Conflicts of interest

The authors declare no conflicts of interest.

References

1. Lindstrom, J.M. *et al.* 1976. Antibody to acetylcholine receptor in myasthenia gravis. Prevalence, clinical correlates, and diagnostic value. *Neurology* **26:** 1054–1059.
2. Hoch, W. *et al.* 2001. Auto-antibodies to the receptor tyrosine kinase MuSK in patients with myasthenia gravis without acetylcholine receptor antibodies. *Nat. Med.* **7:** 365–368.
3. Higuchi, O. *et al.* 2011. Autoantibodies to low-density lipoprotein receptor-related protein 4 in myasthenia gravis. *Ann. Neurol.* **69:** 418–422.
4. Leite, M.I. *et al.* 2007. Myasthenia gravis thymus: complement vulnerability of epithelial and myoid cells, complement attack on them, and correlations with autoantibody status. *Am. J. Pathol.* **171:** 893–905.
5. Hill, M.E. *et al.* 2008. The myasthenia gravis thymus: a rare source of human autoantibody-secreting plasma cells for testing potential therapeutics. *J. Neuroimmunol.* **201–202:** 50–56.
6. Leite, M.I. *et al.* 2005. Fewer thymic changes in MuSK antibody-positive than in MuSK antibody-negative MG. *Ann Neurol.* **57:** 444–448.
7. Klooster, R. *et al.* 2012. Muscle-specific kinase myasthenia gravis IgG4 autoantibodies cause severe neuromuscular junction dysfunction in mice. *Brain* **135:** 1081–1101.
8. Gomez, A.M. *et al.* 2010. Antibody effector mechanisms in myasthenia gravis-pathogenesis at the neuromuscular junction. *Autoimmunity* **43:** 353–370.
9. Diaz-Manera, J. *et al.* 2012. Long-lasting treatment effect of rituximab in MuSK myasthenia. *Neurology* **78:** 189–193.
10. Lifter, J., P.W. Kincade & Y.S. Choi. 1976. Subpopulations of chicken B lymphocytes. *J. Immunol.* **117:** 2220–2225.

11. Miller, J.J., 3rd. 1964. An autoradiographic study of the stability of plasma cell ribonucleic acid in rats. *J. Immunol.* **93:** 250–254.

12. Manz, R.A., A. Thiel & A. Radbruch. 1997. Lifetime of plasma cells in the bone marrow. *Nature* **388:** 133–134.

13. Slifka, M.K. *et al.* 1998. Humoral immunity due to long-lived plasma cells. *Immunity* **8:** 363–372.

14. Radbruch, A. *et al.* 2006. Competence and competition: the challenge of becoming a long-lived plasma cell. *Nat. Rev. Immunol.* **6:** 741–750.

15. DiLillo, D.J. *et al.* 2008. Maintenance of long-lived plasma cells and serological memory despite mature and memory B cell depletion during CD20 immunotherapy in mice. *J Immunol.* **180:** 361–371.

16. Ahuja, A. *et al.* 2008. Maintenance of the plasma cell pool is independent of memory B cells. *Proc. Natl. Acad. Sci. USA* **105:** 4802–4807.

17. Belnoue, E. *et al.* 2012. Homing and adhesion patterns determine the cellular composition of the bone marrow plasma cell niche. *J. Immunol.* **188:** 1283–1291.

18. Minges Wols, H.A. 2002. Plasma cells. In *Encyclopedia of Life Sciences.* Nature Pub. Group. London, New York.

19. Iwakoshi, N.N. *et al.* 2003. Plasma cell differentiation and the unfolded protein response intersect at the transcription factor XBP-1. *Nat. Immunol.* **4:** 321–329.

20. Shaffer, A.L. *et al.* 2004. XBP1, downstream of Blimp-1, expands the secretory apparatus and other organelles, and increases protein synthesis in plasma cell differentiation. *Immunity* **21:** 81–93.

21. Hoyer, B.F. *et al.* 2004. Short-lived plasmablasts and long-lived plasma cells contribute to chronic humoral autoimmunity in NZB/W mice. *J. Exp. Med.* **199:** 1577–1584.

22. Szyszko, E.A. *et al.* 2011. Distinct phenotypes of plasma cells in spleen and bone marrow of autoimmune NOD.B10.H2b mice. *Autoimmunity* **44:** 415–426.

23. Teng, Y.O. *et al.* 2012. Induction of long-term B-cell depletion in refractory rheumatoid arthritis patients preferentially affects autoreactive more than protective humoral immunity. *Arthritis Res. Ther.* **14:** R57.

24. Merrill, J.T. *et al.* 2010. Efficacy and safety of rituximab in moderately-to-severely active systemic lupus erythematosus: the randomized, double-blind, phase II/III systemic lupus erythematosus evaluation of rituximab trial. *Arthritis Rheum.* **62:** 222–233.

25. Hiepe, F. *et al.* 2011. Long-lived autoreactive plasma cells drive persistent autoimmune inflammation. *Nat. Rev. Rheumatol.* **7:** 170–178.

26. Miller, J.J. & L.J. Cole. 1967. The radiation resistance of long-lived lymphocytes and plasma cells in mouse and rat lymph nodes. *J. Immunol.* **98:** 982–990.

27. Perry, D.K. *et al.* 2009. Proteasome inhibition causes apoptosis of normal human plasma cells preventing alloantibody production. *Am. J. Transplant* **9:** 201–209.

28. Miller, J.J., 3rd & L.J. Cole. 1967. Resistance of long-lived lymphocytes and plasma cells in rat lymph nodes to treatment with prednisone, cyclophosphamide, 6-mercaptopurine, and actinomycin D. *J. Exp. Med.* **126:** 109–125.

29. Kane, R.C. *et al.* 2006. United States Food and Drug Administration approval summary: bortezomib for the treatment of progressive multiple myeloma after one prior therapy. *Clin. Cancer Res.* **12:** 2955–2960.

30. Goldberg, A.L. 2011. Bortezomib's scientific origins and its tortuous path to the clinic. In *Bortezomib in the Treatment of Multiple Myeloma.* I.M. Ghobrial, P.G. Richardson & K.C. Anderson, Eds.: 1–27. Birkhäuser Basel.

31. Moreau, P. *et al.* 2011. Subcutaneous versus intravenous administration of bortezomib in patients with relapsed multiple myeloma: a randomised, phase 3, non-inferiority study. *Lancet Oncol.* **12:** 431–440.

32. Bringhen, S. *et al.* 2010. Efficacy and safety of once-weekly bortezomib in multiple myeloma patients. *Blood* **116:** 4745–4753.

33. Vij, R. *et al.* 2012. An open-label, single-arm, phase 2 study of single-agent carfilzomib in patients with relapsed and/or refractory multiple myeloma who have been previously treated with bortezomib. *Br. J. Haematol.*

34. Arastu-Kapur, S. *et al.* 2011. Nonproteasomal targets of the proteasome inhibitors bortezomib and carfilzomib: a link to clinical adverse events. *Clin. Cancer Res.* **17:** 2734–2743.

35. Obeng, E.A. *et al.* 2006. Proteasome inhibitors induce a terminal unfolded protein response in multiple myeloma cells. *Blood* **107:** 4907–4916.

36. Hideshima, T. *et al.* 2002. NF-kappa B as a therapeutic target in multiple myeloma. *J. Biol. Chem.* **277:** 16639–16647.

37. Meister, S. *et al.* 2007. Extensive immunoglobulin production sensitizes myeloma cells for proteasome inhibition. *Cancer Res.* **67:** 1783–1792.

38. Neubert, K. *et al.* 2008. The proteasome inhibitor bortezomib depletes plasma cells and protects mice with lupus-like disease from nephritis. *Nat. Med.* **14:** 748–755.

39. Gomez, A.M. *et al.* 2011. Proteasome inhibition with bortezomib depletes plasma cells and autoantibodies in experimental autoimmune myasthenia gravis. *J. Immunol.* **186:** 2503–2513.

40. Vogelbacher, R. *et al.* 2010. Bortezomib and sirolimus inhibit the chronic active antibody-mediated rejection in experimental renal transplantation in the rat. *Nephrol. Dial Transplant.* **25:** 3764–3773.

41. Meslier, Y. *et al.* 2011. Bortezomib delays the onset of factor VIII inhibitors in experimental hemophilia A, but fails to eliminate established anti-factor VIII IgG-producing cells. *J. Thromb. Haemost.* **9:** 719–728.

42. Ichikawa, H.T. *et al.* 2012. Beneficial effect of novel proteasome inhibitors in murine lupus via dual inhibition of type I interferon and autoantibody-secreting cells. *Arthritis Rheum.* **64:** 493–503.

43. Bontscho, J. *et al.* 2011. Myeloperoxidase-specific plasma cell depletion by bortezomib protects from anti-neutrophil cytoplasmic autoantibodies-induced glomerulonephritis. *J. Am. Soc. Nephrol.* **22:** 336–348.

44. Everly, M.J. *et al.* 2008. Bortezomib provides effective therapy for antibody- and cell-mediated acute rejection. *Transplantation* **86:** 1754–1761.

45. Willcox, H.N., J. Newsom-Davis & L.R. Calder. 1984. Cell types required for anti-acetylcholine receptor antibody synthesis by cultured thymocytes and blood lymphocytes in myasthenia gravis. *Clin. Exp. Immunol.* **58:** 97–106.

46. Willcox, H.N., J. Newsom-Davis & L.R. Calder. 1983. Greatly increased autoantibody production in myasthenia gravis by thymocyte suspensions prepared with proteolytic enzymes. *Clin. Exp. Immunol.* **54:** 378–386.

47. Richardson, P.G. *et al.* 2005. Bortezomib or high-dose dexamethasone for relapsed multiple myeloma. *N. Engl. J. Med.* **352:** 2487–2498.

48. Carson, K.R., L.G. Beckwith & J. Mehta. 2010. Successful treatment of IgM-mediated autoimmune hemolytic anemia with bortezomib. *Blood* **115:** 915.

49. Diwan, T.S. *et al.* 2011. The impact of proteasome inhibition on alloantibody-producing plasma cells in vivo. *Transplantation* **91:** 536–541.

50. Everly, M.J. *et al.* 2010. Protective immunity remains intact after antibody removal by means of proteasome inhibition. *Transplantation* **90:** 1493–1498.

51. Sberro-Soussan, R. *et al.* 2010. Bortezomib as the sole post-renal transplantation desensitization agent does not decrease donor-specific anti-HLA antibodies. *Am. J. Transplant.* **10:** 681–686.

52. Waiser, J. *et al.* 2012. Comparison between bortezomib and rituximab in the treatment of antibody-mediated renal allograft rejection. *Nephrol. Dial Transplant.* **27:** 1246–1251.

53. Danchaivijitr, P., J. Yared & A.P. Rapoport. 2011. Successful treatment of IgG and complement-mediated autoimmune hemolytic anemia with bortezomib and low-dose cyclophosphamide. *Am. J. Hematol.* **86:** 331–332.

54. van der Heijden, J.W. *et al.* 2009. The proteasome inhibitor bortezomib inhibits the release of NFkappaB-inducible cytokines and induces apoptosis of activated T cells from rheumatoid arthritis patients. *Clin. Exp. Rheumatol.* **27:** 92–98.

55. Frohlich, K. *et al.* 2011. Successful use of bortezomib in a patient with systemic lupus erythematosus and multiple myeloma. *Ann. Rheum. Dis.* **70:** 1344–1345.

56. Woodle, E.S., R.R. Alloway & A. Girnita. 2011. Proteasome inhibitor treatment of antibody-mediated allograft rejection. *Curr. Opin. Organ Transplant.* **16:** 434–438.

57. Walsh, R.C. *et al.* 2010. Proteasome inhibitor-based primary therapy for antibody-mediated renal allograft rejection. *Transplantation* **89:** 277–284.

58. Walsh, R.C. *et al.* 2011. Early and late acute antibody-mediated rejection differ immunologically and in response to proteasome inhibition. *Transplantation* **91:** 1218–1226.

59. Hiepe, F. *et al.* 2011. Therapeutic inhibition of proteasomes in systemic lupus erythematosus. *J. Transl. Med.* **9**(Suppl 2)**:** I9.

60. Sanders, D. B. & A. Evoli. 2010. Immunosuppressive therapies in myasthenia gravis. *Autoimmunity* **43:** 428–435.

61. Palace, J., J. Newsom-Davis & B. Lecky. 1998. A randomized double-blind trial of prednisolone alone or with azathioprine in myasthenia gravis. Myasthenia Gravis Study Group. *Neurology* **50:** 1778–1783.

62. Richardson, P.G. *et al.* 2009. Single-agent bortezomib in previously untreated multiple myeloma: efficacy, characterization of peripheral neuropathy, and molecular correlations with response and neuropathy. *J. Clin. Oncol.* **27:** 3518–3525.

63. Cavaletti, G. & A.J. Jakubowiak. 2010. Peripheral neuropathy during bortezomib treatment of multiple myeloma: a review of recent studies. *Leuk. Lymphoma.* **51:** 1178–1187.

64. Kirk, C.J. 2012. Discovery and development of second-generation proteasome inhibitors. *Semin. Hematol.* **49:** 207–214.

65. Podar, K. *et al.* 2011. The selective adhesion molecule inhibitor Natalizumab decreases multiple myeloma cell growth in the bone marrow microenvironment: therapeutic implications. *Br. J. Haematol.* **155:** 438–448.

66. Matsuyama, Y. *et al.* 2011. Successful treatment of a patient with rheumatoid arthritis and IgA-kappa multiple myeloma with tocilizumab. *Intern. Med.* **50:** 639–642.

67. Hunsucker, S.A. *et al.* 2011. Blockade of interleukin-6 signalling with siltuximab enhances melphalan cytotoxicity in preclinical models of multiple myeloma. *Br. J. Haematol.* **152:** 579–592.

68. Lor, K.W. *et al.* 2012. Plerixafor as first- and second-line strategies for autologous stem cell mobilization in patients with non-Hodgkin's lymphoma or multiple myeloma. *Pharmacotherapy* **32:** 596–603.

69. Lonial, S. *et al.* 2012. Elotuzumab in combination with lenalidomide and low-dose dexamethasone in relapsed or refractory multiple myeloma. *J. Clin. Oncol.* **30:** 1953–1959.

70. de Weers, M. *et al.* 2011. Daratumumab, a novel therapeutic human CD38 monoclonal antibody, induces killing of multiple myeloma and other hematological tumors. *J. Immunol.* **186:** 1840–1848.

71. Ikeda, H. *et al.* 2009. The monoclonal antibody nBT062 conjugated to cytotoxic Maytansinoids has selective cytotoxicity against CD138-positive multiple myeloma cells in vitro and in vivo. *Clin. Cancer Res.* **15:** 4028–4037.

72. Hawkey, C.J., J. Newsom-Davis & A. Vincent. 1981. Plasma exchange and immunosuppressive drug treatment in myasthenia gravis: no evidence for synergy. *J. Neurol. Neurosurg. Psychiatr.* **44:** 469–475.

Ann. N.Y. Acad. Sci. ISSN 0077-8923

The role of B cell–activating factor in autoimmune myasthenia gravis

Robert P. Lisak[1] and Samia Ragheb[1,2]

[1]Departments of Neurology, and Immunology and Microbiology, Wayne State University School of Medicine, Detroit, Michigan.
[2]Department of Biomedical Sciences, Oakland University William Beaumont (OUWB) School of Medicine, Rochester, Michigan

Address for correspondence: Robert P Lisak, Department of Neurology, Wayne State University School of Medicine, 8D University Health Center, 4201 St Antoine, Detroit, MI 48201. rlisak@med.wayne.edu

B cell–activating factor (BAFF) is important in the development and maturation of B cells and their progeny—plasma blasts and plasma cells. There is increasing evidence that BAFF is involved in the pathogenesis of several autoimmune diseases including myasthenia gravis. Increased expression of BAFF and receptors for BAFF have been demonstrated in thymus of patients with myasthenia gravis, and an increase in serum levels of BAFF have been reported in patients with myasthenia gravis. While the exact role of BAFF in the pathogenesis of myasthenia gravis is not clear, BAFF and its receptors may provide potential targets for therapy in patients with myasthenia gravis.

Keywords: autoimmunity; BAFF; B cells; cytokines; immunotherapy

Introduction

Autoimmune myasthenia gravis (MG) is a disease mediated by antibodies directed against molecules of the postsynaptic portion of the neuromuscular junction (NMJ), most often skeletal muscle nicotinic acetylcholine receptor (AChR).[1–3] Other patients have antibodies directed against other components of the postsynaptic membrane.[4–10] Approximately 65–75% of patients with MG have changes in their thymus that together are referred to as *germinal center follicular hyperplasia*. Such germinal center follicles appear the same as germinal centers in a typical lymph node during an immune response to an antigen and hence contain B cells, T cells, and dendritic cells. Lymphoid cells from isolated from the thymus[11–13,14] and peripheral blood[14–18] of patients with MG, but not from individuals without MG, are able to synthesize antibodies to acetylcholine receptor. The antibodies produced by thymic and blood lymphocytes seem to be the same between individual patients. Other studies have demonstrated a general increase in activity of B cells from blood and thymus of MG patients.[19–22] The increase in B cell reactivity in the thymic cell population cannot be attributed to sim-ple differences in the T cell population,[22–24] which supports the notion that thymic B cells are activated because of other stimuli.

B cells seem to be able to get to the thymus from the peripheral immune compartments, as thymic lymphocytes from patients with MG and thymic hyperplasia, who received a booster injection of tetanus toxoid (TT) several weeks before undergoing thymectomy, synthesize anti-TT antibodies *in vitro*, whereas thymic cells from patients who did not receive a booster immunization do not.[14] In addition, many patients with MG also have increased incidence of other organ-specific and non-organ-specific autoantibodies, as well as other autoimmune diseases,[3,25–27] supporting the hypothesis that MG patients have increased activity of B cells and their progeny, namely, plasma blasts and plasma cells.

B cell–activating factor (BAFF), alternatively called B-lymphocyte stimulator (BLyS) and a member of the tumor necrosis factor super family (BAFF = TNFSF13b), is an important factor in B cell development and activation.[28,29] Because of its effects on B cells, the possibility that BAFF is playing a role in autoimmunity in patients with MG is important to investigate.[30,31]

doi: 10.1111/j.1749-6632.2012.06842.x

BAFF exists as a transmembrane protein that can be cleaved and thereby becomes the source of soluble BAFF. Myeloid-derived cells are the major sources of BAFF production,[32,33] although BAFF is produced by astrocytes—but not by microglia, which originate from the bone marrow during development—in brains of patients with multiple sclerosis (MS).[34] In the atypical germinal follicle-like structures seen in the meninges of patients with secondary progressive MS (SPMS), BAFF is made by B cells, whereas it is generally expressed in myeloid cells as is seen in lymphoid follicles elsewhere,[35] including in animals with experimental autoimmune encephalomyelitis.[36] In addition, there are instances of B cells appearing to produce BAFF in some autoimmune diseases.[35,37] And although there are studies on control of BAFF secretion in experimental autoimmune myasthenia gravis (EAMG),[38] little is known about control of BAFF secretion in MG itself, including which cytokines might be important for stimulation and inhibition of BAFF secretion. APRIL (a proliferation-inducing ligand), also a member of the TNF superfamily, binds to the BAFF receptors B cell maturation antigen (BCMA) and transmembrane activator and cyclophilin interactor (TACI).[39,40]

There is extensive experimental evidence demonstrating the importance of BAFF in B cell development and function. BAFF-deficient animals show defects in peripheral blood B cells and hypogammaglobulinemia,[41,42] while animals that overexpress BAFF have hypergammaglobulinemia, B cell hyperplasia, lymphoproliferation, enlarged spleens, a disease that resembles certain aspects of systemic lupus erythematosis (SLE), and potentially develop B cell lymphomas.[43,44] In addition to its role in B cell development, BAFF is also important survival factor for B cells. Plasma cells are responsive to BAFF,[45,46] and when overexpressed, BAFF inhibits B cell apoptosis, which seems to involve an increase in the anti-apoptotic Bcl-2 family. BAFF also seems to be particularly potent in the survival of autoimmune B cells, which may be particularly dependent on BAFF.[47,48]

As mentioned above, BAFF interacts with its receptors BAFF receptor (BAFF-R), TACI, and BCMA, which seem to be restricted in expression to cells of the B cell lineage,[40,49–51] although there are data suggesting that TACI and BCMA may be present on other lymphoid cell types.[52,49] BAFF is also apparently able to stimulate B cells via interaction with CD40.[28,29] Interestingly, signaling via BAFF-R causes prosurvival effects, while signaling via TACI produces inhibitory effects under some circumstances.[51–57] Animals that are deficient in BAFF-R have a reduction in peripheral B cells, reduced levels of serum immunoglobulins, lack marginal zones in lymph nodes, and are unable to form germinal follicles, very much like animals that are in deficient in BAFF itself.[58–62] TACI-deficient mice have an increase in hyper-responsive B cells, increased lymphocyte proliferation, and develop autoimmune diseases and B cell lymphomas.[53–57] When BAFF interacts with TACI there is a reduction in the B cell pool in experimental animals. The effect of signaling through TACI is less clear, with evidence for both inhibitory actions with signaling, although mutations can lead to immunoglobulin deficiency, variable immunodeficiency, or IgA deficiency.[55] Thus, TACI may be stimulatory in terminal B cell differentiation and inhibitory in earlier stages of B cell maturation. In contrast, in experimental animals, BCMA deficiency does not seem to result in any obvious abnormalities.[42,63] BCMA is found to be upregulated in germimal follicles and is expressed by plasma blasts, suggesting importance predominately in later phases of B cell differentiation to plasma cells.[45,46] Obviously, then, the differences in effects of signaling through the different BAFF receptors, and the regulation of the receptors at different stages of B cell, plasma blast, and plasma cell development, are important to consider when planning therapy that inhibits either BAFF or one or more of its receptors.

There are several studies that have demonstrated increased serum levels of BAFF, or BAFF production, by circulating blood cells in patients with autoimmune diseases, including SLE, Sjogren's disease, Wegener's granulomatosis, opsoclonus-myoclonus, rheumatoid arthritis (RA), Graves disease, and neuromyelitis optica (NMO).[37,64–71] Elevated levels of BAFF have also been reported in the cerebrospinal fluid (CSF) of some patients with MS and NMO.[69,72]

Increased serum levels of BAFF have been reported by several groups in MG.[73–75] In our studies, for example, BAFF levels were higher in MG patients who had elevated titers of anti-AChR but did not correlate with serum levels of immunoglobulins.[73] In these studies, there were too few anti-MuSK antibody positive patients to comment on whether increased serum BAFF correlated with the presence or absence of serum anti-MuSK antibodies; and BAFF levels did not correlate with severity of disease. There is one report of increase in BAFF-R in peripheral blood of patients with MG,[76] yet another study did not confirm that finding.[77] Thus, the question of BAFF-R expression by blood cells in MG is not settled.

BAFF is found in germinal follicles at sites of inflammation along with the chemokine CXCL13, a major chemotactic factor for B cells. Thus, it is not surprising that BAFF has been reported in macrophages within germinal follicles in the hyperplastic thymus of patients with MG.[76,78] Thymic epithelial cells express CXDL13[79,80] and have been shown to produce CXCL13 *in vitro*.[79] CXCL13 and BAFF are able to act in synergy to help form the germinal center follicles of the hyperplastic thymus.[81] It is also known that lymphotoxin (LT) signaling is important in germinal follicle formation.[82–84]

BAFF-R is upregulated in the thymic germinal centers in MG.[78] And as noted earlier, there is one study reporting an increased frequency of BAFF-R-expressing B cells in the blood of patients with MG, while another study did not find this, nor did it show differences in B cells expression of TACI or BCMA when compared to controls. There is some recent evidence that BAFF may also serve as a costimulant in T cell responses although this work, to date, relates to animal models.[85,86] What role BAFF plays in T cells in humans is not clear but BAFF interaction with T cells seems to be through BAFF-R.[49,85–87]

Several BAFF antagonists exist and treatment of patients with these might offer an additional approach to treatment of patients with MG, particularly those who have failed to have a sufficient response to symptomatic treatments, standard immunosuppressive and immunomodulatory therapies, or where side effects of these treatment modalities have led to dangerous side effects or intolerance of side effects. Belimumab, for example, is a neutralizing anti-BAFF monoclonal antibody (MoAb) that has been shown to be effective in SLE and RA and approved for SLE by the U.S. Federal Drug Administration (FDA).[88–90] Belimumab inhibits signaling through the BAFF-related pathways initiated by BAFF itself but not signaling triggered by APRIL, which shares a receptor with BAFF. Other agents such as several inhibitors of tumor necrosis alpha (TNF-α) and the anti-CD20 MoAb antibody rituximab, which depletes B cells, seem to be more effec-

tive clinically than belimumab in RA. Interestingly, in planning studies of agents that block important immune molecules, blockade of TNF-α worsened patients with MS,[91,92] and induced first episodes of the central nervous system (CNS) and peripheral nervous system (PNS) demyelinating events.[93–98] There is a molecule directed against BAFF-R, but it does not inhibit signaling by BAFF through its other receptors;[99] this molecule is a fusion protein of the extracellular domain of human BAFF-R and the Fc portion of human IgG1 and acts as a decoy that binds to BAFF-R but not the other BAFF or APRIL receptors.[99] Thus the inhibitors of BAFF signaling pathways are relatively selective, which offers an advantage over blocking all BAFF-related receptors.

A final inhibitor of the BAFF pathway is another fusion protein, TACI-Ig, that fuses the extracellular portion of the TACI receptor and Fc of human IgG1. This molecule binds to both BAFF and APRIL, inhibits the effects on cells expressing the receptors for both BAFF and APRIL, and thus is nonselective. This agent, atacicept, is under study for SLE and RA.[100–102] As a cautionary note, atacicept was not only ineffective in a trial of RRMS but also the trial had to be stopped because it was associated with worsening of disease.[103] And while the reason for this is not known, one could speculate that atacicept blocked the other functions of B cells that are important for inhibiting disease activity in MS, or that blocking of the potentially inhibitory TACI receptor-triggered signaling pathway resulted in more pathogenic B cell activity.

In addition to targeting BAFF and/or its receptors, another strategy to affect B cells is to deplete them in patients using the rituximab, a monoclonal antibody directed against CD20 expressed on the surface of B cells. Rituximab, reported in case series, has been used in MG patients resistant or intolerant to other therapies.[104–116] The overall clinical impression is that it is effective—perhaps more so and with longer duration of improvement than other therapies—in patients with anti-MuSK antibodies than in patients who possess anti-AChR antibodies or in patients who lack either anti-MuSK or anti-AChR antibodies (double seronegative patients). An important consideration, however, is that at least in other autoimmune diseases and in lymphomas an increase in serum BAFF levels occurs quickly after the decline in circulating B cells.[117–120] Thus, were the therapeutic effect of rituximab to persist for a longer period of time than in other MG patients, it is interesting to speculate whether there might be a difference in serum BAFF levels after rituximab treatment in the anti-MuSK patients compared to anti-AChR or double seronegative patients. Other potential explanations include that anti-MuSK antibodies are predominately IgG4, whereas anti-AChR antibodies consist of several IgG subisotypes.[121]

Finally, some widely employed treatments for MG may work, in part, by affecting BAFF, including corticosteroids, which may inhibit pathways involved in BAFF production,[122] and intravenous immunoglobulin (IVIg), as anti-BAFF and anti-APRIL activity have been detected in these preparations.[123]

Summary

BAFF seems to be an important factor in the pathogenesis of MG, with potential roles in both the peripheral immune system as well as in the thymus, especially in patients with germinal center follicular hyperplasia. We need to know more about control of BAFF in individuals with autoimmune diseases including MG. Modification or inhibition of BAFF pathways may have potential as treatment in patients who are resistant to, or intolerant of, other treatments, although caution is needed because inhibiting molecules, such as BAFF, and their receptors, proven successful in some immunopathologically mediated/autoimmune diseases, have led to worsening in of some diseases. If BAFF-inhibiting agents are found to be relatively safe, their use could be expanded to early use in patients with anti-AChR, who are likely to have germinal center follicular hyperplasia.

Acknowledgments

The studies of BAFF by the authors was supported by a grant from the Muscular Dystrophy Association, the Parker Webber Chair in Neurology endowment (Wayne State University School of Medicine), and by the Mary Parker Neuroscience Fund (Detroit Medical Center/Wayne State University School of Medicine).

Conflicts of interest

The authors have no potential conflicts of interest related to research on myasthenia gravis and related disorders.

References

1. Appel, S.H., R.R. Almon & N. Levy. 1975. Acetylcholine receptor antibodies in myasthenia gravis. *N. Engl. J. Med.* **293:** 760–761.

2. Lindstrom, J.M., M.E. Seybold, V.A. Lennon, *et al.* 1976. Antibody to acetylcholine receptor in myasthenia gravis. prevalence, clinical correlates, and diagnostic value. *Neurology* **26:** 1054–1059.

3. Ragheb, S. & R. Lisak. 1994. The immunopathogenesis of acquired (autoimmune) myasthenia gravis. In *Handbook of Myasthenia Gravis and Myasthenic Syndromes.* R. Lisak, Ed.: 239–276. New York. Marcel Dekker.

4. McConville, J., M.E. Farrugia, D. Beeson, *et al.* 2004. Detection and characterization of MuSK antibodies in seronegative myasthenia gravis. *Ann. Neurol.* **55:** 580–584.

5. Evoli, A., P.A. Tonali, L. Padua, *et al.* 2003. Clinical correlates with anti-MuSK antibodies in generalized seronegative myasthenia gravis. *Brain* **126:** 2304–2311.

6. Oh, S.J., Y. Hatanaka, S. Hemmi, *et al.* 2006. Repetitive nerve stimulation of facial muscles in musk antibody-positive myasthenia gravis. *Muscle Nerve* **33:** 500–504.

7. Sanders, D.B., K. El-Salem, J.M. Massey, *et al.* 2003. Clinical aspects of MuSK antibody positive seronegative MG. *Neurology* **60:** 1978–1980.

8. Higuchi, O., J. Hamuro, M. Motomura & Y. Yamanashi. 2011. Autoantibodies to low-density lipoprotein receptor-related protein 4 in myasthenia gravis. *Ann. Neurol.* **69:** 418–422.

9. Pevzner, A., B. Schoser, K. Peters, *et al.* 2012. Anti-LRP4 autoantibodies in AChR- and MuSK-antibody-negative myasthenia gravis. *J. Neurol.* **259:** 427–435.

10. Zhang, B., J.S. Tzartos, M. Belimezi, *et al.* 2012. Autoantibodies to lipoprotein-related protein 4 in patients with double-seronegative myasthenia gravis. *Arch. Neurol.* **69:** 445–451.

11. Vincent, A., G.K. Scadding, H.C. Thomas & J. Newsom-Davis. 1978. In-vitro synthesis of anti-acetylcholine-receptor antibody by thymic lymphocytes in myasthenia gravis. *Lancet* **1:** 305–307.

12. Scadding, G.K., A. Vincent, J. Newsom-Davis & K. Henry. 1981. Acetylcholine receptor antibody synthesis by thymic lymphocytes: correlation with thymic histology. *Neurology* **31:** 935–943.

13. Fujii, Y., Y. Monden, J. Hashimoto, *et al.* 1985. Acetylcholine receptor antibody-producing cells in thymus and lymph nodes in myasthenia gravis. *Clin. Immunol. Immunopathol.* **34:** 141–146.

14. Lisak, R.P., A.I. Levinson, B. Zweiman & M.J. Kornstein. 1986. Antibodies to acetylcholine receptor and tetanus toxoid: in vitro synthesis by thymic lymphocytes. *J. Immunol.* **137:** 1221–1225.

15. Lisak, R.P., C. Laramore, B. Zweiman & A. Moskovitz. 1983. In vitro synthesis of antibodies to acetylcholine receptor by peripheral blood mononuclear cells of patients with myasthenia gravis. *Neurology* **33:** 604–608.

16. Lisak, R.P., C. Laramore, A.I. Levinson, *et al.* 1986. Suppressor T cells in myasthenia gravis and antibodies to acetylcholine receptor. *Ann. Neurol.* **19:** 87–89.

17. Lisak, R.P., C. Laramore, A.I. Levinson, et al. 1984. In vitro synthesis of antibodies to acetylcholine receptor by peripheral blood cells: role of suppressor T cells in normal subjects. Neurology **34**: 802–805.

18. Lisak, R.P., A.I. Levinson, B. Zweiman & M.J. Kornstein. 1987. In vitro synthesis of IgG and antibodies to AChR by peripheral and thymic lymphocytes. Ann. N.Y. Acad. Sci. **505**: 39–49.

19. Levinson, A.I., A. Dziarski, R.P. Lisak, et al. 1981. Comparative immunoglobulin synthesis by blood lymphocytes of myasthenics and normals. Ann. N.Y. Acad. Sci. **377**: 385–392.

20. Levinson, A.I., A. Dziarski, R.P. Lisak, et al. 1981. Polyclonal B-cell activity in myasthenia gravis. Neurology **31**: 1198–1201.

21. Levinson, A.I., R.P. Lisak, B. Zweiman & M. Kornstein. 1985. Phenotypic and functional analysis of lymphocytes in myasthenia gravis. Springer Semin. Immunopathol. **8**: 209–233.

22. Levinson, A.I., B. Zweiman, R.P. Lisak, et al. 1984. Thymic B-cell activation in myasthenia gravis. Neurology **34**: 462–468.

23. Levinson, A.I., B. Zweiman & R.P. Lisak. 1990. Pokeweed mitogen-induced immunoglobulin secretory responses of thymic B cells in myasthenia gravis: selective secretion of IgG versus IgM cannot be explained by helper functions of thymic T cells. Clin. Immunol. Immunopathol. **57**: 211–217.

24. Zweiman, B., A.I. Levinson & R.P. Lisak. 1989. Phenotypic characteristics of thymic B lymphocytes in myasthenia gravis. J. Clin. Immunol. **9**: 242–247.

25. Simpson, J.A. 1977. Myasthenia gravis—validation of a hypothesis. Scott. Med. J. **22**: 201–210.

26. Simpson, J.A. 1966. Myasthenia gravis as an autoimmune disease: clinical aspects. Ann. N. Y. Acad. Sci. **135**: 506–516.

27. Simpson, J.F., M.R. Westerberg & K.R. Magee. 1966. Myasthenia gravis. An analysis of 295 cases. Acta. Neurol. Scand. **42**(Suppl 23): 1–7.

28. Moore, P.A., O. Belvedere, A. Orr, et al. 1999. BLyS: member of the tumor necrosis factor family and B lymphocyte stimulator. Science **285**: 260–263.

29. Schneider, P., F. MacKay, V. Steiner, et al. 1999. BAFF, a novel ligand of the tumor necrosis factor family, stimulates B cell growth. J. Exp. Med. **189**: 1747–1756.

30. Mackay, F., P.A. Silveira & R. Brink. 2007. B cells and the BAFF/APRIL axis: fast-forward on autoimmunity and signaling. Curr. Opin. Immunol. **19**: 327–336.

31. Ragheb, S. & R.P. Lisak. 2011. B-cell-activating factor and autoimmune myasthenia gravis. Autoimmune Dis. **2011**: 939520.

32. Nardelli, B., O. Belvedere, V. Roschke, et al. 2001. Synthesis and release of B-lymphocyte stimulator from myeloid cells. Blood **97**: 198–204.

33. Craxton, A., D. Magaletti, E.J. Ryan & E.A. Clark. 2003. Macrophage- and dendritic cell–dependent regulation of human B-cell proliferation requires the TNF family ligand BAFF. Blood **101**: 4464–4471.

34. Krumbholz, M., D. Theil, T. Derfuss, et al. 2005. BAFF is produced by astrocytes and up-regulated in multiple sclerosis lesions and primary central nervous system lymphoma. J. Exp. Med. **201**: 195–200.

35. Serafini, B., M. Severa, S. Columba-Cabezas, et al. 2010. Epstein-Barr virus latent infection and BAFF expression in B cells in the multiple sclerosis brain: implications for viral persistence and intrathecal B-cell activation. J. Neuropathol. Exp. Neurol. **69**: 677–693.

36. Magliozzi, R., S. Columba-Cabezas, B. Serafini & F. Aloisi. 2004. Intracerebral expression of CXCL13 and BAFF is accompanied by formation of lymphoid follicle-like structures in the meninges of mice with relapsing experimental autoimmune encephalomyelitis. J. Neuroimmunol. **148**: 11–23.

37. Chu, V.T., P. Enghard, S. Schurer, et al. 2009. Systemic activation of the immune system induces aberrant BAFF and APRIL expression in B cells in patients with systemic lupus erythematosus. Arthritis Rheum. **60**: 2083–2093.

38. Xiao, B.G., R.S. Duan, H. Link & Y.M. Huang. 2003. Induction of peripheral tolerance to experimental autoimmune myasthenia gravis by acetylcholine receptor-pulsed dendritic cells. Cell Immunol. **223**: 63–69.

39. Mackay, F., P. Schneider, P. Rennert & J. Browning. 2003. BAFF AND APRIL: a tutorial on B cell survival. Annu. Rev. Immunol. **21**: 231–264.

40. Kalled, S.L., C. Ambrose & Y.M. Hsu. 2005. The biochemistry and biology of BAFF, APRIL and their receptors. Curr. Dir. Autoimmun. **8**: 206–242.

41. Bjartmar, C., R.P. Kinkel, G. Kidd, et al. 2001. Axonal loss in normal-appearing white matter in a patient with acute MS. Neurology **57**: 1248–1252.

42. Schiemann, B., J.L. Gommerman, K. Vora, et al. 2001. An essential role for BAFF in the normal development of B cells through a BCMA-independent pathway. Science **293**: 2111–2114.

43. Mackay, F., S.A. Woodcock, P. Lawton, et al. 1999. Mice transgenic for BAFF develop lymphocytic disorders along with autoimmune manifestations. J. Exp. Med. **190**: 1697–1710.

44. Khare, S.D., I. Sarosi, X.Z. Xia, et al. 2000. Severe B cell hyperplasia and autoimmune disease in TALL-1 transgenic mice. Proc. Natl. Acad. Sci. USA **97**: 3370–3375.

45. O'Connor, B.P., V.S. Raman, L.D. Erickson, et al. 2004. BCMA is essential for the survival of long-lived bone marrow plasma cells. J. Exp. Med. **199**: 91–98.

46. Benson, M.J., S.R. Dillon, E. Castigli, et al. 2008. Cutting edge: the dependence of plasma cells and independence of memory B cells on BAFF and APRIL. J. Immunol. **180**: 3655–3659.

47. Lesley, R., Y. Xu, S.L. Kalled, et al. 2004. Reduced competitiveness of autoantigen-engaged B cells due to increased dependence on BAFF. Immunity **20**: 441–453.

48. Thien, M., T.G. Phan, S. Gardam, et al. 2004. Excess BAFF rescues self-reactive B cells from peripheral deletion and allows them to enter forbidden follicular and marginal zone niches. Immunity **20**: 785–798.

49. Ng, L.G., A.P. Sutherland, R. Newton, et al. 2004. B cell-activating factor belonging to the TNF family (BAFF)-R is the principal BAFF receptor facilitating BAFF costimulation of circulating T and B cells. J. Immunol. **173**: 807–817.

50. Bossen, C. & P. Schneider. 2006. BAFF, APRIL and their receptors: structure, function and signaling. *Semin. Immunol.* **18:** 263–275.

51. Mackay, F. & P. Schneider. 2009. Cracking the BAFF code. *Nat. Rev. Immunol.* **9:** 491–502.

52. von Bulow, G.U., J.M. van Deursen & R.J. Bram. 2001. Regulation of the T-independent humoral response by TACI. *Immunity* **14:** 573–582.

53. Yan, M., H. Wang, B. Chan, *et al.* 2001. Activation and accumulation of B cells in TACI-deficient mice. *Nat. Immunol.* **2:** 638–643.

54. Seshasayee, D., P. Valdez, M. Yan, *et al.* 2003. Loss of TACI causes fatal lymphoproliferation and autoimmunity, establishing TACI as an inhibitory BLyS receptor. *Immunity* **18:** 279–288.

55. Castigli, E., S.A. Wilson, L. Garibyan, *et al.* 2005. TACI is mutant in common variable immunodeficiency and IgA deficiency. *Nat. Genet.* **37:** 829–834.

56. Salzer, U., H.M. Chapel, A.D. Webster, *et al.* 2005. Mutations in TNFRSF13B encoding TACI are associated with common variable immunodeficiency in humans. *Nat. Genet.* **37:** 820–828.

57. Sakurai, D., Y. Kanno, H. Hase, *et al.* 2007. TACI attenuates antibody production costimulated by BAFF-R and CD40. *Eur. J. Immunol.* **37:** 110–118.

58. Miller, D.J. & C.E. Hayes. 1991. Phenotypic and genetic characterization of a unique B lymphocyte deficiency in strain A/WySnJ mice. *Eur. J. Immunol.* **21:** 1123–1130.

59. Harless, S.M., V.M. Lentz, A.P. Sah, *et al.* 2001. Competition for BLyS-mediated signaling through Bcmd/BR3 regulates peripheral B lymphocyte numbers. *Curr. Biol.* **11:** 1986–1989.

60. Yan, M., J.R. Brady, B. Chan, *et al.* 2001. Identification of a novel receptor for B lymphocyte stimulator that is mutated in a mouse strain with severe B cell deficiency. *Curr. Biol.* **11:** 1547–1552.

61. Sasaki, Y., S. Casola, J.L. Kutok, *et al.* 2004. TNF family member B cell-activating factor (BAFF) receptor-dependent and -independent roles for BAFF in B cell physiology. *J. Immunol.* **173:** 2245–2252.

62. Shulga-Morskaya, S., M. Dobles, M.E. Walsh, *et al.* 2004. B cell-activating factor belonging to the TNF family acts through separate receptors to support B cell survival and T cell-independent antibody formation. *J. Immunol.* **173:** 2331–2341.

63. Xu, S. & K.P. Lam. 2001. B-cell maturation protein, which binds the tumor necrosis factor family members BAFF and APRIL, is dispensable for humoral immune responses. *Mol. Cell Biol.* **21:** 4067–4074.

64. Groom, J., S.L. Kalled, A.H. Cutler, *et al.* 2002. Association of BAFF/BLyS overexpression and altered B cell differentiation with Sjogren's syndrome. *J. Clin. Invest.* **109:** 59–68.

65. Mariette, X., S. Roux, J. Zhang, *et al.* 2003. The level of BLyS (BAFF) correlates with the titre of autoantibodies in human Sjogren's syndrome. *Ann. Rheum. Dis.* **62:** 168–171.

66. Krumbholz, M., U. Specks, M. Wick, *et al.* 2005. BAFF is elevated in serum of patients with Wegener's granulomatosis. *J. Autoimmun.* **25:** 298–302.

67. Bosello, S., P. Youinou, C. Daridon, *et al.* 2008. Concentrations of BAFF correlate with autoantibody levels, clinical disease activity, and response to treatment in early rheumatoid arthritis. *J. Rheumatol.* **35:** 1256–1264.

68. Fuhlhuber, V., S. Bick, A. Kirsten, *et al.* 2009. Elevated B-cell activating factor BAFF, but not APRIL, correlates with CSF cerebellar autoantibodies in pediatric opsoclonus-myoclonus syndrome. *J. Neuroimmunol.* **210:** 87–91.

69. Okada, K., T. Matsushita, J. Kira & S. Tsuji. 2010. B-cell activating factor of the TNF family is upregulated in neuromyelitis optica. *Neurology* **74:** 177–178.

70. Vadacca, M., D. Margiotta, D. Sambataro, *et al.* 2010. BAFF/APRIL pathway in Sjogren syndrome and systemic lupus erythematosus: relationship with chronic inflammation and disease activity. *Reumatismo* **62:** 259–265.

71. Vannucchi, G., D. Covelli, N. Curro, *et al.* 2012. Serum BAFF concentrations in patients with Graves' disease and orbitopathy before and after immunosuppressive therapy. *J. Clin. Endocrinol. Metab.* **97:** E755–E759.

72. Ragheb, S., Y. Li, K. Simon, *et al.* 2011. Multiple sclerosis: BAFF and CXCL13 in cerebrospinal fluid. *Mult. Scler.* **17:** 819–829.

73. Ragheb, S., R. Lisak, R. Lewis, *et al.* 2008. A potential role for B-cell activating factor in the pathogenesis of autoimmune myasthenia gravis. *Arch. Neurol.* **65:** 1358–1362.

74. Kim, J.Y., Y. Yang, J.S. Moon, *et al.* 2008. Serum BAFF expression in patients with myasthenia gravis. *J. Neuroimmunol.* **199:** 151–154.

75. Scuderi, F., P.E. Alboini, E. Bartoccioni & A. Evoli. 2011. BAFF serum levels in myasthenia gravis: effects of therapy. *J. Neurol.* **258:** 2284–2285.

76. Li, X., B.G. Xiao, J.Y. Xi, *et al.* 2008. Decrease of CD4(+)CD25(high)Foxp3(+) regulatory T cells and elevation of CD19(+)BAFF-R(+) B cells and soluble ICAM-1 in myasthenia gravis. *Clin. Immunol.* **126:** 180–188.

77. Thangarajh, M., L. Kisiswa, R. Pirskanen & J. Hillert. 2007. The expression of BAFF-binding receptors is not altered in multiple sclerosis or myasthenia gravis. *Scand. J. Immunol.* **65:** 461–466.

78. Thangarajh, M., T. Masterman, L. Helgeland, *et al.* 2006. The thymus is a source of B-cell-survival factors-APRIL and BAFF-in myasthenia gravis. *J. Neuroimmunol.* **178:** 161–166.

79. Meraouna, A., G. Cizeron-Clairac, R.L. Panse, *et al.* 2006. The chemokine CXCL13 is a key molecule in autoimmune myasthenia gravis. *Blood* **108:** 432–440.

80. Shiao, Y.M., C.C. Lee, Y.H. Hsu, *et al.* 2010. Ectopic and high CXCL13 chemokine expression in myasthenia gravis with thymic lymphoid hyperplasia. *J. Neuroimmunol.* **221:** 101–106.

81. Aloisi, F. & R. Pujol-Borrell. 2006. Lymphoid neogenesis in chronic inflammatory diseases. *Nat. Rev. Immunol.* **6:** 205–217.

82. Gommerman, J.L. & J.L. Browning. 2003. Lymphotoxin/light, lymphoid microenvironments and autoimmune disease. *Nat. Rev. Immunol.* **3:** 642–655.

83. McCarthy, D.D., L. Summers-Deluca, F. Vu, *et al.* 2006. The lymphotoxin pathway: beyond lymph node development. *Immunol. Res.* **35:** 41–54.

84. Ruddle, N.H. 1999. Lymphoid neo-organogenesis: lympho-toxin's role in inflammation and development. *Immunol. Res.* **19**: 119–125.

85. Sutherland, A.P., L.G. Ng, C.A. Fletcher, *et al.* 2005. BAFF augments certain Th1-associated inflammatory responses. *J. Immunol.* **174**: 5537–5544.

86. Lai Kwan Lam, Q., O. King Hung Ko, B.J. Zheng & L. Lu. 2008. Local BAFF gene silencing suppresses Th17-cell generation and ameliorates autoimmune arthritis. *Proc. Natl. Acad. Sci. USA* **105**: 14993–14998.

87. Huard, B., P. Schneider, D. Mauri, *et al.* 2001. T cell costimulation by the TNF ligand BAFF. *J. Immunol.* **167**: 6225–6231.

88. Baker, K.P., B.M. Edwards, S.H. Main, *et al.* 2003. Generation and characterization of LymphoStat-B, a human monoclonal antibody that antagonizes the bioactivities of B lymphocyte stimulator. *Arthritis Rheum.* **48**: 3253–3265.

89. Espinosa, G. & R. Cervera. 2010. Belimumab, a BLyS-specific inhibitor for the treatment of systemic lupus erythematosus. *Drugs Today* **46**: 891–899.

90. Navarra, S.V., R.M. Guzman, A.E. Gallacher, *et al.* 2011. Efficacy and safety of belimumab in patients with active systemic lupus erythematosus: a randomised, placebo-controlled, phase 3 trial. *Lancet* **377**: 721–731.

91. The Lenercept Multiple Sclerosis Study Group and The University of British Columbia MS/MRI Analysis Group. 1999. TNF neutralization in MS: results of a randomized, placebo-controlled multicenter study. *Neurology* **53**: 457–465.

92. Schwid, S.R. & J.H. Noseworthy. 1999. Targeting immunotherapy in multiple sclerosis: a near hit and a clear miss. *Neurology* **53**: 444–445.

93. van Oosten, B.W., F. Barkhof, L. Truyen, *et al.* 1996. Increased MRI activity and immune activation in two multiple sclerosis patients treated with the monoclonal anti-tumor necrosis factor antibody cA2. *Neurology* **47**: 1531–1534.

94. Enayati, P.J. & K.A. Papadakis. 2005. Association of anti-tumor necrosis factor therapy with the development of multiple sclerosis. *J. Clin. Gastroenterol.* **39**: 303–306.

95. Robinson, W.H., M.C. Genovese & L.W. Moreland. 2001. Demyelinating and neurologic events reported in association with tumor necrosis factor alpha antagonism: by what mechanisms could tumor necrosis factor alpha antagonists improve rheumatoid arthritis but exacerbate multiple sclerosis? *Arthritis Rheum.* **44**: 1977–1983.

96. Chung, J.H., G.P. Van Stavern, L.P. Frohman & R.E. Turbin. 2006. Adalimumab-associated optic neuritis. *J. Neurol. Sci.* **244**: 133–136.

97. Stubgen, J.P. 2008. Tumor necrosis factor-alpha antagonists and neuropathy. *Muscle Nerve* **37**: 281–292.

98. Richez, C., P. Blanco, A. Lagueny, *et al.* 2005. Neuropathy resembling CIDP in patients receiving tumor necrosis factor-alpha blockers. *Neurology* **64**: 1468–1470.

99. Lin, W.Y., Q. Gong, D. Seshasayee, *et al.* 2007. Anti-BR3 antibodies: a new class of B-cell immunotherapy combining cellular depletion and survival blockade. *Blood* **110**: 3959–3967.

100. Carbonatto, M., P. Yu, M. Bertolino, *et al.* 2008. Nonclinical safety, pharmacokinetics, and pharmacodynamics of atacicept. *Toxicol. Sci.* **105**: 200–210.

101. Dall'Era, M., E. Chakravarty, D. Wallace, *et al.* 2007. Re-duced B lymphocyte and immunoglobulin levels after atacicept treatment in patients with systemic lupus erythematosus: results of a multicenter, phase Ib, double-blind, placebo-controlled, dose-escalating trial. *Arthritis Rheum.* **56**: 4142–4150.

102. Tak, P.P., R.M. Thurlings, C. Rossier, *et al.* 2008. Atacicept in patients with rheumatoid arthritis: results of a multicenter, phase Ib, double-blind, placebo-controlled, dose-escalating, single- and repeated-dose study. *Arthritis Rheum.* **58**: 61–72.

103. Hartung, H.-P. & B. Kieseier. 2010. Atacicept: targeting B cells in multiple sclerosis. *Ther. Adv. Neurol. Disord.* **3**: 205–216.

104. Baek, W.S., A. Bashey & G.L. Sheean. 2007. Complete remission induced by rituximab in refractory, seronegative, muscle-specific, kinase-positive myasthenia gravis. *J. Neurol. Neurosurg. Psychiatr.* **78**: 771.

105. Blum, S., D. Gillis, H. Brown, *et al.* 2011. Use and monitoring of low dose rituximab in myasthenia gravis. *J. Neurol. Neurosurg. Psychiatr.* **82**: 659–663.

106. Burusnukul, P., T.D. Brennan & E.J. Cupler. 2010. Prolonged improvement after rituximab: two cases of resistant muscle-specific receptor tyrosine kinase +myasthenia gravis. *J. Clin. Neuromuscul. Dis.* **12**: 85–87.

107. Hain, B., K. Jordan, M. Deschauer & S. Zierz. 2006. Successful treatment of MuSK antibody-positive myasthenia gravis with rituximab. *Muscle Nerve* **33**: 575–580.

108. Lindberg, C. & M. Bokarewa. 2010. Rituximab for severe myasthenia gravis—experience from five patients. *Acta. Neurol. Scand.* **122**: 225–228.

109. Maddison, P., J McConville, M.E. Farrugia, *et al.* 2011. The use of rituximab in myasthenia gravis and Lambert-Eaton myasthenic syndrome. *J. Neurol. Neurosurg. Psychiatr.* **82**: 671–673.

110. Nowak, R.J., D.B. Dicapua, N. Zebardast & J.M. Goldstein. 2011. Response of patients with refractory myasthenia gravis to rituximab: a retrospective study. *Ther. Adv. Neurol. Disord.* **4**: 259–266.

111. Stein, B. & S.J. Bird. 2011. Rituximab in the treatment of MuSK antibody-positive myasthenia gravis. *J. Clin. Neuromuscul. Dis.* **12**: 163–164.

112. Stieglbauer, K., R. Topakian, V. Schaffer & F.T. Aichner. 2009. Rituximab for myasthenia gravis: three case reports and review of the literature. *J. Neurol. Sci.* **280**: 120–122.

113. Thakre, M., J. Inshasi & M. Marashi. 2007. Rituximab in refractory MuSK antibody myasthenia gravis. *J. Neurol.* **254**: 968–969.

114. Wylam, M.E., P.M. Anderson, N.L. Kuntz & V. Rodriguez. 2003. Successful treatment of refractory myasthenia gravis using rituximab: a pediatric case report. *J. Pediatr.* **143**: 674–677.

115. Zaja, F., D. Russo, G. Fuga, *et al.* 2000. Rituximab for myasthenia gravis developing after bone marrow transplant. *Neurology* **55**: 1062–1063.

116. Zebardast, N., H.S. Patwa, S.P. Novella & J.M. Goldstein. 2010. Rituximab in the management of refractory myasthenia gravis. *Muscle Nerve* **41**: 375–378.

117. Lavie, F., C. Miceli-Richard, M. Ittah, *et al.* 2007. Increase of B cell-activating factor of the TNF family (BAFF) after

rituximab treatment: insights into a new regulating system of BAFF production. *Ann. Rheum. Dis.* **66:** 700–703.

118. Pers, J.O., V. Devauchelle, C. Daridon, *et al.* 2007. BAFF-modulated repopulation of B lymphocytes in the blood and salivary glands of rituximab-treated patients with Sjogren's syndrome. *Arthritis Rheum.* **56:** 1464–1477.

119. Pranzatelli, M.R., E.D. Tate, A.L. Travelstead & S.J. Verhulst. 2011. Chemokine/cytokine profiling after rituximab: reciprocal expression of BCA-1/CXCL13 and BAFF in childhood OMS. *Cytokine* **53:** 384–389.

120. Vallerskog, T., M. Heimburger, I. Gunnarsson, *et al.* 2006. Differential effects on BAFF and APRIL levels in rituximab-treated patients with systemic lupus erythematosus and rheumatoid arthritis. *Arthritis Res. Ther.* **8:** R167.

121. Leite, M.I., S. Jacob, S. Viegas, *et al.* 2008. IgG1 antibodies to acetylcholine receptors in 'seronegative' myasthenia gravis. *Brain* **131:** 1940–1952.

122. Zen, M., M. Canova, C. Campana, *et al.* 2011. The kaleidoscope of glucorticoid effects on immune system. *Autoimmun. Rev.* **10:** 305–310.

123. Le Pottier, L., B. Bendaoud, M. Dueymes, *et al.* 2007. BAFF, a new target for intravenous immunoglobulin in autoimmunity and cancer. *J. Clin. Immunol.* **27:** 257–265.

Ann. N.Y. Acad. Sci. ISSN 0077-8923

ANNALS OF THE NEW YORK ACADEMY OF SCIENCES
Issue: *Myasthenia Gravis and Related Disorders*

Functional defect in regulatory T cells in myasthenia gravis

Muthusamy Thiruppathi,[1,2] Julie Rowin,[1] Qin Li Jiang,[1] Jian Rong Sheng,[1,2] Bellur S. Prabhakar,[2] and Matthew N. Meriggioli[1]

[1]Department of Neurology and Rehabilitation, [2]Department of Microbiology and Immunology, College of Medicine, University of Illinois Hospital and Health Sciences System, Chicago, Illinois

Address for correspondence: Matthew N. Meriggioli, MD, Department of Neurology and Rehabilitation, College of Medicine, University of Illinois, 912 S. Wood Street, M/C 796, Chicago, IL 60612. mmeriggioli@gmail.com

Forkhead box P3 (FOXP3) is a transcription factor necessary for the function of regulatory T cells (T_{reg} cells). T_{reg} cells maintain immune homeostasis and self-tolerance and play an important role in the prevention of autoimmune disease. Here, we discuss the role of T_{reg} cells in the pathogenesis of myasthenia gravis (MG) and review evidence indicating that a significant defect in T_{reg} cell *in vitro* suppressive function exists in MG patients, without an alteration in circulating frequency. This functional defect is associated with a reduced expression of key functional molecules, such as FOXP3 on isolated T_{reg} cells, and appears to be more pronounced in immunosuppression-naive MG patients. *In vitro* administration of granulocyte macrophage–colony-stimulating factor (GM-CSF) enhanced the suppressive function of T_{reg} cells and upregulated FOXP3 expression. These findings indicate a clinically relevant T_{reg} cell–intrinsic defect in immune regulation in MG that may reveal a novel therapeutic target.

Keywords: myasthenia gravis; regulatory T cells; FOXP3; GM-CSF

Introduction

Acquired myasthenia gravis (MG) is an autoimmune disorder of the neuromuscular junction in which patients experience fluctuating skeletal muscle weakness that often affects selected muscle groups preferentially. The target of the autoimmune attack in most cases is the skeletal muscle acetylcholine receptor (AChR), but in others, non-AChR components of the neuromuscular junction, such as the muscle-specific receptor tyrosine kinase, are targeted (reviewed in Ref. 1). The precise origin of the autoimmune response in MG is unknown, but abnormalities of the thymus gland (hyperplasia and neoplasia) almost certainly play a role in patients with anti-AChR antibodies,[2,3] and genetic predisposition is also likely to influence which patients develop the disorder.[4–6] High-affinity, anti-AChR antibodies bind to the neuromuscular junction, activate complement, and accelerate AChR destruction, while causing failure of neuromuscular transmission and the resulting myasthenic symptoms (reviewed in Ref. 1). However, autoreactive AChR-specific CD4$^+$ T cells, which can be detected in most MG patients,[7–10] likely play an important role in MG, through cognate interactions with B cells leading to the synthesis of anti-AChR antibodies.[11]

Regulatory T cells and immune tolerance

Immune tolerance to self-antigens is initially achieved during thymic development by the clonal deletion of potentially autoreactive T cells. However, some of these pathogenic cells, including some with reactivity to skeletal muscle AChR, survive clonal deletion in normal individuals and are kept in check by peripheral tolerance mechanisms, most notably by a specialized subset of CD4$^+$ T cells called regulatory T cells (T_{reg} cells).[12] T_{reg} cells are a subpopulation of T cells that act to suppress activation of other immune cells and thereby maintain immune system homeostasis and self-tolerance.[13] Current theories regarding the pathogenesis of autoimmune disease hypothesize that a functional deficiency in T_{reg} cells could result in a failure to suppress autoreactive T cell responses.[14,15]

doi: 10.1111/j.1749-6632.2012.06840.x

Ann. N.Y. Acad. Sci. 1274 (2012) 68–76 © 2012 New York Academy of Sciences.

The thymus gland is the primary source of T$_{reg}$ cells, which constitute approximately 5–10% of the peripheral CD4$^+$ T cell population and play a crucial role in the maintenance of immune homeostasis.[13] T$_{reg}$ cells actively mediate self-tolerance and thus control autoimmunity by suppressing the activation, proliferation, and cytokine production of effector autoreactive T cells that either arise *de novo* or escape thymic deletion.[13,16] The transcription factor forkhead box protein P3 (FOXP3) expressed in CD4$^+$ CD25$^+$ T$_{reg}$ cells is the master regulator for the development and function of these cells.[17,18] FOXP3 gene transfer has been shown to convert naive CD4$^+$ CD25$^-$ T cells into a functional regulatory lymphocyte population, thus demonstrating the pivotal role of FOXP3 in T$_{reg}$ cell biology.[18]

A deficiency or dysfunction of T$_{reg}$ cells has been shown to contribute to the pathogenesis and development of many autoimmune diseases.[19–22] Functional defects have been demonstrated in T$_{reg}$ cells isolated from patients with diverse autoimmune diseases, suggesting that in autoimmunity T$_{reg}$ cell–suppressive capacity may be diminished. It has also recently been reported that the source of the apparent T$_{reg}$ cell dysfunction may not necessarily be primarily intrinsic to T$_{reg}$ cells, and that effector T cells may acquire resistance to T$_{reg}$ cell suppression in certain autoimmune diseases.[19,23–25]

Regulatory T cells and immune regulation in MG

While it is likely that T$_{reg}$ cells exert their effects on T helper cells, thereby regulating B cell function and antibody secretion, there is also evidence that T$_{reg}$ cells may have a direct effect on B cells.[26] Specifically, in MG it may be hypothesized that dysfunctional T$_{reg}$ cells permit the production of anti-AChR autoantibodies, a hypothesis that remains to be specifically tested. Investigators examining the relative frequencies and function of T$_{reg}$ cells in the peripheral circulation and thymi of MG patients have reported conflicting results, including reductions in T$_{reg}$ cell numbers,[27–29] impaired regulatory function,[30] or no defect.[31,32] Aside from measuring T$_{reg}$ cell numbers, and the ability to suppress nonspecific T cell proliferation, more detailed analyses of T$_{reg}$ cell–intrinsic (T$_{reg}$ phenotype, cytokine production, and suppressive function) versus T$_{reg}$ cell–extrinsic factors (T helper/effector cells, dendritic cells) and the ability to suppress specific AChR-induced T cell

proliferation have not been performed. The reported demonstration of a functional impairment of thymic T$_{reg}$ cells in MG patients is an interesting finding and suggests an origin for T$_{reg}$ cell dysfunction in the thymus, possibly owing to thymic pathology (hyperplasia or neoplasia).[33]

Importantly, in all of the studies referenced above, investigators used a single step–enrichment protocol in which T$_{reg}$ cells were identified and isolated by high surface expression of CD25. Unfortunately, the level of expression of CD25 that defines T$_{reg}$ cells has been inconsistently reported in the literature, and CD25 is also expressed by recently activated T cells, resulting in the possible inclusion of effector T cells in isolated T$_{reg}$ cell populations.[34] More recent studies have shown that T$_{reg}$ cells express low or absent levels of the IL-7 receptor α-chain (CD127) and that this expression is inversely correlated with FOXP3 expression and with suppressive function;[35,36] thus, screening for CD127 expression may provide a more precise method for isolating a pure T$_{reg}$ cell population.

Impaired suppressive function of isolated MG T$_{reg}$ cells

We have investigated the existence of a functional defect in CD4$^+$ CD25^{high} CD127$^{low/-}$ T$_{reg}$ cells in MG patients by isolating this population using flow-based sorting and then coculturing the cells with autologous CD4$^+$ CD25$^-$ T responder cells (T$_{resp}$) at different T$_{reg}$:T$_{resp}$ ratios in the presence of irradiated autologous antigen presenting cells (APCs). We performed T cell–proliferation studies (CFSE dilution), by stimulating the cell cultures with anti-CD3 Abs, and analyzed cytokine profiles from cell culture supernatants. We found that the suppressive ability of isolated T$_{reg}$ cells from MG patients (MG T$_{reg}$ cells) was consistently reduced compared to age-matched controls analyzed concurrently.[37] As expected, T$_{resp}$ cells from MG patients produced higher levels of proinflammatory cytokines (IL-6 and IFN-γ) and lower levels of IL-10, compared with controls. Furthermore, when isolated CD4$^+$ CD25^{high} CD127$^{low/-}$ cells (T$_{reg}$ cells) were added to the cultures, IL-6 and IL-17 levels actually increased without alterations in IL-10 levels.[37] This result suggests not only a functional inability of MG T$_{reg}$ cells to suppress the production of proinflammatory cytokines, but also the possibility of production of IL-6 and IL-17 by CD4$^+$ CD25^{high} CD127$^{low/-}$ cells in MG. Along these lines, it has been recently reported that peripheral T$_{reg}$ cells may differentiate into IL-17 producing cells upon T cell receptor stimulation in the presence of IL-6.[38] Thus, enhanced T$_{reg}$ cell plasticity in MG may underlie the observed disturbance in T$_{reg}$ cell suppressive function in MG through functional conversion of cells with a T$_{reg}$ cell phenotype into pathogenic Th17 cells. This phenomenon may be associated with the level of FOXP3 expression within a T cell (see below).

Dysfunctional MG T$_{reg}$ cells express attenuated FOXP3 levels

The expression level of FOXP3 plays a critical role in the development and function of T$_{reg}$ cells. A number of factors, some positive, some negative, collectively drive FOXP3 gene expression and then maintain its expression in T$_{reg}$ cells. Reduced FOXP3 expression in circulating CD4$^+$ CD25$^+$ T cells[33,39] and CD4$^+$ CD25$^+$ thymocytes[33] has been observed in MG patients. We isolated CD4$^+$ CD25^{high} CD127$^{low/-}$ T$_{reg}$ cells from peripheral blood–mononuclear cells (PBMCs) and found no alteration in the reservoir of T$_{reg}$ cells in the peripheral blood of MG patients compared to controls. We confirmed that these cells were largely (>90%) FOXP3-expressing cells (by flow cytometry–based phenotypic analysis) and were highly suppressive in functional suppressor assays.[37] However, we observed a significant downregulation of the relative expression of FOXP3 at the protein and mRNA levels in CD4$^+$ CD25^{high} CD127$^{low/-}$ cells isolated from MG patients compared with healthy controls.[37]

We evaluated the expression of FOXP3-associated proteins, including those responsible for key features of T$_{reg}$ function such as cytotoxic T lymphocyte antigen-4 (CTLA-4). We have shown that a significantly lower percentage of isolated T$_{reg}$ cells from MG patients express CTLA-4,[37] consistent with the impairment of suppressive function when these cells are used in suppressive assays.

MHC II expression on human T$_{reg}$ cells has been reported to identify a distinct population of T$_{reg}$ cells with high FOXP3 expression and with the capability to mediate strong contact-dependent suppression.[40] HLA-DR expressing T$_{reg}$ cells have also been hypothesized to be involved in homeostatic maintenance of T$_{reg}$ cells *in vivo* via presentation of self-antigens,[40] so that a deficiency in this subset of T$_{reg}$ cells may influence tolerance to self-antigens

such as the AChR. Accordingly, we have found that a reduced number of CD4$^+$ CD25^{high} CD127$^{low/-}$ cells express HLA-DR in MG patients.[37]

It should be pointed out that the functional defect reported in MG T$_{reg}$ cells appears to be a global one (i.e., nonspecific) since there is a failure to normally suppress T cell proliferation in response to nonspecific T cell receptor engagement (anti-CD3 antibodies). One may hypothesize that T$_{reg}$ cell suppression of AChR-specific T cells is perturbed in MG, and that restoration of function in this population of T$_{reg}$ cells may be a focused strategy for treatment. The first step to address this possibility would be to investigate whether T$_{reg}$ cells from MG patients have a reduced ability to suppress AChR-reactive T cells. While the number of circulating AChR-specific T cells is low, previous investigators have identified in many MG patients the presence of myasthenogenic AChR peptides that induce T cell proliferation.[41] Based on this work, we synthesized two peptides from the human AChR-α subunit (p195–212 and p257–259), one of which had been determined to induce proliferation of peripheral blood lymphocytes in approximately 70% of patients with MG.[41] These peptides were used in suppression assays performed as described above except that the AChR peptide, rather than anti-CD3, was used for stimulation. To assess T$_{reg}$ cell suppression of AChR-stimulated T cell proliferation, previously activated CD4$^+$ CD25^{high} CD127$^{low/-}$ cells were added to the culture. T cell proliferation of 4.2–15% in response to one of the two AChR peptides was observed and was not significantly suppressed by the addition of MG T$_{reg}$ cells.[37] Little or no proliferation in response to the AChR-α peptide was seen in the age-matched healthy control population. These studies indicate that the observed defect in suppressive function of T$_{reg}$ cells in MG extends to AChR-specific T cell responses.

Defects in *in vitro* T$_{reg}$ cell suppression in autoimmune disease may potentially be explained by T$_{reg}$ cell–intrinsic defects, resistance of T$_{resp}$ cells, or the proinflammatory properties of APCs.[23–25] Our data showing reduced cellular expression of FOXP3 in MG T$_{reg}$ cells argue for a T$_{reg}$ cell–intrinsic defect. To further test this, we cocultured MG T$_{reg}$ cells with T$_{resp}$ from healthy controls, and performed the reverse experiment, to determine the degree of *in vitro* suppression of both of polyclonal and AChR-stimulated T cell proliferation. Both polyclonal and

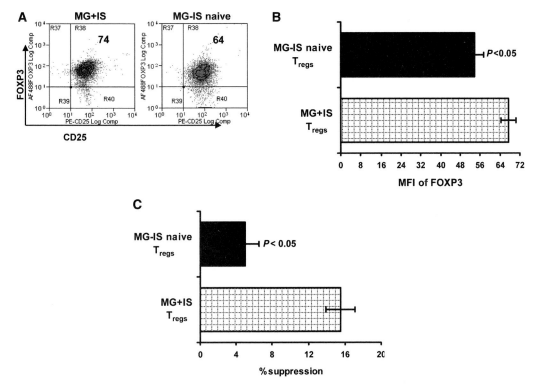

Figure 1. FOXP3 expression and suppressive function of T$_{reg}$ cells in treated versus untreated MG patients. Intensity of FOXP3 expression (MFI = mean fluorescent intensity) in CD4$^+$ CD25^{high} CD127$^{low/-}$ T$_{reg}$ cells. (A) Representative data for immunosuppressive naive (MG – IS naive) and immunosuppressed (MG + IS) subjects. (B) MFI of FOXP3 expression in isolated CD4$^+$ CD25^{high} CD127$^{low/-}$ cells. (C) Percent suppression of T$_{resp}$ cell proliferation by T$_{reg}$ cells. Data in (B) and (C) represent $n = 5$ for MG-IS naive subjects and $n = 12$ for MG-IS subjects. Results are expressed as mean ± SEM.

AChR-activated T$_{resp}$ cells from MG patients could be effectively suppressed using T$_{reg}$ cells isolated from healthy controls, while polyclonal-activated T$_{resp}$ cells from controls were not effectively suppressed using T$_{reg}$ cells isolated from MG patients, which strongly suggests a primary intrinsic defect in isolated T$_{reg}$ cells in MG.[37]

Imbalanced homeostatic composition of circulating T$_{reg}$ cells in MG

While the existing data suggest that the relative number of circulating T$_{reg}$ cells is unchanged in MG patients, the observed T$_{reg}$ cell dysfunction may be linked to an imbalanced homeostatic composition of circulating T$_{reg}$ cell subsets. There are two major types of CD4$^+$ FOXP3$^+$ T$_{reg}$ cells.[42] Natural T$_{reg}$ cells (nT$_{reg}$ cells) constitute a stable subset derived from the thymus and are thought to control reactivity to self-antigens. Induced or adaptive T$_{reg}$ cells (iT$_{reg}$ cells) are less stable, being derived from CD4$^+$

CD25$^-$ T cells in the periphery upon antigen exposure. There is currently no good method for isolating viable nT$_{reg}$ cells for functional studies, since the most reliable method relies on the presence of an epigenetic signature. However, cells recently exiting the thymus, including nT$_{reg}$ cells, may be identified by expression of CD45RA and CD31 ("recent thymic emigrants", RTE). In addition, important biological differences between naive (CD45RA$^+$) and memory (CD45RO$^+$) CD4$^+$ CD25^{high} T$_{reg}$ cells have been described.[43,44] Differences in T$_{reg}$ cell subsets in patients with autoimmune disease (SLE, T1D) compared to controls have also been reported when CD45RA is used to differentiate T$_{reg}$ cell subsets,[45] suggesting that alterations in the relative composition of T$_{reg}$ cell subsets may underlie autoimmunity. Therefore, we have analyzed the frequency of circulating recent thymic emigrant (CD31$^+$) and naive (CD45RA$^+$) CD4$^+$ CD25^{high} CD127$^{low/-}$ T$_{reg}$ cells in MG patients and found that the prevalence of recent thymic emigrant and naive T_{reg} cells is significantly decreased in MG patients compared to healthy controls.[37]

This finding raises the question of whether T_{reg} cells may exhibit multiple differences from healthy controls that are likely to play roles in the complex pathogenesis of MG, including reduced thymic output of naive T_{reg} cells, impaired naive T_{reg} cell suppression, and distinct impairments in specific subsets of memory T_{reg} cells. The reduced percentage of circulating naive and RTE T_{reg} cells is particularly intriguing given the high incidence of thymic pathology (hyperplasia and neoplasia) in MG. Further studies correlating T_{reg} cell subset phenotype and function with thymic pathology will help to better characterize the relationship of circulating T_{reg} cell alterations and thymic T_{reg} cell development.

Are CD4+ CD25^high CD127^low/− T_{reg} cells affected by immunotherapy?

Most MG patients in our studies were treated with prednisone or other immunosuppressive drugs, and thus it is conceivable that these drugs may have an effect on T_{reg} cell function. Subset analyses of T_{reg} cell–suppressive function and FOXP3 expression in MG patients treated with immunosuppressants (IS) compared to those that were immunsuppression naive at the time of blood collection showed that T_{reg} cells from MG patients treated with IS more effectively suppressed T cell proliferation and expressed higher levels of FOXP3 (Fig. 1). In addition, a correlation was also found between manual muscle testing (MMT) scores and T_{reg} cell–suppressive function.[37] These findings agree with those of other investigators[46,47] and suggest that the observed T_{reg}

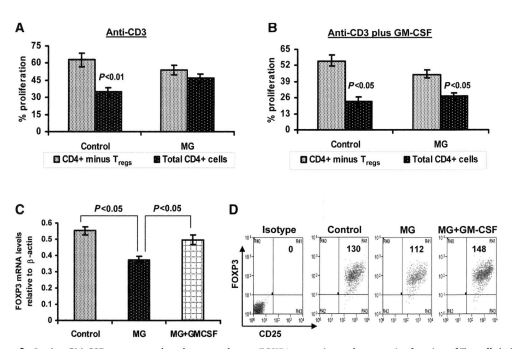

Figure 2. *In vitro* GM-CSF treatment to lymphocytes enhances FOXP3 expression and suppressive function of T_{reg} cells in MG. CFSE-labeled total CD4+ T cells and T_{reg} cell–depleted CD4+ T cells were stimulated with human anti-CD3 alone or anti-CD3 plus GM-CSF in the presence of autologous irradiated APCs. Cultures consisting of total CD4+ cells (black bars) and CD4+ cells after removal of CD4+ CD25^high CD127^low/− cells (gray bars) were compared to evaluate suppressive function of T_{reg} cells. After five days of culture, the percentage of T cell proliferation was analyzed based on CFSE dilution. The bar diagram represents the percentage of T_{resp} cell proliferation in response to anti-CD3 alone (A) and anit-CD3 plus GM-CSF (B) for four MG patients and four healthy controls. (C) FOXP3 mRNA expression as determined by multiplex PCR using isolated CD4+ CD25^high CD127^low/− T_{reg} cells obtained from control subjects, MG patients, and MG patients' PBMCs treated with GM-CSF ($n = 4$ in each group). Results are expressed as relative FOXP3 mRNA expression and as the mean ± SEM. (D) Representative flow cytometry plots illustrate mean florescent intensity of FOXP3 expression within isolated CD4+ CD25^high CD127^low/− T_{reg} cells.

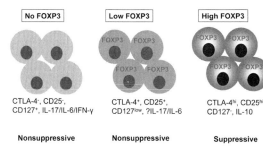

Figure 3. Hypothetical model linking T$_{reg}$ cell–suppressive function to FOXP3 expression level. In this model, high expression of FOXP3 in T cells endows them with enhanced suppressive capacity and a characteristic phenotype. Absence of FOXP3 expression is associated with no suppressive capacity, but reduced FOXP3 expression may result in an intermediate phenotype without suppressive function, and possibly a tendency for enhanced functional plasticity.

cell defects are clinically relevant, and that the beneficial effects of IS therapy are at least partly mediated through enhancement of T$_{reg}$ cell function.

Granulocyte-macrophage–colony-stimulating factor enhances T$_{reg}$ cell function in MG

The expansion of T$_{reg}$ cell numbers for cellular therapy is a common experimental strategy applied to a number of autoimmune conditions.[48,49] Unfortunately, expansion of dysfunctional MG T$_{reg}$ cells is unlikely to provide a therapeutic benefit; instead, the identification of agents that enhance the function of T$_{reg}$ cells would be a more appropriate strategy. Granulocyte-macrophage–colony-stimulating factor (GM-CSF) is an important hematopoietic growth factor and immune modulator that has a profound effect on various circulating immune cells.[50] *In vivo* administration of GM-CSF has been shown to prevent or attenuate autoimmunity in a number of mouse models of autoimmune disease by expanding dendritic cells and inducing an expansion of T$_{reg}$ cells.[51–55] Furthermore, we have used the murine experimental model of MG to demonstrate that the therapeutic administration of GM-CSF produces clinical improvement, an expansion of the numbers of splenic FOXP3$^+$ cells, a suppression of AChR-induced T cell proliferation, diminished production of anti-AChR antibodies, and a reduction of the deposition of IgG and complement at the muscle endplate, resulting in preservation of the normal postsynaptic endplate morphology and functional AChRs.[53,54] More im-

portantly, adoptively transferred GM-CSF–induced T$_{regs}$ potently suppressed ongoing MG in recipient mice, confirming their critical role in GM-CSF's effects.[55]

Based on these preclinical studies, we have investigated the effects of GM-CSF treatment in a case of refractory myasthenic crisis.[56] Clinical improvement in this case was associated with expansion in the circulating numbers of FOXP3$^+$ cells, increase in FOXP3 expression levels in CD4$^+$ CD25^{high} CD127$^{low/-}$ T$_{reg}$ cells, early improvement in T$_{reg}$ cell–suppressive capacity for AChR-α–induced T cell proliferation, and subsequent enhancement in T$_{reg}$ cell suppression of polyclonal T cell proliferation.[56] Although the use of multiple immunosuppressive drugs may have contributed to these findings, the observed effects on T$_{reg}$ cells are consistent with preclinical studies.

We have also performed studies examining the *in vitro* effects of GM-CSF in T cell proliferation/suppression assays from MG patients and healthy controls. Total CD4$^+$ and/or CD4$^+$ CD25^{high} CD127$^{low/-}$ T$_{reg}$ cell–depleted CD4$^+$ T cells were cultured with autologous APCs in the presence of anti-CD3 or anti-CD3 plus GM-CSF. We found that the addition of GM-CSF to lymphocyte cultures ameliorated the suppressive defect in MG T$_{reg}$ cells (Fig. 2A and B) and markedly enhanced expression of FOXP3 in MG T$_{reg}$ cells at the mRNA and protein levels (Fig. 2C and D). This suggests that GM-CSF may be effectively used as an enhancer of T$_{reg}$ cell–suppressive function, as has been reported for a number of other agents (i.e., rapamycin, vitamin D analogues).[57,58] Additional studies are needed to confirm these findings, define the requirements for GM-CSF's *in vitro* effects, and also determine its actions on non-T$_{reg}$ cells.

Conclusions

Defective immune regulation present in patients with MG is characterized by defects in suppressive function and low expression of FOXP3 in CD4$^+$ CD25^{high} CD127$^{low/-}$ cells. T$_{reg}$ cell–mediated suppression of both polyclonal and autoantigen (AChR)-specific T cell responses is impaired and may correlate with disease severity, being notably less severe in the subgroup of patients treated with immunosuppressive drugs. This defect primarily resides within the population of CD4$^+$ CD25^{high} CD127$^{low/-}$ cells, which display reduced or unstable FOXP3 expression. While it has been generally thought that FOXP3 expression is an "on–off switch" endowing T lymphocytes with suppressive ability, emerging evidence, including our own work showing an association between attenuated FOXP3 expression in T$_{reg}$ cells and human MG, suggests a paradigm in which alterations in FOXP3 expression in lymphocytes may lead to loss of immune tolerance in a dose-dependent manner (Fig. 3). Furthermore, GM-CSF has a profound *in vitro* beneficial effect on T$_{reg}$ cell function as well as FOXP3 expression, and further investigations of the mechanisms responsible for these effects are warranted.

In sum, investigation of the nature and subset localization of the T$_{reg}$ cell defect in MG may reveal critical factors that regulate immune responses in MG and other autoimmune diseases, leading to the identification of novel therapeutic targets.

Acknowledgments

This work was funded by the NIH (National Institute of Neurologic Disorders and Stroke, K08NS058800, MNM; and National Institute of Allergy and Infectious Diseases, RO1 AI 058190, BSP); the Muscular Dystrophy Association (MDA 185924, MNM and MDA 157286, JRS); and by the University of Illinois at Chicago (UIC) Center for Clinical and Translational Science (CCTS), Award Number UL1RR029879 from the National Center for Research Resources. The content is solely the responsibility of the authors and does not necessarily represent the official views of the National Center for Research Resources or the National Institutes of Health.

Conflicts of interest

The authors declare no competing financial interests.

References

1. Meriggioli, M.N. & D.B. Sanders. 2009. Autoimmune myasthenia gravis: emerging clinical and biological heterogeneity. *Lancet Neurol.* **8:** 475–490.
2. Berrih, S., E. Morel, C. Gaud, *et al.* 1984. Anti-AChR antibodies, thymic histology, and T cell subsets in myasthenia gravis. *Neurology* **34:** 66–71.
3. Roxanis, I., K. Micklem & N. Willcox. 2001. True epithelial hyperplasia in the thymus of early-onset myasthenia gravis: implications for immunopathogenesis. *J. Neuroimmunol.* **112:** 163–173.
4. Giraud, M., C. Vandiedonck & H.J. Garchon. 2008. Genetic factors in autoimmune myasthenia gravis. *Ann. N.Y. Acad. Sci.* **1132:** 180–192.
5. Landoure, G., M.A. Knight, H. Stanescu, *et al.* 2012. A candidate gene for autoimmune myasthenia gravis. *Neurology* **79:** 342–347.
6. Maniaol, A.H., A. Elsais, A.R. Lorentzen, *et al.* 2012. Late onset myasthenia gravis is associated with HLA DRB1*15:01 in the Norwegian population. *PLoS One.* **7**(5): e36603. Epub 2012 May 9.
7. Protti, M.P., A. A. Manfredi, C. Straub, *et al.* 1990. Immunodominant regions for T helper-cell sensitization on the human nicotinic receptor alpha subunit in myasthenia gravis. *Proc. Natl. Acad. Sci. USA* **87:** 7792–7796.
8. Wang, Z.Y., D. K. Okita, J. Jr. Howard, *et al.* 1998. T-cell recognition of muscleacetylcholine receptor subunits in generalized and ocular myasthenia gravis. *Neurology* **50:** 1045–1054.
9. Abramsky, O., A. Aharonov, C. Webb & S. Fuchs. 1975. Cellular immune response to acetylcholine receptor rich-fraction, in patients with myasthenia gravis. *Clin. Exp. Immunol.* **19:** 11–16.
10. Richman, D.P., J.P. Antel, J.W. Patrick & B.G.W. Arnason. 1979. Cellular immunity to acetylcholine receptor in myasthenia gravis: relationship to histocompatibility type and antigenic site. *Neurology* **29:** 291–296.
11. Hohlfeld, R., I. Kalies, B. Kohleisen, *et al.* 1986. Myasthenia gravis: stimulation of anti-receptor autoantibodies by autoreactive T cell lines. *Neurology* **36:** 618–621.
12. Bouneaud, C., P. Kourilsky & P. Buosso. 2000. Impact of negative selection on the T cell repertoire reactive to a self peptide: a large fraction of T cell clones escapesclonal deletion. *Immunity* **13:** 829–840.
13. Workman, C.J., A.L. Szymczak-Workman, L.W. Collison, *et al.* 2009. Thedevelopment and function of regulatory T cells. *Cell. Mol. Life Sci.* **66:** 2603–2622.
14. Baecher-Allan, C. & D.A. Hafler. 2006. Human regulatory T cells and their role in autoimmune disease. *Immunol. Rev.* **212:** 203–216.
15. Torgerson, T.R. 2006. Regulatory T cells in human autoimmune diseases. *Springer Semin. Immunopathol.* **28:** 63–76.
16. Sakaguchi, S., M. Miyara, C.M. Costantino, *et al.* 2010. FOXP3+ regulatory T cells in the human immune system. *Nat. Rev. Immunol.* **10:** 490–500.
17. Fontenot, J.D., M.A. Gavin & A.Y. Rudensky. 2003. FOXP3 programs the development and function of CD4+CD25+ regulatory T cells. *Nat.Immunol.* **4:** 330–336.
18. Hori, S., T. Nomura & S. Sakaguchi. 2003. Control of regulatory T cell development by the transcription factor FOXP3. *Science* **299:** 1057–1061.
19. Buckner, J.H. 2010. Mechanisms of impaired regulation by CD4(+)CD25(+)FOXP3(+) regulatory T cells in human autoimmune diseases. *Nat. Rev. Immunol.* **10:** 849–859.
20. Moes, N., F. Rieux-Laucat, B. Begue, *et al.* 2010. Reduced expression of FOXP3 and regulatory T-cell function in severe forms of early-onset autoimmune enteropathy. *Gastroenterology* **139:** 770–778.
21. Valencia, X.C., G. Yarboro, P. Illei, *et al.* 2007. Deficient CD4$^+$CD25^{high} T regulatory cell function in patients with

active systemic lupus erythematosus. *J. Immunol.* **178:** 2579–2588.

22. Venken, K., N. Hellings, M. Thewissen, *et al.* 2008. Compromised CD4$^+$CD25^{high} regulatory T-cell function in patients with relapsing-remitting multiple sclerosis is correlated with a reduced frequency of FOXP3-positive cells and reduced FOXP3 expression at the single-cell level. *Immunology* **123:** 79–89.

23. Venigalla, R.K., T. Tretter, S. Krienke, *et al.* 2008. Reduced CD4+,CD25- T cell sensitivity to the suppressive function of CD4+,CD25high,CD127-/low regulatory T cells in patients with active systemic lupus erythematosus. *Arthritis Rheum.* **58:** 2120–2130.

24. Vargas-Rojas, M.I., J.C. Crispín, Y. Richaud-Patin, *et al.* 2008. Quantitative and qualitative normal regulatory T cells are not capable of inducing suppression in SLE patients due to T-cell resistance. *Lupus* **17:** 289–294.

25. Walker, L.S. 2009. Regulatory T cells overturned: the effectors fight back. *Immunology* **126:** 466–474.

26. Iikuni, N., E.V. Lourenco, B.H. Hahn, *et al.* 2009. Regulatory T cells directly suppress B cells in systemic lupus erythematosis. *J. Immunol.* **183:** 1518–1522.

27. Fattorossi, A., A. Battaglia, A. Buzzonetti, *et al.* 2005. Circulating and thymic CD4+CD25+ T regulatory cells in myasthenia gravis: effect of immunosuppressive treatment. *Immunology* **116:** 134–141.

28. Li, X., B.G. Xiao, J.Y. Xi, *et al.* 2008. Decrease of Foxp3+ regulatory T cells and elevation of CD19+BAFF-R+ B cells and soluble ICAM-1 in myasthenia gravis. *Clin. Immunol.* **126:** 180–188.

29. Masuda, M., M. Matsumoto, S. Tanaka, *et al.* 2010. Clinical implication of peripheral CD4+ CD25+ regulatory T cells and Th17 cells in myasthenia gravis patients. *J. Neuroimmunol.* **225:** 123–131.

30. Zhang, Y., H. Wang, L. Chi, *et al.* 2009. The role of FoxP3+CD4+CD25hi Tregs in the pathogenesis of myasthenia gravis. *Immunol. Lett.* **122:** 52–57.

31. Huang, Y.M., R. Pirskanen, R. Giscombe, *et al.* 2004. Circulating CD4+CD25 +and CD4+CD25+Tcells in myasthenia gravis and in relation to thymectomy. *Scand. J. Immunol.* **59:** 408–414.

32. Matsui, N., S. Nakane, F. Saito, *et al.* 2010. Undiminished regulatory T cells in the thymus of patients with myasthenia gravis. *Neurology* **74:** 816–820.

33. Balandina, A., S. Lécart, P. Dartevelle, *et al.* 2005. Functional defect of regulatory CD4(+)CD25+ T cells in the thymus of patients with autoimmune myasthenia gravis. *Blood* **105:** 735–741.

34. Lim, A.Y., P. Price, M.W. Beilharz, *et al.* 2006. Cell surface markers of regulatory T cells are not associated with increased forkheadbox p3 expression in blood CD4+ T cells from HIV-infected patients responding to antiretroviral therapy. *Immunol. Cell. Biol.* **84:** 530–536.

35. Seddiki, N., B. Santner-Nanan, J. Martinson, *et al.* 2006. Expression of interleukin (IL)-2 and IL-7 receptors discriminates between human regulatory and activated T cells. *J. Exp. Med.* **203:** 1693–1700.

36. Liu W., A.L. Putnam, Z. Xu-Yu, *et al.* 2006. CD127 expression inversely correlates with FOXP3 and suppressive function of human CD4+ T reg cells. *J. Exp. Med.* **203:** 1701–1711.

37. Thiruppathi, M., J. Rowin, B. Ganesh, *et al.* 2012. Impaired regulatory function in circulating CD4$^+$CD25^{high}CD127$^{low/-}$T cells in patients with myasthenia gravis. *Clin. Immunol.* **145:** 209–223.

38. Voo, K.S., Y.H. Wang, F.R. Santori, *et al.* 2009. Identification of IL-17-producing FOXP3+ regulatory T cells in humans. *Proc. Natl. Acad. Sci. USA* **106:** 4793–4798.

39. Xu, W.H., A.M. Zhang, M.S. Ren, *et al.* 2012. Changes of Treg-associated molecules on CD4(+)CD25(+) Treg cells in myasthenia gravis and effects of immunosuppressants. *J. Clin. Immunol.* **32:** 975–983.

40. Baecher-Allan, C., E. Wolf & D.A. Hafler. 2006. MHC class II expression identifies functionally distinct human regulatory T cells. *J. Immunol.* **176:** 4622–4631.

41. Brocke, S., C. Brautbar, L. Steinman, *et al.* 1988. In vitro proliferative responses and antibody titers specific to human acetylcholine receptor synthetic peptides in patients with myasthenia gravis and relation to HLA class II genes. *J. Clin. Invest.* **82:** 1894–1900.

42. Miyara, M., Y. Yoshioka, A. Kitoh, *et al.* 2009. Functional delineation and differentiation dynamics of human CD4+ T cells expressing the FoxP3 transcription factor. *Immunity* **30:** 899–911.

43. Sakaguchi, S., T. Yamaguchi, T. Nomura, *et al.* 2008. Regulatory T cells and immune tolerance. *Cell.* **133:** 775–787.

44. Hoffmann, P., R. Eder, T.J. Boeld, *et al.* 2006. Only the CD45RA +subpopulation of CD4+CD25high T cells gives rise to homogeneous regulatory T-cell lines upon in vitro expansion. *Blood* **108:** 4260–4267.

45. d'Hennezel, E., E. Yurchenko, E. Sgouroudis, *et al.* 2011. Single-cell analysis of the human T regulatory population uncovers functional heterogeneity and instability within FOXP3+ cells. *J. Immunol.* **186:** 6788–6797.

46. Luther, C., E. Adamopoulou, C. Stoeckle, *et al.* 2009. Prednisolone treatment induces tolerogenic dendritic cells and a regulatory milieu in myasthenia gravis patients. *J. Immunol.* **183:** 841–848.

47. Kessel, A., H. Ammuri, R. Peri, *et al.* 2007. Intravenous immunoglobulin therapy affects T regulatory cells by increasing their suppressive function. *J. Immunol.* **179:** 5571–5575.

48. Hoffman P., R. Eder, L.A. Kunz-Schughart, *et al.* 2004. Large-scale in vitro expansion of polyclonal human CD4+CD25high regulatory T cells. *Blood* **104:** 895–903.

49. Earle, K.E., Q. Tang, X. Zhou, *et al.* 2005. In vitro expanded human CD4+CD25+ regulatory T cells suppress effector T cell proliferation. *Clin. Immunol.* **115:** 3–9.

50. Hamilton, J.A. 2002. GM-CSF in inflammation and autoimmunity. *Trends Immunol.* **23:** 403–408.

51. Ganesh, B.B., D.M. Cheatem, J.R. Sheng, *et al.* 2009. GMCSF-induced CD11c+CD8a- -dendritic cells facilitate FOXP3+ and IL-10 +regulatory T cell expansion resulting in suppression of autoimmune thyroiditis. *Int. Immunol.* **21:** 269–282.

52. Gaudreau, S., C. Guindi, M. Menard, *et al.* 2007. Granulocyte-macrophage colony stimulating factor prevents diabetes development in NOD mice by inducing tolerogenic

dendritic cells that sustain the suppressive function of regulatory T cells. *J. Immunol.* **179:** 3638–3647.

53. Sheng, J.R., L.C. Li, B.B. Ganesh, *et al.* 2006. Suppression of experimental autoimmune myasthenia gravis (EAMG) by granulocyte-macrophage colony-stimulating factor (GM-CSF) is associated with an expansion of FOXP3+ regulatory T cells. *J. Immunol.* **177:** 5296–5306.

54. Sheng, J.R., L.C. Li, B.B. Ganesh, *et al.* 2008. Regulatory T cells induced by GM-CSF suppress ongoing experimental myasthenia. *Clin. Immunol.* **128:** 172–180.

55. Sheng, J.R., T. Muthusamy, B.S. Prabhakar, *et al.* 2011. GM-CSF-induced regulatory T cells selectively inhibit anti-acetylcholine receptor-specific immune responses in experimental myasthenia gravis. *J. Neuroimmunol.* **240–241:** 65–73.

56. Rowin, J., M. Thiruppathi, E. Arhebamen, *et al.* 2012. Granulocyte macrophage colony-stimulating factor treatment of a patient in myasthenic crisis: Effects on regulatory T cells. *Muscle Nerve* **46:** 449–453.

57. Adorini, L. & G. Penna. 2009. Dendritic cell tolerogenicity: a key mechanism in immunomodulation by vitamin D receptor agonists. *Hum. Immunol.* **70:** 345–352.

58. Battaglia, M., A. Stabilini, B. Migliavacca, *et al.* 2006. Rapamycin promotes expansion of functional CD4+CD25+FOXP3+ regulatory T cells of both healthy subjects and type 1 diabetic patients. *J. Immunol.* **177:** 8338–8347.

Ann. N.Y. Acad. Sci. ISSN 0077-8923

ANNALS OF THE NEW YORK ACADEMY OF SCIENCES

Issue: *Myasthenia Gravis and Related Disorders*

Jitter analysis with concentric needle electrodes

Erik Stålberg

Department of Clinical Neurophysiology, Uppsala University, Uppsala, Sweden

Address for correspondence: Erik Stålberg, Department of Clinical Neurophysiology, University Hospital, S-75185 Uppsala, Sweden. stalberg.erik@gmail.com

Because of certain restrictions in medical praxis, reusable materials are only allowed in some countries. This also applies to electrodes for electromyography; the special single-fiber electromyography electrode must be replaced. This article gives some details of the possibilities of using an alternative—a small concentric needle electrode. Practical hints, reference values, and the application in diagnostic work for myasthenia gravis are summarized.

Keywords: concentric needle electrode; single fiber EMG electrode; jitter; neuromuscular transmission

Introduction

Single-fiber electromyography (SFEMG) is an established method for the study of motor unit microphysiology. It has a unique recording selectivity that allows various studies of the motor unit (MU) microphysiology, such as neuromuscular jitter, muscle fiber organization (fiber density (FD)), muscle fiber propagation velocity, and also reflex studies on a single cell level. The SFEMG electrode (SFE) has a relatively high cost and must be sterilized; however, it can be reused many times, keeping the cost per examination down. To prolong its survival and to guarantee its performance quality, it requires regular maintenance (inspection under the microscope for burs at the tip, and passing a weak electric current for electrolytic cleaning).

The neuromuscular jitter has a well-validated role in the diagnostic evaluation of patients with a suspected myasthenic condition. Further, additional SFEMG parameters allow for the evaluation of other conditions. The jitter represents the time variability that occurs in the motor end-plate at consecutive discharges. With volitional activation, action potentials from two muscle fibers belonging to the same MU are identified by triggering one of them; their combined jitter is displayed in the nontriggering component. When electrical stimulation of the motor axon is used to activate the MU, the jitter from individual motor end-plates is measured as the time variability between the stimulus and the spike under study at consecutive discharges. Since many countries have restrictions for reusable material in medicine, including EMG electrodes, it is necessary to find an acceptable surrogate for the SFE that fulfills the criteria for quality and price. No such disposable SFE has been developed yet, and a concentric needle electrode (CNE) has been the nearest alternative. Even several decades ago, individual spike components of motor unit potentials (MUPs) recorded with these electrodes were enhanced by low-cut filtering (the so-called high-pass filter limits were increased from 500 Hz, which is the standard for SFE, to 3,000 Hz) to visualize the shape variability at consecutive discharges,[1] though this technique was never proposed for the quantitative study of the neuromuscular jitter.

What is the alternative to using SFEMG electrodes for jitter analysis?

The best alternative to using SFEMG electrodes would be a new, inexpensive SFE, but the development of such electrodes has not been successful so far. Another possibility would be to extract individual single-fiber spike components from the MUP recorded with conventional EMG electrodes by means of advanced signal analysis. This has been shown to be feasible,[2] but the method has not reached a level of routine use.

doi: 10.1111/j.1749-6632.2012.06775.x

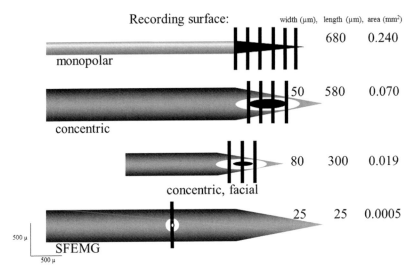

Figure 1. EMG electrodes: monopolar, conventional concentric, SFEMG, and facial concentric electrodes with measures of recording surfaces inserted. Muscle fibers in direct contact with the electrode surface are indicated, using an average fiber density.

Presently, one practical alternative is to use the smallest possible disposable CNE, a so-called facial electrode.[3] Conventional CNEs have an oval recording area; the most commonly used has a recording surface of 0.070 μm², whereas the facial CNE has a recording surface of 0.019 μm² (Fig. 1). Although it has been used to measure jitter,[4–6] the monopolar electrode is not recommended for this because it has a large recording surface (typically 0.240 μm²), and the reference electrode may be far away from the active recording tip and therefore not able to actively suppress remote activity. Figure 1 illustrates that the SFE recording surface may be in close contact with at most one muscle fiber, with another one or two within its uptake area, while the facial electrode is close to up to three fibers, with another three to five within its uptake area. The conventional concentric electrode is in close contact with four fibers, and another five to ten lie within its uptake area. The monopolar electrode has even more fibers in the recording area.

To further improve selectivity, signal filtering is used. Low frequencies that are mainly generated by remote activity are suppressed by a high-pass filter (low-cut filtering), for example, at 1,000 Hz, although other high-pass filter settings can be used. It should be noted that all filtering distorts the signal to some degree. With settings of 2,000 Hz or higher, the low frequencies of the signal are progressively suppressed, making the signal sharper and with a lower amplitude. This will result in a reduced signal-to-noise ratio, which is undesirable. In addition, the original shape is lost and the fast changes in the signal are enhanced. There is also a risk of artifactual generation of extra phases ("ringing"), which may be confused with signal spikes. A feature such as inflection points in the signal ("shoulders"), which is an important indicator of summation of activity from other muscle fibers, disappear. A filter setting of 1,000 Hz seems to give a good balance between the desired effect of low frequency suppression with a reasonably preserved original signal shape and an acceptable signal-to-noise ratio.

What is the difference between facial needle electrode and SFEMG electrode recordings?

With the SFE, there is a very high probability that the recorded signal represents electrical activity from just one fiber. This likelihood varies somewhat among muscles, depending on the organization of the MU. With the facial CNE, there is a higher probability that the recorded signal is a summation from two or more muscle fibers, making it particularly difficult to detect when individual spikes appear nearly simultaneous.

This summation phenomenon is the main problem with using CNE recordings for jitter analysis. The jitter, which should be measured between signals from individual muscle fibers, is now measured between summated components from many fibers in CNE recordings. Therefore, the concept of jitter may be violated.

What is the problem with jitter analysis from summated spikes?

There are at least two situations where problems may arise when analyzing jitter from summated spikes. The first is the situation of signals "riding" on each other (Fig. 2A), which makes the reference point for time measurement uncertain. This is particularly the case if an amplitude-level technique is used for time interval measurements. Such signals cannot be used for jitter measurements, especially if the peaks are separated by less than 150 μsec. If signal peaks are used for time interval measurements, the error is much less (Fig. 2B). Although signal noise may influence the results, peak measurements are preferred for analyzing signals riding on each other.

The other situation affecting jitter analysis is when the composite single-fiber action potentials (SFAPs) are so close together that they create a spike-like component with a "shoulder" or a notch on its rising slope (Fig. 3). The jitter of the summated spike is less than that of any composed individual signal. Even if a measurement is made between a clean SFAP and such a composite signal, the calculated

jitter is reduced. To some extent, this error depends on the temporal relationship between the summating signals in addition to the method of analysis. In any case, the operator must try to obtain as clean signals as possible. Signals that are not apparently disturbed by activity from other fibers in the MU are called apparent single fiber action potentials (ASFAPs).

Jitter recordings during electrical stimulation

In the same way that jitter can be measured with the SFE with electrical stimulation, CNE recording can also be used with electrical activation. Here, there is even a greater risk of signal summation than with voluntary activation. With volitional activity, signals from different MUs can usually be separated by selective triggering, relying on differences in their amplitudes. With electrical stimulation, typically more than one axon is stimulated, and the resulting signal is the sum of different MUPs and thus more complex than with volitional activation. In some muscles, especially large limb muscles, analysis can be quite difficult. MUP spikes are more separated in facial muscles, which have smaller MUs, likely more dispersed end-plates, and shorter duration SFAPs. Therefore, the signals in facial muscles are more "desynchronized" than those from large limb muscles, and stimulation and recording positions can be optimized in these muscles to give separable spikes that are acceptable for jitter analysis.

What are the criteria for acceptable signals for jitter recordings?

Two criteria for signals that are acceptable for jitter recordings will be considered. The first is the definition of an acceptable individual spike for measurement, and the second is the criterion for an acceptable recording for jitter analysis.

Criteria for acceptable spikes

The classical definition of a single-fiber action potential is that it has a short and smooth rising phase with a duration of <300 μsec and a constant shape at consecutive discharges. Can these criteria be transferred to signals recorded with CNE? The answer is no, since the larger recording area gives somewhat lower amplitudes, and depending on the orientation of the muscle fiber across the electrode surface, also a theoretically somewhat longer rise time.

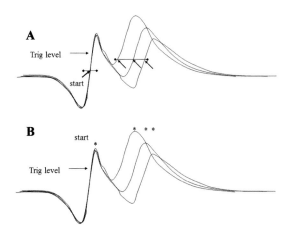

Figure 2. Time measurements using amplitude level (A) and peak detection (B) in signals riding on each other. (A) Using the amplitude-level method, the measuring point (arrows) is defined as the crossing between the given amplitude (horizontal line) and the signal. With a riding signal, this will refer to different parts of the signal rising phase of the signal. (B) When peaks (asterisks) are used for measurement, the interval between the signals is much less influenced by the riding effect.

However, the criteria of a smooth rising phase without notches or shoulders holds true as well as the requirement of a constant signal shape at consecutive discharges. These criteria can best be invoked by observing a number of superimposed discharges (Fig. 3).

In practice, interference from another fiber in the beginning of the signal, that is, close to the positive peak or after a clean negative peak in the falling phase, can be accepted when the peak trigger method is used for analysis. For the amplitude level method, the main part of the rising phase must be clean. These criteria have evolved over the last few years in our laboratory and others. No consensus has formally been reached at this time.

The criteria for jitter measurements between individual spikes

First, all spikes must fulfill the above definition of acceptable spikes (ASFAPs). Second, the mean distance between spikes must exceed 150 μsec, otherwise there is too much interference between spikes.

For electrical stimulation, both with SFE and with CNE, special criteria must be fulfilled before the jitter can be classified as abnormal. First, the individual signals must be clean as defined above. Second, each accepted component chosen for analysis must be tested for supraliminal stimulation. Note that a liminal stimulation will give a large jitter, which then decreases to its correct value when the stimulus intensity is increased even by less than 1 mA. With

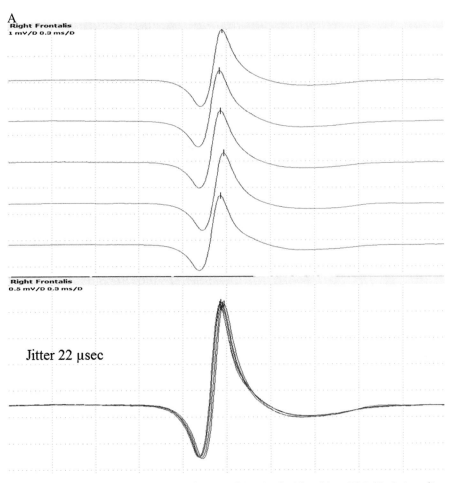

Figure 3. Signals using electrical stimulation. (A) Frontalis, normal jitter in a healthy subject. (B) Orbicularis oculi, normal. Signal with one ASFAP (the first, accepted) and one with a slight shoulder (second, not accepted). (C) Extensor digitorum. The recording consists of 4 spike-like components. The first is clearly a summation signal with shoulders or almost notches (trace 1), seen best in superimposed mode. Note that in trace 3 there is a combination of components that make the summated signal look like a clean signal.

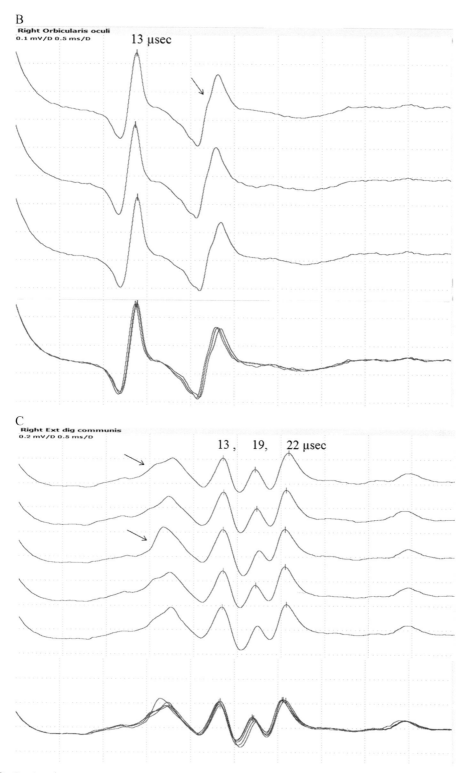

Figure 3. *Continued*

this maneuver, there is a risk that a new axon is recruited, in turn giving a large jitter. Thus, for the spike to be used for analysis, it must be confirmed that it is stimulated above threshold.

Practical aspects

A major advantage of the CNE is that the electrode tip is always sharp, which is not necessarily the case with SFE, unless they are well maintained. This also means that they are easy to insert into the muscle. A personal impression is that the CNE is better tolerated than the SFE, which has been shown in a separate study.[7] This is partly due to the tip, but also to the fact that the outer diameter of a SFE is 0.5 mm, whereas the facial CNE is 0.3 millimeters.

A disadvantage of the CNE is related to its sharpness and smoothness. Compared with the SFE, it is more difficult to keep in a constant recording position, particularly during electric stimulation. The CNE is not "directional" and has no marking on the holder or cable indicating the position of the tip bevel. Thus, one cannot get guidance to optimize the recording position by rotating the electrode, as is the case with the SFE.

Some experienced SFEMG analysts find that it takes more time to get acceptable clean signals with the CNE than with SFE; more signals have to be omitted and more time is devoted to checking signal quality.

Reference values

A few studies that have obtained reference values for CNE jitter in healthy subjects have been published.[8–14] These reference values vary between studies and differ somewhat from the values obtained in a large multicenter study with the SFE (Table 1).[15] This can be due to differences in the material size, uncertain definitions, different electrodes, and different analysis methods. The last factor is more important for CNE signals, which are more prone to have riding signals or summation signals than with clean, well-separated SFAPs. Therefore, any multicenter study must start with well-defined methodological criteria.

So far only a few studies have compared jitter values with SFE and CNE in the same muscle. Ertaş et al.[13] found very similar jitter values with the two electrodes in a sample of 10 healthy subjects. Our own unpublished study with a mixed patient sample showed that those with jitter within or close to normal limits, had 3–5 μsec lower jitter with CNE.

Volitional and electrical activation in the extensor digitorum (ED) muscle have also been compared. The difference between the two activation techniques was similar to other published reports using the SFE.

In general, the jitter values seem to be somewhat lower with the CNE than with the SFE, but this differs by muscle.

Table 1. Jitter values from healthy controls in different studies using different electrodes during volitional activation

Electrode	Muscle	Subjects	MCD (μs)	95%	Number pairs	All pairs (μs)	95%	Ref.
SFEMG	ED	Multicenter		35.9[a]	Multicenter		52.5[a]	15
Monopolar	ED	41	22.4 ± 2.8[b]	28.0	820	22.0 ± 5.6[b]	33.2	4
CN	ED	10			200	23.3 ± 8.0	39.3	13
CN	ED	20	30.7 ± 3.7	38.1	453	30.6 ± 9.2	49.0	16
CN	ED	67	23.6 ± 3.1[b]	29.7	1340	23.5 ± 7.3[b]	38.2	12
CN	OOc	20	29.1 ± 3.9	36.9	484	28.8 ± 10.5	49.8	16
SFEMG	OOc	Multicenter		40.9[a]	Multicenter		55.0[a]	15
CN	OOc	50	24.7 ± 3.1[b]	31.0	1000	24.7 ± 7.1[b]	39.0	12
CN	Frontalis	23			460	29.1 ± 12.0	53.1	17

[a]Age dependent, values given for 50 years; [b]not age dependent.
ED, extensor digitorum muscle; OOc, orbicularis oculi muscle.

Usefulness in diagnosing neuromuscular disturbances

There are only a few studies directly comparing diagnostic sensitivity between CNE and SFE in the same patients. Farrugia et al.[7] found no significant difference in jitter values for the two techniques. Ertaş et al.[13] found clearly increased and similar jitter in 10 patients with myasthenia gravis (MG), with the same diagnostic outcome for the two electrodes. Our own experience is that the SFE and CNE studies give very similar conclusions in diagnosing MG, provided that correct reference values are used. An increasing number of studies report the usefulness of CNE jitter measurements in MG. In a retrospective analysis of 56 consecutive MG patients,[16] with positive acetylcholine receptor (AChR) antibody titer and the clinical features of MG, the sensitivity was 96.4%.

In a prospective study using electrical stimulation in 20 clinically diagnosed MG patients with AChR antibodies (75%) and decrement (80%), the combined CNE studies in ED and frontalis muscles showed abnormal jitter recordings in 93.7%

of the patients with generalized MG and 75% of those with ocular MG.[10] Example of two recordings using electrical stimulation is shown in Figures 4 and 5.

In a study of sensitivity and specificity, 51 patients with probably MG were tested.[17] Jitter analysis diagnostic sensitivity was 0.67 and specificity 0.96. The positive and negative predictive values were 0.93 and 0.76, respectively. The authors considered abnormal CNE jitter "extremely useful" for confirming the diagnosis of MG, but with limited utility in excluding the diagnosis.

Specificity is comparable between SFE and CNE in the sense that an increased jitter is not equal to MG, but indicates disturbed neuromuscular transmission. Therefore, other parameters need to be added to get a full neurophysiological picture.

The future of jitter analysis

Ultimately, we hope to return to making viable SFAP recordings using disposable SFEs, as CNE is not as useful as the SFE in basic research for assessing the

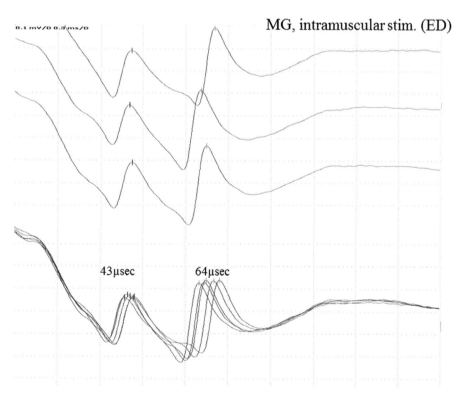

MG, intramuscular stim. (ED)

0.1 mV/D 0.3 ms/D

43 μsec   64 μsec

Figure 4. MG intramuscular axonal stimulation from extensor digitorum. Jitter values indicated. (Courtesy of J. Kouyoumdjian.)

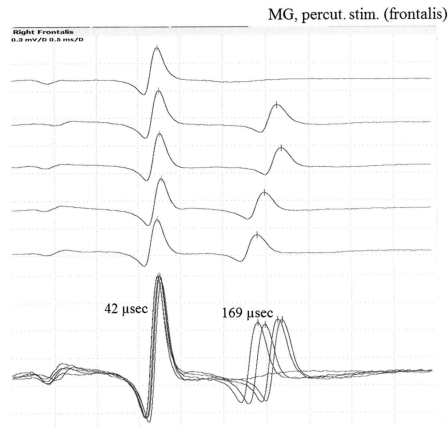

Figure 5. MG, percutaneous stimulation from frontalis. One end-plate has a moderately increased jitter, the other shows intermittent blocking and a large jitter. (Courtesy of J. Kouyoumdjian.)

function of single muscle fibers, individual motor end-plates, or single axons. The signal quality, the cumulated knowledge in the field, the possibility to perform fiber density measurements, and the possibility for further studies of the microphysiology of the MU, makes the return of the SFE highly desired. Until then, many investigators may have to make do with other electrodes, and, presently, the smallest routine CNE seems to be the best alternative. In addition, there is a great need to continue to define the criteria for acceptable signals and to conduct more multicenter studies examining a range of muscles to establish reference values. We anticipate that the CNE, in the hands of trained electromyographers, will prove to play an important role in the clinical diagnosis of disturbed neuromuscular transmission.

Conflicts of interest

The author declares no conflicts of interest.

References

1. Payan, J. 1978. The blanket principle: a technical note. *Muscle Nerve* **1:** 423–426.
2. Stashuk, D.W. 1999. Detecting single fiber contributions to motor unit action potentials. *Muscle Nerve* **22:** 218–229.
3. Stålberg, E. & D.B. Sanders. 2009. Jitter recordings with concentric needle electrodes. *Muscle Nerve* **40:** 331–339.
4. Buchman, A.S. & M. Garratt. 1992. Determining neuromuscular jitter using a monopolar electrode. *Muscle Nerve* **15:** 615–619.
5. Wiechers, D.O. 1985. Single fiber electromyography with a standard monopolar electrode. *Arch. Phys. Med. Rehabil.* **66:** 47–48.
6. Clarke, S. & A. Eisen. 1985. Electromyographic jitter measured using a monopolar electrode. *Neurol.* **35:** S1–69.
7. Farrugia, M.E., A.I. Weir, M. Cleary, *et al.* 2009. Concentric and single fiber needle electrodes yield comparable jitter results in myasthenia gravis. *Muscle Nerve* **39:** 579–585.
8. Kouyoumdjian, J.A. & E. Stålberg. 2012. Concentric needle jitter in stimulated frontalis in 20 healthy subjects. *Muscle Nerve* **45:** 276–278.

9. Kouyoumdjian, J.A. & E. Stålberg. 2011. Concentric needle jitter on stimulated Orbicularis Oculi in 50 healthy subjects. *Clin. Neurophysiol.* **122:** 617–622.

10. Kouyoumdjian, J.A., A.C. Fanani & E. Stålberg. 2011. Concentric needle jitter on stimulated frontalis and extensor digitorum in 20 myasthenia gravis patients. *Muscle Nerve* **44:** 912–918.

11. Kouyoumdjian, J.A. & E. Stålberg. 2008. Concentric needle single fiber electromyography: comparative jitter on voluntary-activated and stimulated Extensor Digitorum Communis. *Clin. Neurophysiol.* **119:** 1614–1618.

12. Kouyoumdjian, J.A. & E. Stålberg. 2008. Reference jitter values for concentric needle electrodes in voluntarily activated extensor digitorum communis and orbicularis oculi muscles. *Muscle Nerve* **37:** 694–699.

13. Ertaş, M., M.B. Baslo, N. Yildiz, *et al.* 2000. Concentric needle electrode for neuromuscular jitter analysis. *Muscle Nerve* **23:** 715–719.

14. Cattaneo, L., L. Cucurachi & G. Pavesi. 2007. Concentric needle recording of neuromuscular jitter in the temporalis muscle. *Neurophysiol. Clin.* **37:** 50–51.

15. Gilchrist, J., P.E. Barkhaus, V. Bril, *et al.* 1992. Single fiber EMG reference values: a collaborative effort. *Muscle Nerve* **15:** 151–161.

16. Sarrigiannis, P.G., R.P. Kennett, S. Read & M.E. Farrugia. 2006. Single-fiber EMG with a concentric needle electrode: validation in myasthenia gravis. *Muscle Nerve* **33:** 61–65.

17. Benatar, M., M. Hammad & H. Doss-Riney. 2006. Concentric-needle single-fiber electromyography for the diagnosis of myasthenia gravis. *Muscle Nerve* **34:** 163–168.

Ann. N.Y. Acad. Sci. ISSN 0077-8923

ANNALS OF THE NEW YORK ACADEMY OF SCIENCES

Issue: *Myasthenia Gravis and Related Disorders*

Management challenges in muscle-specific tyrosine kinase myasthenia gravis

Amelia Evoli,[1] Paolo E. Alboini,[1] Ana Bisonni,[2] Alessia Mastrorosa,[1] and Emanuela Bartoccioni[3]

[1]Institute of Neurology, Catholic University, Rome, Italy. [2]Department of Neurology, Hospital Italiano de Buenos Aires, Buenos Aires, Argentina. [3]Institute of General Pathology, Catholic University, Rome, Italy

Address for correspondence: Amelia Evoli, Institute of Neurology, Catholic University, Largo F. Vito 1, 00168 Roma, Italy. a.evoli@rm.unicatt.it

Myasthenia gravis with antibodies to muscle-specific tyrosine kinase (MuSK-MG) is generally considered a severe disease because of the associated weakness distribution with prevalent involvement of bulbar muscles and a rapidly progressive course and early respiratory crises. Its treatment can be unrewarding, owing to poor response to acetylcholinesterase inhibitors in most patients, disease relapses in spite of high-dose immunosuppression, and development of permanent bulbar weakness. High-dose prednisone plus plasma exchange is the recommended approach for treating rapidly progressive bulbar weakness. In the disease management, oral steroids proved effective, plasma exchange produced marked, albeit short-term, improvement, while conventional immunosuppressants were comparatively less effective. Rituximab is a promising treatment for refractory MuSK-MG; in uncontrolled studies, nearly all treated patients achieved significant improvement with substantial decrease of medication. It is yet to be clarified whether the early use of rituximab could prevent the permanent bulbar weakness, which constitutes a relevant disability in these patients.

Keywords: anti-MuSK antibodies; myasthenia gravis; MuSK-positive myasthenia gravis; rituximab

Introduction

Serum antibodies (Abs) against the muscle-specific tyrosine kinase (MuSK) indicate a clinical form of myasthenia gravis (MuSK-MG) that differs in many ways from the far more common disease associated with antiacetylcholine receptor Abs (AChR-MG). A rather focal clinical phenotype with predominant cranial weakness,[1] rare thymus abnormalities with apparently no response to thymectomy,[2,3] and poor response to acetylcholinesterase inhibitors (AChE-I),[4] are all well-known clinical characteristics of MuSK-MG. In contrast to anti-AChR Abs, which mostly belong to IgG1 and IgG3 subclasses,[5] Abs to MuSK are mostly of IgG4 isotype[6] and are thought to exert their pathogenic effect through direct interference with the protein signaling pathway.[7]

Treatment is thought to be less effective than in typical MG, and the last few years have seen a number of clinical reports on difficult-to-treat MuSK-MG cases. There are several reasons why the disease management can be challenging. First, symptoms are usually severe with a high rate of respiratory crises.[8,9] Second, not only do most patients fail to improve on symptomatic drugs, but the response to conventional immunosuppressive therapy also appears less satisfactory than in AChR-MG.[10] Last, a proportion of MuSK-MG patients develop permanent weakness and muscle atrophy in spite of long-term treatment.[11] Here, we analyze these aspects, on the basis of our own experience and in light of other authors' reports.

Clinical aspects of MuSK-MG

Typically, anti-MuSK Abs are associated with generalized disease, although they have rarely been reported in patients with isolated ocular symptoms.[12] In contrast to AChR-MG, which shows remarkable

doi: 10.1111/j.1749-6632.2012.06781.x

clinical variability, in most patients, MuSK-MG is characterized by predominant involvement of bulbar, neck, and respiratory muscles. Such a phenotype is quite typical and has been observed worldwide.[8,9,13–15] Notably, it is consistent with the weakness pattern in experimental MuSK-MG,[16] where an intrinsic low-level MuSK expression can make certain muscles more susceptible to the Ab effect.[17]

Most patients with fully developed disease complain of dysarthria and dysphagia, secondary to tongue and pharyngeal dysfunction, associated with facial and neck weakness; ocular symptoms are usually present, although not disabling; and limb weakness is relatively less severe and inconsistent. The disease is graded as moderate to severe in the great majority of cases.[10] Accordingly, in a recent study on 110 MuSK-MG patients, the maximum MGFA (Myasthenia Gravis Foundation of America) clinical class[18] was III or greater in 85% and IV or greater in 44% of the patients.[19]

Respiratory involvement is frequent and tends to occur early in the disease course. A higher frequency of myasthenic crises has been reported in MuSK-MG in comparison with AChR-MG[9,20] and AChR/MuSK-negative MG.[1,21] The proportion of patients who suffered from respiratory failure ranged from 25%[22] to 48%[23] in different series (see Table 1), although the actual crisis rate may even have been underestimated in these studies, considering that repeated crises are not rare in these patients.[24,25] Respiratory failure is generally due to diaphragm dysfunction associated with airway collapse caused by oropharyngeal weakness. However, in some patients, vocal cord paralysis, which is a very unusual finding in AChR-MG, contributes to respiratory dysfunction.[26,27]

MuSK-MG is generally characterized by an acute onset and a rapidly progressive course. However, some patients may have mild to moderate disease for months or even years and then progress to persistent bulbar weakness.[19] Exacerbation phases are common, in particular in the first years from onset, and can occur in the absence of apparent triggering factors, in patients on full-dose immunosuppressive treatment.[11] Serial Ab testing on individual patients have shown a correlation between clinical fluctuations and variations of serum anti-MuSK Ab titer[28,29] that appears to be related to changes in specific IgG4 concentrations.[30]

A proportion of MuSK-MG patients develops permanent cranial and bulbar muscle dysfunction, with facial weakness and dysarthria, associated with atrophy of tongue and facial muscles.[1] In a combined survey from Catholic University (Rome, Italy) and Duke Medical Center (Durham, NC),[19] 25 of 110 patients (23%) had fixed bulbar weakness, which was disabling in eight cases with a myopathic face, and severe speech impairment. At present, muscle atrophy is rare in AChR-MG, being mostly restricted to nonimmunosuppressed patients with severe long-standing disease. On the other hand, bulbar muscle wasting appears to be significantly more common in MuSK-MG,[31] where it can be an early finding[32] occurring in treated and untreated patients[33] and which can be partially reversed by treatment.[34]

Disease management with standard treatment

It is generally accepted that current treatment for MG is very effective and can restore normal life conditions in the great majority of patients.[35] Here, we discuss the extent to which this statement applies to MuSK-MG and the role of different therapeutic options in the disease management.

It has long been known that the response to AChE-Is is generally unsatisfactory in MuSK-MG.[8–11,13] Furthermore, standard pyridostigmine doses frequently induce muscle cramps and fasciculations, and some patients even experience worsening of weakness and cholinergic crises.[1,4] An explanation of cholinergic hypersensitivity in MuSK-MG patients has recently been provided by Kawakami *et al.*, who demonstrated that anti-MuSK

Table 1. Frequency of respiratory crises in MuSK-MG

Series	Ref.	No. of Patients	Patients with crises (%)
Deymeer *et al.*	9	32	11 (34%)
Evoli *et al.*	11	57	21 (37%)
Lavrnic *et al.*	8	17	6 (35%)
Pasnoor *et al.*	13	53	18 (34%)
Sanders *et al.*	22	12	3 (25%)
Wolfe *et al.*	23	21	10 (48%)

NOTE: Studies including at least 10 patients were considered.

Abs interfere with MuSK-ColQ binding, thus reducing AChE concentration at the neuromuscular junction.[36] However, nonresponsiveness to AChE-Is is by no means an absolute rule as 32% of the patients in a large series[19] showed satisfactory response to and good tolerance of pyridostigmine. Interestingly, these subjects had a more stable disease course and very rarely developed muscle atrophy in comparison with AChE-I nonresponsive cases.[19] In practice, at least in patients with definite improvement on the edrophonium test, pyridostigmine could be tried at low doses, with subsequent dosage adjusted according to the clinical response. On the other hand, in the absence of clear records of positive response, AChE-I should be avoided in all patients with severe bulbar weakness or impending respiratory crisis.[11]

Immunosuppression is the mainstay treatment in all forms of MG. This is particularly true in MuSK-MG, where weakness severity and poor response to AChE-Is imply prompt and aggressive treatment. Accordingly, the proportion of patients treated with immunosuppressive therapy has been reported to be higher in MuSK-MG than in the other disease subtypes,[37] ranging from 95% to 100% in different patient series.[21] There is general consensus that MuSK-MG responds well to steroid treatment.[21] High-dose prednisone (1–1.5 mg/kg of body weight/day) associated with plasma exchange has proved very effective in treating severe bulbar weakness and respiratory crises and is the therapy of choice of exacerbation phases, like in other forms of MG.[10] However, during steroid dosage tapering, these patients often complain of increased weakness or suffer from severe disease relapses. Azathioprine, cyclosporine A, and mycophenolate mofetil have been largely used as steroid-sparing agents. Although Sanders *et al.* observed a good response to mycophenolate,[38] immunosuppressants are thought to be comparatively less effective in MuSK-MG than in other MG patients.[1,8,21] In our experience, treatment with either azathioprine or cyclosporine did not significantly add to steroid effectiveness in a high proportion of patients (who remained dependent on prednisone) and did not prevent development of muscle atrophy.[11]

Two reports have described the resolution of tongue atrophy in MuSK-MG following high-dose steroids[34] and in combined treatment with prednisone and mycophenolate,[39] respectively. Moreover, the frequency of muscle wasting in our re-

cent study[19] was lower than in a previous report,[1] probably on account of more aggressive and earlier treatment. From these observations, it seems that early, high-dose therapy can prevent or effectively treat muscle atrophy in these patients, whereas in our experience, steroid treatment at lower dosage was much less effective even when associated with azathioprine or cyclosporine.[11]

Plasma exchange and intravenous immunoglobulin (IVIG) are generally considered equally effective in MG.[40] Most MuSK-MG patients respond well and often dramatically to plasma exchange. In addition, clinical improvement has a rapid onset,[10] suggesting a functional effect of MuSK Abs, which is particularly valuable for patients with life-threatening weakness. On the other hand, according to recent reports IVIG appears to be less effective in MuSK-MG rather than in AChR-MG, with response rates ranging from 11% to 46%.[10,13,21] Finally, the role of thymectomy in management of the disease remains highly controversial. Very few patients have achieved remission after thymectomy,[8,13,14] and most studies have failed altogether to show a better outcome in thymectomized compared to unthymectomized patients both in terms of remission rate and need for immunosuppressive therapy.[11,21]

MuSK-MG is generally considered a hard-to-treat condition, with a less satisfactory outcome in comparison to AChR-MG.[10,21] Such an appraisal is justified by the consideration that MuSK-MG patients, though undoubtedly responsive to immunosuppressive therapy (in particular, to high-dose prednisone), remain, for the most part, dependent on treatment are often left with disabling weakness and suffer from frequent disease relapses.[11,19] This situation accounts for the relatively high rate of patients with refractory disease in this population.

Management of refractory disease

A large number of case reports and small patient series have recently dealt with the management of MuSK-MG that is refractory to conventional treatment. In our and other clinicians' experience, the usefulness of plasma-exchange in patients with frequent disease relapses appears to be significantly limited by the short-lasting effect. In these cases, in spite of concomitant immunosuppressive treatment, the clinical response to plasma exchange tends to become shorter with time, sometimes lasting no longer than two weeks.[11–42] On the other hand, three Japanese patients previously unresponsive to thymectomy, steroids, and tacrolimus, and dependent on plasma exchange, achieved long-term improvement with IVIG treatment.[41,42]

Rebooting the immune system with high-dose cyclophosphamide (50 mg/kg for ideal body weight/daily for four days) has thus far been tried in only a few MuSK-MG patients. It resulted in marked clinical improvement lasting 1–1.5 years and was associated with reduction in specific Ab titers.[24,43,44] One of these patients, who eventually suffered from a clinical relapse, acquired responsiveness to immunosuppressive agents that had previously been ineffective.[44]

In the last few years a breakthrough in the management of refractory MG has been the use of rituximab, a chimeric anti-CD20 monoclonal Ab, that has increasingly popular for the treatment of different autoimmune diseases.[45] In small open-label studies, rituximab proved effective in all forms of MG, and especially in MuSK-MG.[46,47] More than forty patients who received rituximab for refractory MuSK-MG have been reported in the English literature (see Table 2). Treatment was performed with four to six infusions of 375 mg/m^2 weekly in most cases,[19,24,25,46–53] with two infusions of 1,000 mg four weeks apart in a single patient[54] and with a low-dose regimen of 1,000 mg (divided into two doses) in

three cases.[55] All but one[24] patient improved. Clinical response was as early as two weeks[51] and long lasting; most patients achieved optimal control of their disease and were able to discontinue or significantly reduce immunosuppressive treatment and no serious side effects were observed.[19,46–55] Interestingly, a recent study reported a persistent clinical response to a single cycle of rituximab in MuSK-MG, while 54% of the AChR-MG patients suffered from disease relapses requiring reinfusions. Moreover, a significant reduction in serum Ab titers was observed only the MuSK-MG group.[47] The greater efficacy of rituximab in MuSK-MG is possibly related to the disease being mediated by IgG4 Abs. Good response to rituximab has been reported in conditions such as pemphigus, in which IgG4 plays a relevant pathogenic role,[56] and in the so-called IgG4-related disease (IgG4-RD), a multiorgan fibroinflammatory disorder characterized by tissue infiltration with plasma cells bearing IgG4.[57] Like MuSK-MG, IgG4-RD responds well to prednisone, at least in the first stages, while disease flares are frequent during prednisone dosage tapering.[58] Rituximab infusion was followed, in these patients, by prompt clinical improvement associated with a sharp and specific reduction of serum IgG4 concentration.[57,58] The authors hypothesized that B cell depletion, induced by rituximab, disrupts the generation of short-lived IgG4-producing plasma cells.[58]

Table 2. Characteristics of response to rituximab in MuSK-MG

Series	Ref.	MuSK$^+$ patients	Follow-up	Status after rituximab
Baek *et al*	49	1	6 months	CSR(1)
Blum *et al.*	55	3	4–47 months	CSR(1); PR(2)
Burusnukul *et al.*	50	2	21–24 months	CSR(2)
Diaz-Manera *et al.*	47	6	4–60 months	CSR(2); PR(2); MM(2)
Hain *et al.*	48	1	12 months	I(1)
Guptill *et al.*	19	6	2–40 months	PR(2); MM(2); I(2)
Lebrum *et al.*	51	3	18 months (mean)	I(3)
Lin *et al.*	24	1	NR	UNC(1)
Maddison *et al.*	46	3	12–48 months	CSR(1); I(2)
Nowak *et al.*	53	8	12–24 months	CSR(3); PR(2); MM(3)
Stein *et al.*	54	2	14–18 months	PR(2)
Thakre *et al.*	25	1	13 months	PR(1)
Zebardast *et al.*	52	4	NR	CSR(3); MM(1)

NOTE: CSR, complete stable remission; PR, pharmacological remission; MM, minimal manifestations; I, improved; UNC, unchanged; (patient number); NR, not reported.

Rituximab appears to be a safe and promising treatment and has been proposed as an early therapeutic option in MuSK-MG patients with unsatisfactory response to steroids.[47] This viewpoint seems to be justified given the relatively high proportion of patients who remain dependent on high-dose prednisone. However, lack of high-level evidence, possible reporting biases, and potentially severe side effects are all reasons for concern and point to the need for assessing efficacy and safety data in prospective trials. Moreover, it must still be determined whether early treatment with rituximab may prevent the development of permanent weakness and muscle atrophy, which constitutes a relevant disability in these patients.

Conflicts of interest

The authors declare no conflicts of interest.

References

1. Evoli, A. *et al.* 2003. Clinical correlates with anti-MuSK antibodies in generalized seronegative myasthenia gravis. *Brain* **126:** 2304–2311.
2. Lauriola, L. *et al.* 2005. Thymus changes in anti-MuSK-positive and -negative myasthenia gravis. *Neurology* **64:** 536–538.
3. Leite, I. *et al.* 2005. Fewer thymic changes in MuSK antibody-positive than in MuSK antibody negative MG. *Ann. Neurol.* **57:** 444–448.
4. Hatanaka, Y. *et al.* 2005. Nonresponsiveness to anticholinesterase agents in patients with MuSK-antibody-positive MG. *Neurology* **65:** 1508–1509.
5. Vincent, A. 2002. Unravelling the pathogenesis of myasthenia gravis. *Nat. Rev. Immunol.* **2:** 797–804.
6. McConville, J. *et al.* 2004. Detection and characterization of MuSK antibodies in seronegative myasthenia gravis. *Ann. Neurol.* **55:** 580–584.
7. Mori, S. *et al.* 2012. Divalent and monovalent autoantibodies cause dysfunction of MuSK by distinct mechanisms in a rabbit model of myasthenia gravis. *J. Neuroimmunol.* **244:** 1–7.
8. Lavrnic, D. *et al.* 2005. The features of myasthenia gravis with autoantibodies to MuSK. *J. Neurol. Neurosurg. Psychiatry* **76:** 1099–1102.
9. Deymeer, F. *et al.* 2007. Clinical comparison of anti-MuSK-vs anti-AChR-positive and seronegative myasthenia gravis. *Neurology* **68:** 609–611.
10. Guptill, J.T. & D.B. Sanders. 2010. Update on muscle-specific tyrosine kinase antibody positive myasthenia gravis. *Curr.Opin. Neurol.* **23:** 530–535.
11. Evoli, A. *et al.* 2008. Response to therapy in myasthenia gravis with anti-MuSK antibodies. *Ann. N. Y. Acad. Sci.* **1132:** 76–83.
12. Hanisch, E., K. Eger & S. Zierz. 2006. MuSK-antibody positive pure ocular myasthenia gravis. *J. Neurol.* **253:** 659–660.
13. Pasnoor, M. *et al.* 2010. Clinical findings in MuSK-antibody positive myasthenia gravis: a U.S. experience. *Muscle Nerve* **41:** 370–374.
14. Kostera-Pruszczyk, A. *et al.* 2008. MuSK-positive myasthenia gravis is rare in Poland. *Eur. J. Neurol.* **15:** 720–724.
15. Chang, T. *et al.* 2009. MuSK-antibody-positive myasthenia gravis in a South-Asian population. *J. Neurol. Sci.* **284:** 33–35.
16. Mori, S. *et al.* 2012. Antibodies against muscle-specific kinase impair both presynaptic and postsynaptic functions in a murine model of myasthenia gravis. *Am. J. Pathol.* **180:** 798–810.
17. Punga, A.R. *et al.* 2011. Muscle-selective synaptic disassembly and reorganization in MuSK antibody positive MG mice. *Exp. Neurol.* **230:** 207–217.
18. Jaretzki, A. *et al.* 2000. Myasthenia gravis: recommendations for clinical research standards. Task force of the Medical Scientic Advisory Board of the Myasthenia Gravis Foundation of America. *Neurology* **55:** 16–23.
19. Guptill, J.F., D.B. Sanders & A. Evoli. 2011. Anti-MuSK antibody myasthenia gravis: clinical finding and response to therapy in two large cohorts. *Muscle Nerve* **44:** 36–40.
20. Nemoto, Y. *et al.* 2005. Patterns and severity of neuromuscular transmission failure in seronegative myasthenia gravis. *J. Neurol. Neurosurg. Psychiatry* **76:** 714–718.
21. Oh, S.J. 2009. Muscle-specific receptor tyrosine kinase antibody positive myasthenia gravis current status. *J. Clin. Neurol.* **5:** 53–64.
22. Sanders, D.B. *et al.* 2003. Clinical aspects of MuSK antibody positive seronegative myasthenia gravis. *Neurology* **60:** 1978–1980.
23. Wolfe, G.I., J.R. Trivedi & S.J. Oh. 2007. Clinical review of muscle specific tyrosine kinase-antibody positive myasthenia gravis. *J. Clin. Neuromusc. Dis.* **8:** 217–224.
24. Lin, P.T. *et al.* 2006. High-dose cyclophosphamide in refractory myasthenia gravis with anti-MuSK antibodies. *Muscle Nerve* **33:** 433–435.
25. Thakre, M., J. Inshasi & M. Marashi. 2007. Rituximab in refractory MuSK antibody myasthenia gravis. *J. Neurol.* **254:** 968–969.
26. Hara, K. *et al.* 2007. Vocal cord paralysis in myasthenia gravis with anti-MuSK antibodies. *Neurology* **68:** 621–622.
27. Sylva, M., A.J. van der Kooi & W. Grolman. 2008. Dyspnoea due to vocal fold abduction paresis in anti-MuSK myasthenia gravis. *J. Neurol. Neurosurg. Psychiatry* **79:** 1083–1084.
28. Bartoccioni, E. *et al.* 2006. Anti-MuSK antibodies: correlation with myasthenia gravis severity. *Neurology* **67:** 505–507.
29. Ohta, K. *et al.* 2007. Clinical and experimental features of MuSK antibody positive MG in Japan. *Eur. J. Neurol.* **14:** 1029–1034.
30. Niks, E.K. *et al.* 2008. Clinical fluctuations in MuSK myasthenia gravis are related to antigen-specific IgG4 instead of IgG1. *J. Neuroimmunol.* **195:** 151–156.
31. Farrugia, M.E. *et al.* 2006. MRI and clinical studies of facial and bulbar involvement in MuSK antibody-associated myasthenia gravis. *Brain* **129:** 1481–1492.
32. Zouvelou, V. *et al.* 2011. MRI evidence of early muscle atrophy in MuSK positive myasthenia gravis. *J. Neuroimaging* **21:** 303–305.
33. Moon, S-Y., S-S. Lee & Y-H. Hong. 2011. Muscle atrophy in muscle-specific tyrosine kinase (MuSK)-related myasthenia gravis. *J. Clin. Neurosci.* **18:** 1274–1275.

34. Takahashi, H. *et al.* 2010. Is tongue atrophy reversible in anti-MuSK myasthenia gravis? Six-year observation. *J. Neurol. Neurosurg. Psychiatry* **81:** 701–702.

35. Gold, R. & C. Schneider-Gold. 2008. Current and future standards in the treatment of myasthenia gravis. *Neurotherapeutics* **5:** 535–541.

36. Kawakami, Y. *et al.* 2011. Anti-MuSK autoantibodies block binding of collagen Q to MuSK. *Neurology* **77:** 1819–1826.

37. Sanders, D.B. & A. Evoli. 2010. Immunosuppressive therapies in myasthenia gravis. *Autoimmunity* **43:** 428–435.

38. Sanders, D.B., J. Massey & V.C. Juel. 2007. Muscle antibody positive myasthenia gravis: response to treatment in 31 patients. *Neurology (asbtract)* **68:** A299.

39. Sanders, D.B. & V.C. Juel. 2008. MuSK-antibody positive myasthenia gravis. Questions from the clinic. *J. Neuroimmunol.* **201–202:** 85–89.

40. Gaidos, P. *et al.* 1997. Clinical trial of plasma exchange and high dose immunoglobulin in myasthenia gravis. *Ann. Neurol.* **41:** 789–796.

41. Takahashi, H. *et al.* 2006. High-dose intravenous immunoglobulin for the treatment of MuSK antibody positive seronegative myasthenia gravis. *J. Neurol. Sci.* **247:** 239–241.

42. Shibata-Hamaguchi, A. *et al.* 2007. Long-term effect of intravenous immunoglobulin on anti-MuSK antibody-positive myasthenia gravis. *Acta Neurol. Scand.* **116:** 406–408.

43. Drachman, D.B., R.J. Jones & R.A. Brodsky. 2003. Treatment of refractory myasthenia: "rebooting" with high-dose cyclophosphamide. *Ann. Neurol.* **5:** 29–34.

44. Drachman, D.B. *et al.* 2008. Rebooting the immune system with high-dose cyclophosphamide for treatment of refractory myasthenia gravis. *Ann. N. Y. Acad. Sci.* **1132:** 305–314.

45. Townsend, M.J., J.G. Monroe & A.C. Chan. 2010. B cell targeted therapies in human autoimmune diseases: an updated perspective. *Immunol. Rev.* **237:** 264–283.

46. Maddison, P. *et al.* 2011. The use of rituximab in myasthenia gravis and Lambert-Eaton myasthenic syndrome. *J. Neurol. Neurosurg. Psychiatry* **82:** 671–673.

47. Dìaz-Manera, J. *et al.* 2012. Long-lasting treatment effect of rituximab in MuSK myasthenia. *Neurology* **78:** 189–193.

48. Hain, B. *et al.* 2009. Successful treatment of MuSK antibody-positive myasthenia gravis with rituximab. *Muscle Nerve* **33:** 575–580.

49. Baek, W.S., A. Bashey & G.L. Sheean. 2007. Complete remission induced by rituximab in refractory, seronegative, muscle-specific, kinase-positive myasthenia gravis. *J. Neurol. Neurosurg. Psychiatry* **78:** 771.

50. Burusnukul, P., T.D. Brennan & E.J. Cupler. 2010. Prolonged improvement after rituximab: two cases of resistant muscle-specific receptor tyrosine kinase+ myasthenia gravis. *J. Clin. Neuromuscular Dis.* **12:** 85–87.

51. Lebrun, C. *et al.* 2009. Successful treatment of refractory generalized myasthenia gravis with rituximab. *Eur. J. Neurol.* **16:** 246–250.

52. Zebardast, N. *et al.* 2010. Rituximab in the management of refractory myasthenia gravis. *Muscle Nerve* **41:** 375–378.

53. Novack, R.J. *et al.* 2011. Response of patients with refractory myasthenia gravis to rituximab: a retrospective study. *Ther. Adv. Neurol. Disord.* **4:** 259–266.

54. Stein, B. & S.J. Bird. 2011. Rituximab in the treatment of MuSK antibody-positive myasthenia gravis. *J. Clin. Neuromuscular Dis.* **12:** 163–164.

55. Blum, S. *et al.* 2011. Use and monitoring of low-dose rituximab in myasthenia gravis. *J. Neurol. Neurosurg. Psychiatry* **82:** 659–663.

56. Kasperkiewicz, M. *et al.* 2011. Rituximab for treatment-refractory pemphigus and pemphigoid: a case series of 17 patients. *J. Am. Acad. Dermatol.* **65:** 552–558.

57. Stone, J.H., Y. Zen & V. Deshpande. 2012. IgG4-related disease. *N. Engl. J. Med.* **366:** 539–551.

58. Khosroshahi, A. *et al.* 2010. Rituximab therapy leads to rapid decline of serum IgG4 levels and prompt clinical improvement in IgG4-related systemic disease. *Arthritis Rheum.* **62:** 1755–1762.

Ann. N.Y. Acad. Sci. ISSN 0077-8923

ANNALS OF THE NEW YORK ACADEMY OF SCIENCES

Issue: *Myasthenia Gravis and Related Disorders*

Antibodies identified by cell-based assays in myasthenia gravis and associated diseases

Angela Vincent, Patrick Waters, M. Isabel Leite, Leslie Jacobson, Inga Koneczny, Judith Cossins, and David Beeson

Nuffield Department of Clinical Neurosciences, and Weatherall Institute of Molecular Medicine, University of Oxford, John Radcliffe Hospital, Oxford, United Kingdom

Address for correspondence: Angela Vincent, Nuffield Department of Clinical Neurosciences, and Weatherall Institute of Molecular Medicine, University of Oxford, John Radcliffe Hospital, Oxford Ox3 9DU, UK. angela.vincent@ndcn.ox.ac.uk.

We have established cell-based assays for the improved detection of acetylcholine receptor (AChR) and muscle-specific kinase (MuSK) antibodies in myasthenia gravis. This approach has enabled us to demonstrate antibodies to "clustered" AChRs in patients who were previously AChR antibody negative and can also be used to distinguish between adult and fetal AChR antibodies in mothers of babies with arthrogryposis multiplex congenita. We summarize our recent evidence for the pathogenicity of MuSK and clustered AChR antibodies using *in vivo* models. Cell-based assays are now also being used for the detection of other antibodies, such as those directed to components of the VGKC/CASPR2/LGI1 complex in Morvan's syndrome, and to AQP4 antibodies in neuromyelitis optica; both of these diseases can be associated with MG and sometimes thymoma. The cell-based method is time consuming but has many advantages and may provide a gold standard for the future in the detection of pathogenic autoantibodies in patients with immune-mediated diseases.

Keywords: acetylcholine receptor; MuSK; VGKC; VGKC-complex; cell-surface antigen

Introduction

The increasing number of antibody-mediated diseases, with diverse target antigens, demand diagnostic antibody assays that are sensitive, specific for pathogenic extracellular epitopes, and that distinguish between different forms of a disease or syndrome. Although the majority of patients with myasthenia gravis (MG) have antibodies detected by radioimmunoprecipitation assay (RIA) of solubilized muscle acetylcholine receptors (AChR) labeled with $[^{125}I]$ alpha-bungarotoxin, as first demonstrated by Lindstrom *et al.* in 1976,[1] up to 20% of patients with generalized MG (GMG) and 50% of those with ocular MG (OMG) are negative in the RIA. This assay, performed in solution phase, is not specific for extracellular epitopes, and it does not distinguish between antibodies to the fetal and adult forms of the AChR, which can be relevant to maternally mediated fetal or neonatal disorders. Moreover, a proportion of sera RIA negative for

AChR antibodies have antibodies to MuSK and a few to LRP4 (see Cossins *et al.* and others in this volume), so these also need to be measured separately in many cases.

We have performed cell-based assays for each of these antibodies. These assays involve expressing the antigen on the surface of live human embryonic kidney (HEK) cells by DNA transfection, and measurement of antibody binding by indirect immunofluorescence. The approach and examples of two MuSK antibody-positive sera are shown in Figure 1A and B, and the correlation between the cell-based assay (CBA) and the RIA is clearly apparent in Figure 1C. Here, we will summarize our recent data on antibodies in myasthenia and associated conditions that have depended on the use of CBAs.

Detection of antibodies that only bind to AChRs that are clustered

We were struck by the fact that a proportion of patients without detectable AChR antibodies, even

doi: 10.1111/j.1749-6632.2012.06789.x

Ann. N.Y. Acad. Sci. 1274 (2012) 92–98 © 2012 New York Academy of Sciences.

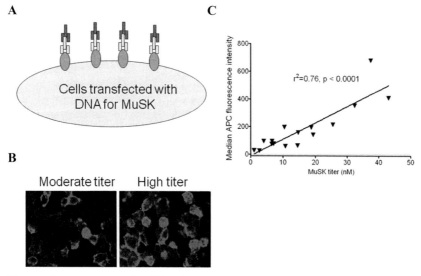

Figure 1. (A). Diagramatic representation of a cell-based assay for MuSK antibodies. (B). Examples of MuSK antibodies binding to transfected cells detected by antihuman IgG (red). (C). MuSK antibodies measured by FACS (vertical axis) correlate with radioimmunoprecipitation of [^{125}I] MuSK in individual patients. Results are representative of those described in Refs. 12 and 5.

using our modified RIAs,[2] had a clinical picture very similar to that of AChR Ab-positive MG (AChR-MG) patients, and many had thymic lymphocytic infiltrates that distinguished them from typical MuSK-Ab MG (MuSK-MG) patients who usually have very few such infiltrates.[3,4] One possibility was that the AChR/MuSK antibody-negative patients might have antibodies that could not bind effectively to AChRs in solution but were only able to bind strongly to AChRs that are clustered tightly on the cell surface as they are at the neuromuscular junction. To investigate this possibility, we transfected HEK cells with DNA for each of the human muscle AChR subunits together with DNA for rapsyn, the AChR-clustering protein. This showed that up to 60% of the previously seronegative AChR patients had antibodies to clustered AChRs,[5] suggesting that tight packing of AChRs on the cell surface allows divalent binding of the antibodies to adjacent molecules.

One of the advantages of using cell-based methods is that the pathogenic potential of the antibodies can also be investigated. We found that the clustered AChR antibodies were predominantly IgG1 subclass and could activate complement on the surface of the HEK cells.[5] This indicated that these antibodies should be pathogenic *in vivo*.

Clustered-AChR antibodies have also been investigated in ocular MG. They were present in up to 40% of the ocular MG patients, were IgG1 subclass, and were able to deposit complement components on the surface of the cells. Importantly, they were often specific for the adult form of the AChR and did not bind detectably to the fetal form. The intensity (scored visually) of the complement deposition, as well as the intensity of the IgG antibody binding, was found to correlate well with neuromuscular transmission defects; single fiber electromyography investigation of the obicularis oculi of the individual patients on the same day as the serum was also obtained,[6] again strongly suggesting pathogenicity.

Pathogenicity of clustered AChR antibodies

To demonstrate that the clustered-AChR antibodies were pathogenic, we performed passive transfer studies by injection of IgG purified from plasma of two previously seronegative MG patients with generalized disease whose plasma contained antibodies binding to clustered AChRs.[6] We first confirmed that the antibodies also bound strongly to mouse AChRs expressed and clustered on HEK cells and then injected with 10–50 mg/day for up to five days into wild-type or complement-regulator deficient mice. The mice did not show any evidence of weakness, but the miniature endplate potential amplitudes were significantly reduced at the diaphragm neuromuscular junctions; the reductions

Table 1. Comparison of active immunization and passive transfer models of MG in mice[a]

Antigen	Active immunization with antigen	Passive transfer with human IgG antibodies to antigen	References
Clustered AChR	Not attempted	MEPPs reduced Quantal content slightly increased	Jacob *et al.*[6]
AChR	MEPPs reduced Quantal content increased	MEPPs reduced Quantal content increased	Plomp *et al.*;[7] Viegas *et al.*[13]
MuSK	MEPPs reduced Quantal content not increased	MEPPs reduced Quantal content not increased	Klooster *et al.*;[14] Viegas *et al.*[13]

[a]The data from these publications, particularly the direct comparisons undertaken in Refs. 13 and 6, emphasize the upregulation of quantal content in AChR-MG and the lack of upregulation in quantal content in MuSK-MG. MEPPS, miniature endplate potential amplitudes.

for each IgG preparation were not different from the reduction seen with injection of IgG purified from plasma of a typical AChR antibody-positive patient.[6] Interestingly, the quantal content (number of packets of acetylcholine released per impulse) was higher overall in both the clustered AChR-IgG–injected and AChR-IgG–injected mice than in the controls, reflecting the increase in quantal content that has previously been reported in both AChR-MG and in animal models of MG.[7] The results are summarized in Table 1.

Antibodies distinguishing adult and fetal AChRs

The clustered AChR antibodies in generalized MG bound equally to clustered fetal or adult AChRs in almost all patients, but in ocular MG, the majority of the antibodies only bound to clustered adult AChR as mentioned above.[6] The importance of using adult AChRs in assays for MG has been known for many years and previously led to improvements in assay sensitivities.[8] In other cases, however, it is antibodies to the fetal AChR that are important. During pregnancy, IgG antibodies cross the placenta in increasing amounts resulting in levels of IgG antibodies in the fetus that are similar to the mothers' levels by the time of delivery. A small proportion of mothers with MG have babies with neonatal MG due to the transfer of AChR antibodies, but these usually decrease over a few weeks and the babies improve. Even less often, the baby develops fetal paralysis during pregnancy and is born, or stillborn, with fixed joints and other deformities described as arthrogryposis multiplex congenital (AMC). These rare cases have been

found in consecutive pregnancies of individual MG mothers, strongly suggesting that they are caused by maternal antibodies; moreover, they are not always associated with maternal MG.[9] We showed previously that in these few patients the AChR antibodies were mainly fetal specific and inhibited the function of the fetal AChR, while having no effect on the function of the adult AChR.[9,10] The antibodies were pathogenic as demonstrated in maternal-to-fetal transfer studies in mice.[11]

Over the intervening years, we have been asked to investigate serum from other mothers, both with and without MG, who had histories of AMC in their babies, sometimes after the first affected pregnancy. The sera are first tested by RIAs for AChR and MuSK antibodies, but the CBAs have proved useful in distinguishing clearly between adult and fetal AChR antibodies, and also looking for MuSK antibodies. Figure 2 shows maternal serum binding to fetal AChR, but only very weakly to adult AChR,

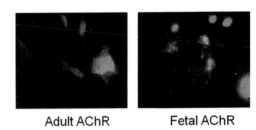

Adult AChR   Fetal AChR

Figure 2. Binding of serum from a mother of consecutive babies affected by arthrogryposis multiplex congential showing very weak binding to adult AChR (left) but strong binding to fetal AChR (right). In this case, the HEK cells have been transfected with enhanced green fluorescent protein as well as the different AChR subunits and rapsyn. Results are representative of those shown in Refs. 10 and 5.

Table 2. Antibodies to AChR and MuSK in mothers of fetal or neonatal AMC[a]

Age	Number of AMC offspring	MG?	AChR RIA	AChR CBA	MuSK RIA	MuSK CBA
28	3	No MG	< 0.2	None	Negative	Positive
32	4	MG	19.1	Fetal>adult	Negative	Negative
35	4	No MG	32.4	Fetal>adult	Negative	Negative

[a]Examples of three mothers, two without clinical evidence of MG, in whom consecutive pregnancies were complicated by fetal arthrogryposis multiplex congenital (AMC). RIA, radiommunoprecipation assay; CBA, cell-based assay. Antibodies distinguishing between adult and fetal receptors in AMC are described in detail in Riemersma.[10]

and Table 2 summarizes data from three representative cases.

Antibodies to MuSK

Most patients with MuSK antibodies are clearly positive on the RIA for MuSK, which is widely available. But CBAs are also useful because MuSK is expressed very strongly in HEK cells (see Fig. 1B), and there is a good correlation between the two techniques, particularly when the binding to the MuSK-HEK cells is measured quantitatively by FACS (Fig. 1C).[12] In a few cases, we have found MuSK antibodies by cell-based assay that were not detected by RIA.[5,6]

There is now ample evidence that MuSK antibodies are pathogenic with several animal models presented by others in this volume and elsewhere. We carefully compared the effects of MuSK immunization with passive injection of MuSK-MG IgG. The miniature endplate potential amplitudes were reduced in both models suggesting that active immunization provides a good model for the human disease (Table 1). Interestingly, with MuSK immunizations, the quantal contents were not increased compared with the significant increase found when we immunized against AChRs,[13] and in contrast to the results with passive transfer of the clustered-AChR antibodies,[6] Table 1). This suggests that MuSK antibodies are able to interfere with the compensatory increase in presynaptic release (see also Refs. 4 and 14) that occurs in typical MG.

Antibodies in diseases associated with MG

Antibodies to VGKC-complex proteins
Antibodies to voltage-gated potassium channels (VGKC) were first identified by radioimmunoprecipitation of [^{125}I]-dendrotoxin-VGKCs solubilized from rabbit brain tissue in the 1990s.[15,16] These antibodies were found only in a proportion of patients

with neuromyotonia but were frequently positive in those with thymoma, most of whom had coexisting symptoms of MG.[17] Some patients had MG and neuromyotonia without thymoma.

Following these observations, higher titers of VGKC antibodies were detected in Morvan's syndrome[18] and in a form of limbic encephalitis.[19,20] It was only over the last few years that it has become clear that the "VGKC" antibodies are mainly directed toward membrane or associated proteins that complex with the VGKCs themselves.[21] Thus antibodies to LGI1, CASPR2, or Contactin-2 can be shown to immunoprecipitate VGKCs from mammalian brain tissue extracts (see Fig. 3 for a diagram of the VGKC complex). In order to explore the contributions of these antibodies to the "VGKC" antibodies (now usually known as VGKC-complex antibodies), we and others established cell-based assays for the complex proteins.[21,22] In general, LGI1 antibodies are most common in limbic encephalitis and in a newly defined seizure disorder called faciobrachial dystonic seizures.[23]

CASPR2 antibodies are present at very high titers in a the majority of patients with Morvan's syndrome, particularly in patients with thymomas and MG.[24] These patients develop combinations of insomnia, autonomic dysfunction, and peripheral nerve hyperexcitability. Although very rare, this condition can be misdiagnosed as schizophrenia;[25] it has been noted that more patients are interested in these antibodies, and the availability of antibody tests increases. At present only CBAs are available for testing these antibodies.

AQP4 antibodies
One of the most clinically important uses of the cell-based assay is in the diagnosis of neuromyelitis optica and its distinction from multiple sclerosis and other demyelinating disorders. Antibodies to

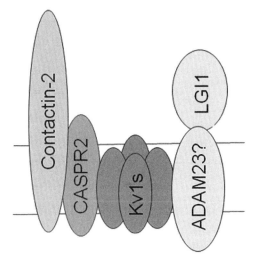

Figure 3. Diagramatic representation of the VGKC complex. Voltage-gated potassium channel Kv1 subunits form a tetramer in the neuronal membrane. These interact strongly with other membrane and associated proteins such as CASPR2 and Contactin-2. LGI1 is also part of the VGKC complex but interacts via another protein, possibly ADAM23. Antibodies to any of these proteins can immunoprecipitate [^{125}I] dendrotoxin-labelled VGKCs. The model is based on data in Refs. 21 and 22.

aquaporin-4 (AQP4) were first described by Lennon *et al.* in 2005,[26] and the detection of these antibodies quickly found its way into clinical practice. Although several different approaches have been tried,[27] a recent multicenter study of coded serum samples showed that the cell-based assay, particularly when combined with FACS analysis, had the best sensitivity and specificity.[28]

The development of neuromyelitis optica in patients with existing or previous histories of myasthenia gravis has been recognized for some time, but whether this was a coincidental association or of etiological significance, and in particular the role of the thymus, was not clear. Altogether, 26 patients with the two diseases have now been reported from two multicenter studies.[29,30] The MG almost always presents first, is relatively mild, and has been treated successful with thymectomy (in most cases, but not necessarily) and immunotherapies. The neuromyelitis optica usually begins subsequently, with a median lag between the two diseases of 16 years.[30] Considering the relative incidences of each of the two diseases in the United Kingdom, we calculated that the two together occur 70 times more frequently than by chance, but one has to appreciate that this might be due to shared genetic factors (e.g., HLA) rather than any shared precipitating cause.

Advantages of cell-based assays

The work described here illustrates many of the studies on specific antibodies that are now becoming incorporated into routine practice for the diagnosis of autoantibody-mediated diseases, which respond to immunotherapies, and which can be found, even if rarely, in patients with MG (Table 3). Although other types of assays are available for several of these antigens, the cell-based assays have many advantages. The antigen is expressed on a mammalian cell surface in a membrane environment, will

Table 3. Antibodies in MG and associated diseases that can be measured by cell-based assays

Disease	Cell-based assay	Incidence in MG	Association with thymic pathology	References
Myasthenia negative for AChR or MuSK antibodies by immuno-precipitation	Clustered AChR	Up to 50%	Evidence of thymic lymphocytic infiltration in many with generalized MG	Leite *et al.*;[5] Jacob *et al.*[6]
	MuSK high expression	Low percentage	None known	Leite *et al.*;[5] Jacob *et al.*[6]
Neuromyotonia	CASPR2 or LGI1	Fairly rare	Thymoma common	Irani *et al.*[21]
Morvan's syndrome	CASPR2 or LGI1	Rare	Thymoma common	Irani *et al.*[23]
Neuromyelitis optica	AQP4 M23 isoform	Rare but 70 times higher than by chance	Not known	Waters *et al.*;[31] Waters *et al.*;[28] Leite *et al.*;[29] Jarius *et al.*[30]

therefore be glycosylated appropriately, and should be in a native conformation. Only extracellular epitopes will be detected if the cells are live and unpermeabilized when the patient's antibodies are applied. By contrast, other assays such as enzyme-linked immunoassays frequently use recombinant proteins produced in bacterial or insect expression systems that are not correctly folded and where antibodies to intracellular epitopes, which are unlikely to be pathogenic, are detected. Another advantage of the cell-based, transient-transfection method is that high expression levels can be obtained on the cell surface by including a clustering protein, thus increasing the chances of bivalent antibody binding with improved sensitivity, as shown for clustered AChRs. Some antigens also express very strongly, for instance, cells expressing the M23 isoform of AQP4 not only express more antigen, but also present dense arrays of the antigen leading to detection of higher titers and greater sensitivity.[28] Modifications of the assays with different isoforms of the antigen or by using different class or subclass-specific second antibodies can lead to direct comparison of fine specificities and IgG subclasses, or classes.[31] Moreover, by expressing antigens fused to enhanced green fluorescent protein (EGFP), it is possible to develop solubilized fluorescent-immunoprecipitation assays that can be used for serial analysis of samples from individual patients as shown, for instance, for AQP4[32] or glycine receptor[33] antibodies. Finally both the cell-based and fluorescence immunoprecipitation assays can be applied in countries where radioactivity is not permitted.[34]

The main problem is that these assays are labor intensive. However, biochips of fixed HEK cells expressing different antigens placed together for testing each serum are beginning to be available for some of the CNS antigens. This or other multiplex methodologies should make it possible in the future to provide simultaneous sensitive assays for antibodies to fetal and adult AChRs, MuSK, LRP4, CASPR2, and other antigens in a single test.

Conflicts of interest

The authors declare no conflicts of interest.

References

1. Lindstrom, J.M., M.E. Seybold, V.A. Lennon, *et al.* 1976. Antibody to acetylcholine receptor in myasthenia gravis. Prevalence, clinical correlates, and diagnostic value. *Neurology* **26**: 1054–1059.

2. Beeson, D., L. Jacobson, J. Newsom-Davis & A. Vincent. 1996. A transfected human muscle cell line expressing the adult subtype of the human muscle acetylcholine receptor for diagnostic assays in myasthenia gravis. *Neurology* **47**: 1552–1555.

3. Leite, M.I., P. Strobel, M. Jones, *et al.* 2005. Fewer thymic changes in MuSK antibody-positive than in MuSK antibody-negative MG. *Ann. Neurol.* **57**: 444–448.

4. Lauriola, L., F. Ranelletti, N. Maggiano, *et al.* 2005. Thymus changes in anti-MuSK-positive and -negative myasthenia gravis. *Neurology* **64**: 536–538.

5. Leite, M.I., S. Jacob, S. Viegas, *et al.* 2008. IgG1 antibodies to acetylcholine receptors in 'seronegative' myasthenia gravis. *Brain* **131**(Pt 7): 1940–1952.

6. Jacob, S., S. Viegas, M.I. Leite, *et al.* 2012. Presence and pathogenic relevance of antibodies to clustered acetylcholine receptor in ocular and generalized myasthenia gravis. *Arch. Neurol.* **69**: 994–1001.

7. Plomp, J.J., G.T. Van Kempen, M.B. De Baets, *et al.* 1995. Acetylcholine release in myasthenia gravis: regulation at single end-plate level. *Ann. Neurol.* **37**: 627–636.

8. MacLennan, C., D. Beeson, A.M. Buijs, *et al.* 1997. Acetylcholine receptor expression in human extraocular muscles and their susceptibility to myasthenia gravis. *Ann. Neurol.* **41**: 423–431.

9. Vincent, A., C. Newland, L. Brueton, *et al.* 1995. Arthrogryposis multiplex congenita with maternal autoantibodies specific for a fetal antigen. *Lancet* **346**: 24–25.

10. Riemersma, S., A. Vincent, D. Beeson, *et al.* 1996. Association of arthrogryposis multiplex congenita with maternal antibodies inhibiting fetal acetylcholine receptor function. *J. Clin. Invest.* **98**: 2358–2363.

11. Jacobson, L., A. Polizzi, G. Morriss-Kay & A. Vincent. 1999. Plasma from human mothers of fetuses with severe arthrogryposis multiplex congenita causes deformities in mice. *J. Clin. Invest.* **103**: 1031–1038.

12. McConville, J., M.E. Farrugia, D. Beeson, *et al.* 2004. Detection and characterization of MuSK antibodies in seronegative myasthenia gravis. *Ann. Neurol.* **55**: 580–584.

13. Viegas, S., L. Jacobson, P. Waters, *et al.* 2012. Passive and active immunization models of MuSK-Ab positive myasthenia: electrophysiological evidence for pre and postsynaptic defects. *Exp. Neurol.* **234**: 506–512.

14. Klooster, R., J.J. Plomp, M.G. Huijbers, *et al.* 2012. Muscle-specific kinase myasthenia gravis IgG4 autoantibodies cause severe neuromuscular junction dysfunction in mice. *Brain* **135**(Pt 4): 1081–1101.

15. Shillito, P., P.C. Molenaar, A. Vincent, *et al.* 1995. Acquired neuromyotonia: evidence for autoantibodies directed against K +channels of peripheral nerves. *Ann. Neurol.* **38**: 714–722.

16. Hart, I.K., C. Waters, A. Vincent, *et al.* 1997. Autoantibodies detected to expressed K+ channels are implicated in neuromyotonia. *Ann. Neurol.* **41**: 238–246.

17. Hart, I.K., P. Maddison, J. Newsom-Davis, *et al.* 2002. Phenotypic variants of autoimmune peripheral nerve hyperexcitability. *Brain* **125**(Pt 8): 1887–1895.

18. Liguori, R., A. Vincent, L. Clover, *et al.* 2001. Morvan's syndrome: peripheral and central nervous system and

cardiac involvement with antibodies to voltage-gated potassium channels. *Brain* **124**(Pt 12): 2417–2426.

19. Buckley, C., J. Oger, L. Clover, *et al.* 2001. Potassium channel antibodies in two patients with reversible limbic encephalitis. *Ann. Neurol.* **50**: 73–78.

20. Vincent, A., C. Buckley, J.M. Schott, *et al.* 2004. Potassium channel antibody-associated encephalopathy: a potentially immunotherapy-responsive form of limbic encephalitis. *Brain* **127**(Pt 3): 701–712.

21. Irani, S.R., S. Alexander, P. Waters, *et al.* 2010. Antibodies to Kv1 potassium channel-complex proteins leucine-rich, glioma inactivated 1 protein and contactin-associated protein-2 in limbic encephalitis, Morvan's syndrome and acquired neuromyotonia. *Brain* **133**: 2734–2748.

22. Lai, M., M.G. Huijbers, E. Lancaster, *et al.* 2010. Investigation of LGI1 as the antigen in limbic encephalitis previously attributed to potassium channels: a case series. *Lancet Neurol.* **9**: 776–785.

23. Irani, S.R., P. Pettingill, K.A. Kleopa, *et al.* 2012. Morvan syndrome: clinical and serological observations in 29 cases. *Ann. Neurol.* **72**: 241–255.

24. Irani, S.R., A.W. Michell, B. Lang, *et al.* 2011. Faciobrachial dystonic seizures precede Lgi1 antibody limbic encephalitis. *Ann. Neurol.* **69**: 892–900.

25. Spinazzi, M., V. Argentiero, L. Zuliani, *et al.* 2008. Immunotherapy-reversed compulsive, monoaminergic, circadian rhythm disorder in Morvan syndrome. *Neurology* **71**: 2008–2010.

26. Lennon, V.A., T.J. Kryzer, S.J. Pittock, *et al.* 2005. IgG marker of optic-spinal multiple sclerosis binds to the aquaporin-4 water channel. *J. Exp. Med.* **202**: 473–477.

27. Waters, P. & A. Vincent. 2008. Detection of anti-aquaporin-4 antibodies in neuromyelitis optica: current status of the assays. *Int. MS J.* **15**: 99–105.

28. Waters, P.J., A. McKeon, M.I. Leite, *et al.* 2012. Serologic diagnosis of NMO: a multicenter comparison of aquaporin-4-IgG assays. *Neurology* **78**: 665–671

29. Leite, M.I., E. Coutinho, M. Lana-Peixoto, *et al.* 2012. Myasthenia gravis and neuromyelitis optica spectrum disorder: a multicenter study of 16 patients. *Neurology* **78**: 1601–1607.

30. Jarius, S., F. Paul, D. Franciotta, *et al.* 2012. Neuromyelitis optica spectrum disorders in patients with myasthenia gravis: ten new aquaporin-4 antibody positive cases and a review of the literature. *Mult. Scler.* **18**: 1135–1143.

31. Waters, P., S. Jarius, E. Littleton, *et al.* 2008. Aquaporin-4 antibodies in neuromyelitis optica and longitudinally extensive transverse myelitis. *Arch. Neurol.* **65**: 913–919.

32. Jarius, S., F. Aboul-Enein, P. Waters, *et al.* 2008. Antibody to aquaporin-4 in the long-term course of neuromyelitis optica. *Brain* **131**(Pt 11): 3072–3080.

33. Hutchinson, M., P. Waters, J. McHugh, *et al.* 2008. Progressive encephalomyelitis, rigidity, and myoclonus: a novel glycine receptor antibody. *Neurology* **71**: 1291–1292.

34. Yang, L., S. Maxwell, M.I. Leite, *et al.* 2011. Non-radioactive serological diagnosis of myasthenia gravis and clinical features of patients from Tianjin, China. *J Neurol Sci.* **301**: 71–76.

Ann. N.Y. Acad. Sci. ISSN 0077-8923

The MG composite: an outcome measure for myasthenia gravis for use in clinical trials and everyday practice

Ted M. Burns

Department of Neurology, University of Virginia, Charlottesville, Virginia

Address for correspondence: Ted M. Burns, M.D., Department of Neurology, University of Virginia, PO Box 800394, Charlottesville, VA 22908. tmb8r@virginia.edu

The myasthenia gravis composite (MGC) was constructed by selecting the best performing items from three commonly used, MG-specific scales. The response categories of the items were subsequently weighted for importance. The MGC, which takes less than five minutes to complete, is made up of three ocular, three bulbar, one respiratory, one neck, and two limb items. After its construction, the MGC was validated in an 11-center scale validity study. During the validation study, which included test–retest analysis, it was determined that a 3-point improvement in MGC score reliably indicates clinical improvement. A 3-point improvement in MGC also appears to be meaningful to the patient. Rasch analysis of the MGC confirmed that all 10 items belong and can be summed to provide a total score, and that the weights given to the response categories of the items are appropriate.

Keywords: MG composite; myasthenia gravis; outcome measures; MGC; MG

Introduction

Myasthenia gravis (MG) is a chronic, autoimmune disorder of neuromuscular junction transmission that manifests with fluctuating, fatigable weakness.[1] Patients with MG may experience varying degrees of ptosis, diplopia, dysarthria, dysphagia, chewing weakness, respiratory weakness, facial weakness, and axial and limb weakness. Most of the outcome measures used in clinical trials for estimating disease status in MG have been multiple-item ordinal scales.[2–21] For example, the quantitative myasthenia gravis scale (QMG)[2,4,5,7,9,12] has been in use in clinical trials for over two decades and has performed well in this setting.[22–26] However, the QMG, like many other ordinal scales for MG, is rarely used in everyday practice because it takes approximately 20 min and requires equipment. Rather, in the everyday practice setting, clinicians largely rely on gestalt impressions of disease severity. At follow-up visits, the impression of change in disease status is often generated by comparisons of serial examinations and symptom severities. This practice has worked well for MG but has limitations, including (1) that any "snapshot" examination is limited by the fluc-tuating and fatigable nature of MG and the inability to observe chewing and swallowing weakness at the bedside and (2) that the impression generated from symptoms relies on imperfect physician and patient recall and review of descriptive narratives in the medical records. Also, patients are sometimes seen serially by different treating physicians. With these limitations in mind, user-friendly, MG-specific outcome measures may be able to play an important role in everyday practice because they may offer more reliability, precision, and scope, including estimates of the status of functional domains (e.g., ocular or bulbar subscores). Furthermore, as payers and policy makers increasingly insist on the demonstration of performance and "value" of care,[27,28] particularly for expensive treatments, such as intravenous immunoglobulin,[29] it seems likely that standardized, user-friendly outcome measures will play bigger roles in patient care, for example, by demonstrating efficacy of a treatment plan. It was with these thoughts in mind that the "MG composite" (MGC) scale was constructed to provide clinicians and investigators with a user-friendly ordinal scale for MG that could be used in both everyday practice and also clinical trials.[15]

doi: 10.1111/j.1749-6632.2012.06812.x

Table 1. MG composite scale

MG composite scale				
Ptosis, upward ease (physician examination)	>45 seconds = 0	11–45 seconds = 1	1–10 seconds = 2	Immediate = 3
Double vision on lateral gaze, left or right (physician examination)	>45 seconds = 0	11–45 seconds = 1	1-10 seconds = 3	Immediate = 4
Eye closure (physician examination)	Normal = 0	Mild weakness (can be forced open with effort) = 0	Moderate weakness (can be forced open easily) = 1	Severe weakness (unable to keep eyes closed) = 2
Talking (patient history)	Normal = 0	Intermittent slurring or nasal speech = 2	Constant slurring or nasal but can be understood = 4	Difficult to understand speech = 6
Chewing (patient history)	Normal = 0	Fatigue with solid food = 2	Fatigue with soft food = 4	Gastric tube = 6
Swallowing (patient history)	Normal = 0	Rare episode of choking or trouble swallowing = 2	Frequent trouble swallowing, for example, necessitating changes in diet = 5	Gastric tube = 6
Breathing (thought to be caused by MG)	Normal = 0	Shortness of breath with exertion = 2	Shortness of breath at rest = 4	Ventilator dependence = 9
Neck flexion or extension (weakest) (physician examination)	Normal = 0	Mild weakness = 1	Moderate weakness (i.e., ~50% weak, ±15%) = 3	Severe weakness = 4
Shoulder abduction (physician examination)	Normal = 0	Mild weakness = 2	Moderate weakness (i.e., ~50% weak, ±15%) = 4	Severe weakness = 5
Hip flexion (physician examination)	Normal = 0	Mild weakness = 2	Moderate weakness (i.e., ~50% weak, ±15%) = 4	Severe weakness = 5

NOTE: Please note that "moderate weakness" for neck and limb items should be construed as weakness that equals roughly 50% ± 15% of expected normal strength. Any weakness milder than that would be "mild," and any weakness more severe than that would be classified as "severe."

Selection of items for the MGC

To construct the MGC (Table 1), the best performing items from the QMG, MG-manual muscle test (MG-MMT),[10] and MG-activities of daily living (MG-ADL)[6,21] scales were selected for each of 10 functional domains (e.g., talking, breathing, and upper limb strength).[15] Item performance from these three scales was based on each item's performance during two randomized, controlled trials of

patients with seropositive, generalized MG.[23,24] Test item performance was judged by considering score distributions, item responsiveness, and correlations with a measure of quality of life. The items were selected by considering what both patients and physicians found important and meaningful. From the patient's perspective, items were selected if they correlated well with the MG-QOL15[18] and were responsive and concordant with the patient's global assessment of response at week 12 in the Aspreva trial.[23] From the physician's perspective, items were chosen if responsive and concordant with the physician's global assessment of response at week 12 in both trials. Furthermore, the physician perspective was important for choosing the functional domains, the number of items selected from each domain, and the weighting of the response categories of the 10 items. During the construction of the MGC, we were mindful to keep to a minimum the number of items in the scale so that our scale was user friendly and not a burden to patients and others. Minimizing the number of items also ensured that each individual item of the MGC was of substantial weight relative to the other items and the total score.

The MGC takes less than five minutes to complete (Table 1). It is made up of three ocular (if one classifies eye closure as ocular), three bulbar, one respiratory, one neck, and two limb items, and thus it differs from the QMG and MMT, which have a greater representation of upper and lower extremity strength items. Some of the items chosen came from the physician examination (MG-MMT, QMG) and others from the patient history (MG-ADL). The MGC differs from most scales in that it is a hybrid of physician-reported and patient-reported test items. This combination, however, is especially appropriate for an MG outcome measure for three major reasons: (1) MG manifests with fluctuating and fatigable symptoms and signs, which consequently limits the utility of measuring disease status solely based on a "snapshot" examination; (2) manifestations of MG are evident not only to the physician but also to the patient (and others), and thus patient-reported measures of symptoms must be considered in assessing disease severity; and (3) dysfunction in chewing and swallowing are almost certainly more evident to the patient than to the physician.[15]

Weighting of the response categories of the items of the MGC

The three rating scales (e.g., QMG) from which the MGC test items were selected use sequential integer scoring, 0–3 (or 0–4 for the MMT). Given that it is almost certain that some functional domains impaired by MG (e.g., talking) carry more weight than others (e.g., eyelid strength), we felt that another important step in constructing our MGC was to assign weighted scores to each response category of each item. The response categories of the ten items were weighted by querying 36 MG spe-

cialists from 10 countries with over 600 cumulative years experience caring for patients with MG. For the weighting step, MG specialists were asked to consider "quality-of-life, health risk, prognosis, estimated item validity and reliability, and any other factors you think are important" when assigning scores.[15] The weighting step resulted in an ordinal scale with items individually weighted to reflect their significance. We found confirmation of the appropriateness of weighting in the relatively tight standard deviations for the assigned weights and from modern psychometric analysis of the items of the MGC, performed through Rasch analysis, discussed later.

Validation of the MGC

Validity testing of the MGC was conducted in 2008–2009 at 11 neuromuscular centers (9 in the United States and 2 in Europe) during the routine care of adults with MG.[16] Before validation, the neck flexion test item of the original MGC was modified to include neck extension testing (worse score recorded). Also, after learning that <1% of ocular score times was between 46 and 60 seconds, the ocular test items were modified so that 45 seconds was the maximum duration of testing. One hundred seventy-five MG patients were enrolled at 11 sites and 151 patients were seen in follow-up. The mean age at visit 1 was 58 years, and the mean disease duration was seven years. Fifty-three percent were men and 47% were women. The mean time between visits 1 and 2 was 4.7 months. Breakdown by current MGFA Class at visit 1 was 22% class I, 41% class II, 19% class III, 3% class IV. Fifteen percent of patients were in remission (class 0) at visit 1. None were intubated and ventilated at visit 1, but 14.3% had experienced at least one prior episode of myasthenic crisis. Seventy-eight percent of patients were acetylcholine receptor antibody positive (AChR+), and 7% were muscle-specific tyrosine kinase–positive (MuSK+). Ten percent of patients had negative serology for at least AChR (often both AChR and MuSK). Serological status was unknown for 5%. Of the 175 subjects, 142 (82%) were follow-up outpatients, 23 (13%) were newly diagnosed, and 8 (5%) were hospitalized for MG at the time of the evaluation. A total of 110 of 175 (63%) patients were taking pyridostigmine at the time of their first visit.

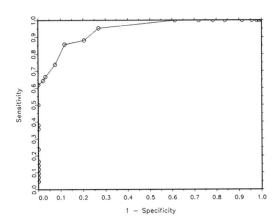

Figure 1. Receiver–operator characteristics (ROC) curve of the MGC, using physician impression of improvement plus improvement in MG-QOL15 score at visit 2 as the criterion of improvement. The area under the ROC curve is 0.94, suggesting high accuracy of the MGC.[16]

Table 2. Comparison of sensitivities and specificities of the MG-MMT, MG-ADL, and MGC

	Sensitivity	Specificity
MGC score change	($n = 42$)	($n = 93$)
−3	85.7	88.2
−2	88.1	79.6
−1	95.2	73.1
MG-MMT score change	($n = 23$)	($n = 48$)
−3	60.9	93.8
−2	82.6	83.3
−1	82.6	66.7
MG-ADL score change	($n = 23$)	($n = 51$)
−3	65.2	92.2
−2	78.3	82.4
−1	95.7	68.6

NOTE: Comparison of sensitivities and specificities of the MG-MMT, MG-ADL, and MGC at various cut-points, using physician impression of improvement plus improvement in MG-QOL15 score at visit 2 as the criterion of improvement, from the multicenter scale validity study. A 3-point improvement in the MGC appears to offer the best trade-off in terms of sensitivity and specificity, and compares favorably to the MG-MMT and MG-ADL.[16]

The total MGC scores showed excellent concurrent validity with other MG-specific scales.[16] At visit 1, the total MGC score had a correlation of 0.68 (95% CI: 0.59, 0.75) with the MG-QOL15 total, 0.85 (95% CI: 0.77, 0.90) with the MG-ADL total score, and 0.80 (95% CI: 0.72, 0.86) with the MG-MMT total score. Nearly identical correlations were observed at visit 2. The mean score of the MGC was 7.6 at visit 1 and 5.6 at visit 2. Figure 1 demonstrates the receiver–operator characteristics (ROC) curve for the MGC using the physician impression of improvement plus improvement in MG-QOL15 score (visit 2–visit 1) as the criterion for improvement, demonstrating high accuracy of the MGC. The QMG scale was not included in our scale validity study[16] because of the time it takes to complete and concern that this would hurt subject enrollment. Thus, correlations of the MGC and QMG do not exist for our scale validity cohort. However, in a larger, more recent study out of Japan, the Pearson correlation coefficient of the MGC and QMG was $r = 0.88$ ($P < 0.0001$) in 640 patients (see Ref. 30; and personal communication of preliminary data). In this Japanese cohort, the correlation of two-year changes in QMG and MGC was $r = 0.66$ ($P < 0.0001$). Bivariate regression analysis using both two-year changes in QMG and MGC as variables to determine the superiority of one compared to the other regarding the effects on changes in MG-QOL15-J demonstrated that MGC showed somewhat better results (coefficient, 0.3626; $P = 0.0034$) compared with QMG (0.3209; $P =$

0.0363) (personal communication of preliminary data).

Using the physician impression of improvement and improvement in the MG-QOL15 score as the gold standard for improvement in the scale validity study,[16] sensitivity and specificity were determined for many changes in score, after which it was felt that the trade-offs between sensitivity and specificity were most optimal at a 3-point cut-point. The sensitivities and specificities for the MGC compared favorably with the MG-ADL and MG-MMT (Table 2). In the subgroup of patients with initial MGC scores of 5 or more, the sensitivity of a 3-point change in MGC was 94.6% ($n = 42$) and the specificity was 80.0% ($n = 45$). In the group with initial MGC score of 7 or more, the sensitivity and specificity were 100% and 81%, respectively. Furthermore, 3-point improvement in the MGC appeared to be meaningful to the patient, as indicated by improved MG-QOL15 scores. Of the 49 patients with a ≥3 point improvement in the MGC score, the mean change in MG-QOL15 total score was −12.2 (SD = 11.4), compared to a mean MG-QOL15 change of −2.5 (SD = 8.7) among the 49 patients with a drop in the MGC of <3 points, and a mean MG-QOL15 change of +1.1 (SD = 8.8) points among the 37 patients whose MGC score increased (worsened) from visit 1 to visit 2. Test–retest reliability testing of the MGC also supports a 3-point cut-point to indicate change as acceptable. Test–retest reliability was performed on 38 patients at the University of Virginia by having the patient evaluated on the same day by two neurologists, each blinded to the other's findings. The MGC score never differed by more than 4 points between evaluators; it was within 3 points in 95%. The test–retest reliability coefficient was 98%, with a lower 95% confidence interval of 97%, indicative of excellent test–retest reliability. Score differences for individual test items were most frequent for ptosis (6/38) and double vision (6/38), followed by neck strength (3/38) testing.

Behavior of each item of the MGC relative to the other items and estimates of the item's relative contribution to the total score could not be determined by the conventional psychometric analyses discussed earlier. Moreover, the exact amount of change between ordinal response categories (i.e., 1, 2, 3...) could not be examined using these conventional methods. Thus, we carried out Rasch analysis to further interrogate the MGC.[31] As brief background, Rasch analysis allows for the investigation of how well items or questions combine to measure an ability or trait. The Rasch model compares item "difficulty" (e.g., probability the item on a scale was scored abnormal or normal) and person "ability" (e.g., disease severity) on a common logarithmic scale from the responses given to each item within a specific probabilistic framework. We applied Rasch analysis to the MGC in order to (1) identify misfitting items and examine their effects on unidimensionality of the MGC; (2) explore item difficulty and person ability range, knowing that an ideal outcome measure is expected to cover a larger ability range and as a result can differentiate between different levels of disability in a wider range of the disease; (3) investigate category response functioning and item weighting, expecting category responses (i.e., normal, mild weakness, etc.) of each item to be in the appropriate order with appropriate spacing; and (4) investigate the appropriateness of the weighted values for the response categories, as seen through the "lens" of the Rasch model. The results indicated that the ten items belong together and can be

summed for a total MGC score (Figure 2). One item, diplopia, demonstrated borderline misfitting. However, the effect of this in terms of the dimensionality of the MGC was very small and removal of this item from the MGC was thought to damage the content and clinical validity of the MGC. A second finding of the Rasch analysis was an overall absence of item order distortion between response categories (i.e., 1 is worse than 0, 2 is worse than 1, etc.) and relatively equal distances between category measures. The one minor exception for this characteristic was for the item "ptosis" where the severe response category ("immediate" ptosis) had similar values as the moderate category (ptosis after 1–10 seconds). This finding did not surprise us because our earlier test–retest reproducibility study of the MGC demonstrated that when disagreement occurred between two independent assessments, it was most often for the timed ocular items, including ptosis (6 of 38 assessments). The source of disagreement between the two examiners was occasionally a simple disagreement about an observation and at other times was related to the fatigable nature of the manifestations of MG (i.e., the examination changes). A third finding of our Rasch analysis was the similarity in weight assignments for the response categories of the items of the MGC, which was remarkable considering that the two methods employed to estimate weights were so different. For the Rasch analysis, the relationships between patient "ability" (i.e., disease severity) and item "difficulty" (i.e., the probability the item was scored abnormal or normal) were analyzed to calculate the weights of the response categories, whereas in our earlier assignment of weights, we asked 36 MG specialists to consider "quality-of-life, health risk, prognosis, estimated item validity and reliability, and any other factors you think are important" when assigning scores. It is worth mentioning that the weights for the "eye closure" category responses were quite different, but this turned out to be mostly an artifact of the unique assignment of values for "eye closure," with "normal" and "mild" weakness both assigned 0 points and the assignment of any points only occurring at moderate or severe eye closure weakness. A fourth finding of the Rasch analysis, observed from the item difficulty and polarity assessments of the items of the MGC, was the demonstration of moderate to large positive point-measure correlations of the item difficulties—with ability levels captured by these items. For patients

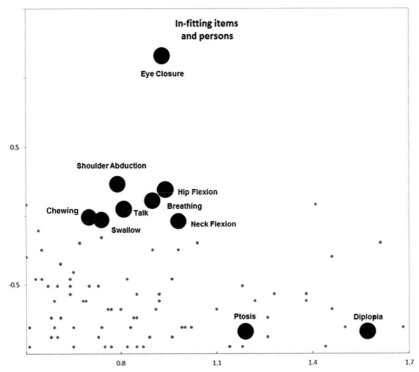

Figure 2. Summary of two different concepts of Rasch statistics in one graph: (1) Vertical axis: position of each MGC item (black circle) on vertical axis correlates with its relative "difficulty" for scoring item as abnormal for the MG patient cohort. Similarly, position of each patient (red dot) on the same axis correlates with degree of person "ability" (i.e., indicator of disease severity in MGC). Vertical axis units represent logarithmic probabilities. (2) Horizontal axis: position of each MGC item on horizontal axis represents the degree of correlation between MGC items and the outcome measure (known as "item fit"). Horizontal axis units represent χ^2 t-statistics values. Items closer to the meridian better "fit" a unidimensional scale. Overall, MGC items cover a good range of disease severity for symptomatic patients (vertical axis). No item measured a significantly different concept than what MGC measures as total (horizontal axis).[31]

not in remission, our analysis demonstrated that the MGC is able to differentiate different levels of disease severity.

Caveats

One criticism of the MGC has been that it does not assess neck or limb neuromuscular endurance/fatigue. Instead, the items for neck and limb strength, selected from the MG-MMT, involve more routine muscle strength testing. Whether this criticism reflects a limitation of the MGC is not entirely settled at this time and may warrant more study. At this time, what argues against inclusion of limb and neck endurance testing is the data from the Muscle Study Group trial of mycophenolate mofetil,[24] which indicated that strength assessments of limbs and neck from the MG-MMT performed better than their counterparts in the QMG scale that assess endurance.[16] For example, in the Muscle

Study Group trial of patients with mild to moderate generalized MG, of subjects with global improvement in MG at week 12, MG-MMT shoulder abduction improved >60% of the time compared to 25% for QMG arms outstretched. Also, subject global impression of change at week 12 was in the opposite direction of MG-MMT shoulder abduction 1.4% of the time versus 8.5% for the QMG arms outstretched. Similar findings were observed for lower extremity testing. Quality-of-life correlations also favored the MG-MMT items. In light of these data, combined with the subsequent psychometric analyses validating the items of the MGC, the substantial influence of subject effort and examiner encouragement on limb and neck endurance results and the ease of routine muscle testing compared to endurance testing, inclusion of the MG-MMT items seems to be appropriate and sufficient, although further study of this issue is welcomed. It is worth noting that endurance/fatigue are assessed for ocular and bulbar items of the MGC. One other caveat about the MGC is that the initial selection of items, which focused heavily on item responsiveness to clinical change, was based on data from a cohort of MG patients with mild or moderate, generalized disease. And while the validation process occurred in a cohort that included asymptomatic, ocular-only, and generalized MG patients of varying severity, it is worth remembering that the MGC has not been specifically validated for unique subgroups of MG patients, such as in ocular-only patients.

Discussion

The notable attributes of the MGC include that (1) the test items were rigorously selected through a process that assessed item performance during two randomized, controlled trials involving >250 generalized MG patients; (2) the MGC covers the 10 important functional domains most frequently affected by MG; (3) the proportion of bulbar and respiratory items to total number of items (4/10) is appropriate given the clinical importance of these domains; (4) the test items are appropriately weighted; (5) the MGC is easy to administer, taking less than five minutes to complete, without the need for any equipment; (6) it is easy to interpret, taking seconds to calculate a total score. Also, the assessment of each of the ten test items provides immediate insight into the status of that particular functional domain; (7) the MGC is reliable, as evidenced by the results of our test–retest assessment; (8) the MGC has been validated in a multicenter cohort of >150 patients; and (9) Rasch analysis of the MGC provides more modern psychometric validation of the scale and demonstrates that, among other things, the weighted item scores can be summed into a total score that reflects overall disease severity.

In 2012, a Task Force of the Medical Scientific Advisory Board (MSAB) of the Myasthenia Gravis Foundation of America (MGFA) recommended using the MGC as the quantitative measure for determining improvement and worsening for patients with generalized MG.[32] This recommendation was based on deliberations during and related to two consensus conferences, held in Durham, North Carolina, and Stresa, Italy, in 2010–2011. The MGC was favored by the Task Force over the QMG, for example, because the MGC is weighted for clinical significance and incorporates patient-reported outcomes. However, the Task Force encouraged future study of existing measures and development of new measures.

In summary, the MGC can be used in both everyday practice and in clinical trials. As it seems likely that user-friendly measures will play more important roles in everyday practice in the future, the MGC is well positioned to efficiently demonstrate outcomes of various treatments for patients with MG. For clinical trials, the MGC can be used as a quantitative measure of clinical status and of clinical change, with a 3-point improvement in MGC score reliably indicating clinical improvement. A 3-point improvement in MGC also appears to be meaningful to the patient, as evidenced by a mean improvement in MG-QOL15 score of >12 points for those patients who had a ≥3-point improvement in the MGC. It is encouraged that future study of the MGC be directed at improving its performance, possibly even through modification of the scale. It is also encouraged that future study eventually result in the development of a new, better measure. For now at least, its use in everyday practice and clinical trials is encouraged.

Acknowledgments

The author wants to acknowledge and thank his colleagues who helped develop and validate the MG Composite, especially Don Sanders, M.D., Mark Conaway, Ph.D., Reza Sadjadi, M.D., Gary Gutter, Ph.D., and others in the MG Composite and MG-QOL15 Study Group. He would also like to thank Professor Kimiaki Utsugisawa and his colleagues for their interesting work and for sharing some of their early results about the performance of the MGC in Japan.

Conflicts of interest

The author declares no conflicts of interest.

References

1. Meriggioli, M.N. & D.B. Sanders. 2009. Autoimmune myasthenia gravis: emerging clinical and biological heterogeneity. *Lancet Neurol.* **8:** 475–490.

2. Tindall, R.S.A., J.A. Rollins, J.T. Phillips, *et al.* 1987. Preliminary results of a double-blind, randomized, placebo-controlled trial of cyclosporine in myasthenia gravis. *N. Engl. J. Med.* **316:** 719–724.

3. Mantegazza, R., C. Antozzi, D. Pelucchetti, *et al.* 1988. Azathioprine as a single drug or in combination with steroids in the treatment of myasthenia gravis. *J. Neurol.* **235:** 449–453.

4. Tindall, R.S.A., J.T. Phillips, J.A. Rollins, *et al.* 1993. A clinical therapeutic trial of cyclosporine in myasthenia gravis. *Ann. N.Y. Acad. Sci.* **681:** 539–551.

5. Barohn, R.J., D. McIntire, L. Herbelin, *et al.* 1998. Reliability testing of the quantitative myasthenia gravis score. *Ann. N.Y. Acad. Sci.* **841:** 769–772.

6. Wolfe, G.I., L. Herbelin, S.P. Nations, *et al.* 1999. Myasthenia gravis activities of daily living profile. *Neurology* **52:** 1487–1489.

7. Jaretzki, A., R.J. Barohn, R.M. Ernstoff, *et al.*; for the Task Force of the Medical Scientific Advisory Board of the Myasthenia Gravis Foundation of America. 2000. Myasthenia gravis: recommendations for clinical research standards. *Neurology* **55:** 16–23.

8. Sharshar, T., S. Chevret, M. Mazighi, *et al.* 2000. Validity and reliability of two muscle strength scores commonly used as endpoints in assessing treatment of myasthenia gravis. *J. Neurol.* **247:** 286–290.

9. Barohn, R.J. 2003. Standards of measurement in myasthenia gravis. *Ann. N.Y. Acad. Sci.* **998:** 432–439.

10. Sanders, D.B., B. Tucker-Lipscomb & J.M. Massey. 2003. A simple manual muscle test for myasthenia gravis: validation and comparison with the QMG score. *Ann. N.Y. Acad. Sci.* **998:** 440–444.

11. Gajdos, P., T. Sharshar & S. Chevret. 2003. Standards of measurements in myasthenia gravis. *Ann. N.Y. Acad. Sci.* **998:** 445–452.

12. Bedlack, R.S., D.L. Simel, H. Bosworth, *et al.* 2005. Quantitative myasthenia gravis score: assessment of responsiveness and longitudinal validity. *Neurology* **64:** 1968–1970.

13. Padua, L., G. Galassi, A. Ariatti, *et al.* 2005. Myasthenia gravis self-administered questionnaire: development of regional domains. *Neurol. Sci.* **25:** 331–336.

14. Farrugia, M.E., M.D. Robson, L. Clover, *et al.* 2006. MRI and clinical studies of facial and bulbar muscle involvement in MuSK antibody-associated myasthenia gravis. *Brain* **129:** 1481–1492.

15. Burns, T.M., M.R. Conaway, G.R. Cutter & D.B. Sanders. 2008. The construction of an efficient evaluative instrument for myasthenia gravis: the MG Composite. *Muscle Nerve* **38:** 1553–1562.

16. Burns, T.M., M.R. Conaway, D.B. Sanders, *et al.* 2010. The MG composite: a valid and reliable tool for myasthenia gravis. *Neurology* **74:** 1434–1440.

17. Burns, T.M. 2010. A history of outcome measures in myasthenia gravis. *Muscle Nerve* **42:** 5–13.

18. Burns, T.M., C.K. Grouse, M.R. Conaway, *et al.* 2010. Construct and concurrent validation of the MG-QOL15 in the practice setting. *Muscle Nerve* **41:** 219–226.

19. Farrugia, M.E., H. Harle, C. Carmichael & T.M. Burns 2011. The oculobulbar facial respiratory score is a tool to assess bulbar function in myasthenia gravis patients. *Muscle Nerve* **43:** 329–334.

20. Burns, T.M., C.K. Grouse, M.R. Conaway, *et al.* 2011. The MG-QOL15 for following the health-related quality of life for patients with myasthenia gravis. *Muscle Nerve* **43:** 14–18.

21. Muppidi, S., G.I. Wolfe, M. Conaway, *et al.* 2011. MG-ADL: still a relevant outcome measure. *Muscle Nerve* **44:** 721–731.

22. Zinman, L. & V. Bril. 2008. IVIG treatment for myasthenia gravis. Effectiveness, limitations, and novel therapeutic strategies. *Ann. N.Y. Acad. Sci.* **1132:** 264–270.

23. Sanders, D.B., I.K. Hart, R. Mantegazza, *et al.* 2008. An international, phase III, randomized trial of mycophenolate mofetil in myasthenia gravis. *Neurology* **71:** 400–406.

24. Muscle Study Group. 2008. A trial of mycophenolate mofetil with prednisone as initial immunotherapy in myasthenia gravis. *Neurology* **71:** 394–399.

25. Wolfe, G.I., R.J. Barohn, D.B. Sanders, *et al.* 2008. Comparison of outcome measures from a trial of mycophenolate mofetil in myasthenia gravis. *Muscle Nerve* **38:** 1429–1433.

26. Barth, D., M. Nabavi Nouri, E. Ng, *et al.* 2011. Comparison of IVIg and PLEX in patients with myasthenia gravis. *Neurology* **76:** 2017–2023.

27. Tompkins, C.P., A.R. Higgins & G.A. Ritter. 2009. Measuring outcomes and efficiency in medicare value-based purchasing. *Health Affairs* **28:** w251–w261.

28. Miller, T.P., T.A. Brennan & A. Milstein 2009. How can we make more progress in measuring physicians' performance to improve the value of care? *Health Affairs* **28:** 1429–1437.

29. Guptill, J.T., B.K. Sharma, A. Marano, *et al.* 2012. Estimated cost of treating myasthenia gravis in an insured U.S. population. *Muscle Nerve* **45:** 363–366.

30. Matsuda, M., K. Utsugisawa, S. Sukuki, *et al.* 2012. The MG-QOL15 Japanese version: validation and associations with clinical factors. *Muscle Nerve* **46:** 166–173.

31. Sadjadi, R., M. Conaway, G.R. Cutter, *et al.* 2012. Psychometric evaluation of the MG Composite using Rasch analysis. *Muscle Nerve* **45:** 820–825.

32. Benatar, M., D.B. Sanders, T.M. Burns, *et al.* 2012. Recommendations for myasthenia gravis clinical trials. *Muscle Nerve* **45:** 909–917.

Ann. N.Y. Acad. Sci. ISSN 0077-8923

ANNALS OF THE NEW YORK ACADEMY OF SCIENCES
Issue: *Myasthenia Gravis and Related Disorders*

Patient registries: useful tools for clinical research in myasthenia gravis

Fulvio Baggi,[1] Renato Mantegazza,[1] Carlo Antozzi,[1] and Donald Sanders[2]

[1]Istituto Neurologico Carlo Besta, Milan, Italy. [2]Duke University Medical Center, Durham, North Carolina

Address for correspondence: Fulvio Baggi, Neurologia IV, Istituto Neurologico Carlo Besta, via Celoria 11, Milan 20133, Italy. baggi@istituto-besta.it

Clinical registries may facilitate research on myasthenia gravis (MG) in several ways: as a source of demographic, clinical, biological, and immunological data on large numbers of patients with this rare disease; as a source of referrals for clinical trials; and by allowing rapid identification of MG patients with specific features. Physician-derived registries have the added advantage of incorporating diagnostic and treatment data that may allow comparison of outcomes from different therapeutic approaches, which can be supplemented with patient self-reported data. We report the demographic analysis of MG patients in two large physician-derived registries, the Duke MG Patient Registry, at the Duke University Medical Center, and the INNCB MG Registry, at the Istituto Neurologico Carlo Besta, as a preliminary study to assess the consistency of the two data sets. These registries share a common structure, with an inner core of common data elements (CDE) that facilitate data analysis. The CDEs are concordant with the MG-specific CDEs developed under the National Institute of Neurological Disorders and Stroke Common Data Elements Project.

Keywords: myasthenia gravis; patient registries; common data elements; clinical trial

Introduction

Patient registries are based on clinical information collected in a systematic way and regularly updated. Patient registries should be of mutual value to both patients and clinicians. Selected information may also be retrieved by a health system for public health reporting, geographic surveys, budgeting, and epidemiological studies.[1] Patient registries are essential in clinical research for evaluating patient outcomes. To achieve this goal, they should be based primarily on clinical data collected from observations on a selected population. Moreover, registries can facilitate the management of patients, especially if they are available electronically. This requires that they are designed, developed, and implemented in collaboration between clinicians and the hospital IT service. Data entry is usually performed by the clinician or by trained nurses or residents, collecting detailed longitudinal clinical information from in and outpatients. The clinical, biological, and immunological information that can be collected in registries over several decades is particularly useful in the design and development of clinical trials. Moreover, by analyzing disease progression and responses to different treatment strategies, registries can uniquely provide comparative data for the epidemiological analysis of a disease that may improve its outcome.

In this article we report our analysis of two large physician-derived patient registries, the Duke Myasthenia Gravis (MG) Patient Registry (Durham, NC) and the Istituto Neurologico Carlo Besta (INNCB) MG Registry (Milan, Italy), which together, as of March 2012, have collected information on more than 2,700 MG patients. As a preliminary analysis, we assessed the consistency of the collected data and report the demographic characterization and clinical classification of MG at entry for the two MG populations.

The Duke MG Patient Registry

Since 1980, data on all patients who have been seen in the myasthenia gravis clinic at Duke University Medical Center have been stored in the Duke

doi: 10.1111/j.1749-6632.2012.06771.x

MG Patient Registry. Approximately 60 new patients with MG, congenital myasthenic syndromes, or Lambert–Eaton myasthenic syndrome (LEMS) are seen in this clinic each year, and patients with these diseases make approximately 550 clinic visits per year. In 2002, this database was approved by the Duke Institutional Review Board as a research registry, the MG Data Registry. Patients give signed consent to have their clinical information stored in the registry, which is maintained in accordance with institutional research requirements and U.S. standards to protect personal health information as established by the Health Information Portability and Accountability Act (HIPAA).

Different classification and disease severity scales have been used since 1980; the following scales are currently used: MGFA Clinical Class and Post-Intervention Status,[2] MG-Manual Muscle Testing,[3] and MG-Composite.[4]

At each visit, a report is printed and information in the registry is updated—this provides incentive to the physicians to keep the registry information accurate and updated. As of March 2012, the registry contained information on 1,545 patients with neuromuscular disease: 1,310 with confirmed MG, 110 with Lambert–Eaton myasthenic syndrome, 20 with congenital myasthenia, and 105 with possible or probable MG. Sixteen percent of males and 22.5% of females were African American.

The INNCB MG Patient Registry

A registry for MG patients was developed in 1986, and only MG cases have been included. As of March 2012, the INNCB MG Registry contained information on 1,204 MG patients and 7,571 clinic visits. Mean follow-up time of the MG patients was 5.2 years (range 0.2–29.6 years). Geographic lo-

calization (actual residence) of the patients was as follows: north Italy, 72.8%; center Italy, 8.9%; and south Italy, 18.3%. MG patients living in the Lombardy region constituted 44.4%. Almost all patients (98.2%) were of Caucasian origin. The INNCB MG registry has been adapted over time in order to include different MG classifications and evaluation protocols: the Osserman classification,[5] the INNCB MG clinical scale,[6] the Myasthenia Gravis Foundation of America (MGFA) clinical classification (since 2000),[2] and the MG Composite scale (since 2011).[4,7] The INNCB-MG Patient Registry is kept according to INNCB personal data protection procedures, and in agreement with the Italian laws.

Comparison of the MG patient registries

Both registries are longitudinal, thus enabling assessment of clinical status of each patient over time. Analysis of the databases' structures revealed that 95/167 data elements are unique for the Duke MG Registry, 90/162 data elements are unique for the INNCB MG Registry, and 72 data elements are common to both. All analyses have been performed on anonymized data sets, and independently by the two centers.

By merging the two databases, clinical information was obtained on more than 2,500 MG patients, of whom 2,305 had sufficient data for demographic analysis. Some patients from both clinics (8.3%) were excluded because of missing data (e.g., dates of birth or of disease onset were incomplete, or MGFA classification was reported only as II or III or IV, without subclassification).

Clinical characteristics of the two MG populations are reported in Table 1, in which MG patients have been grouped on the basis of antibody serology and the presence of thymoma. The main difference

Table 1. Clinical characteristics of the MG populations in the Duke and INNCB MG clinics, grouped by antibody serology and the presence of thymoma

	Duke		INNCB	
	N° (%)	F:M	N° (%)	F:M
MG patients	1300 (100%)	0.94	1005 (100%)	1.88
AChR-ab positive, without thymoma	806 (62.0%)	0.93	603 (60.0%)	1.91
AChR-ab negative	354 (27.2%)	1.30	177 (17.6%)	2.93
MuSK-ab positive	41 (3.2%)	9.25	55 (5.5%)	4.00
Thymomatous MG	99 (7.6%)	1.02	170 (16.9%)	1.05

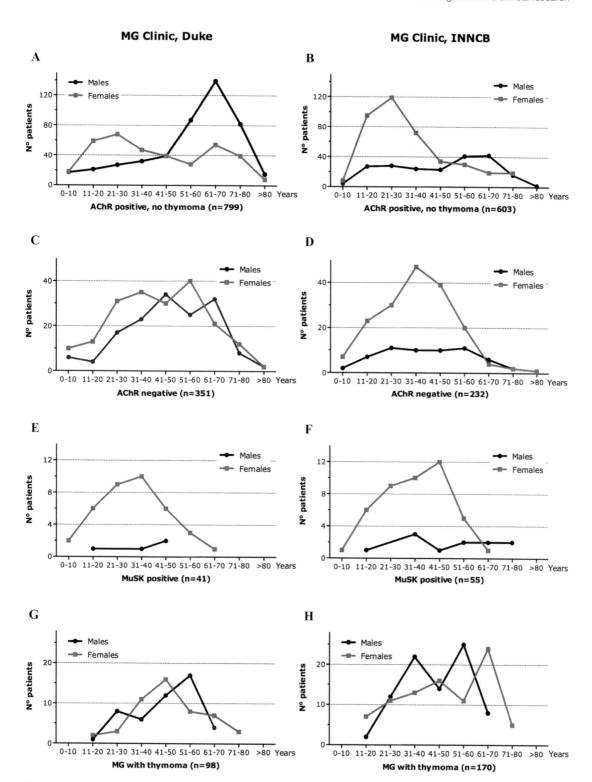

Figure 1. The age of symptom onset among female (gray line) and male (black line) MG patients seen in the MG clinic at Duke (panels A, C, E, G) and INNCB (panels B, D, E, H). Patients are grouped according to the following clinical subgroups: AChR-ab positive (A, B), AChR-ab negative (C, D), MuSK-ab positive (E, F), and thymomatous MG (G, H).

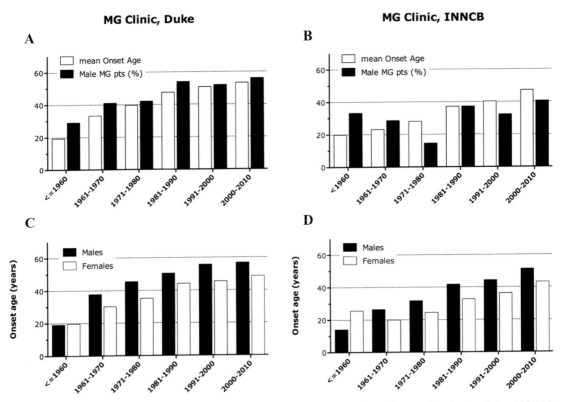

Figure 2. MG patients (Duke MG clinic, panels A and B; INNCB MG clinic, panels B, D) grouped by the decade in which MG symptoms began. The mean age at onset (empty bars) and the percentage of affected males (black bars) are shown in panels A and B. Mean ages at onset for females (empty bars) and males (black bars) are shown in panels C and D.

was in the female:male (F:M) ratios, which were 1.88 for INNCB MG patients and 0.94 for the Duke MG patients. Women predominated in the INNCB acetylcholine receptor antibody (AChR-ab) positive (F:M = 1.91) and AChR-ab negative (F:M = 2.93) patients. On the contrary, the F:M ratio was 9.25 in the Duke MuSK antibody (MuSK-ab) positive patients and 4.0 for the same group seen at the INNCB Clinic. F:M ratios were almost identical in thymomatous MG patients (1.02, Duke and 1.05, INNCB); it should be noted that the frequency of thymomatous MG was higher in the INNCB MG population (16.9%) compared with 7.6% at Duke.

Age at onset of MG symptoms in females and in males is shown in Figure 1. Data are presented for the following MG subclasses: AChR-ab positive (panels A and B), AChR-ab negative (panels C and D), MuSK-ab positive (panels E and F), and thymomatous MG (panels G and H). There were no differences in the onset age distribution of thymomatous (Fig. 1G and H) or MuSK-ab MG (Fig. 1E

and F) seen at the two clinics: in the latter group, females predominated with a peak incidence in the fourth and fifth decades in both populations. On the other hand, the distribution of onset age of AChR-ab negative MG differed between the two populations (Fig. 1C and D), with a marked female peak at 31–40 years in the INNCB cohort only, while no differences related to gender were seen in the Duke cohort. A more striking difference was seen in the distribution of onset age for AChR-ab–positive MG patients (Fig. 1A and B), where males predominated in the Duke cohort (peak incidence 61–70 years) and females in the INNCB cohort (peak incidence at 21–30 years). The total number of males with disease onset between the ages of 51 and 70 were 308 (Duke) and 99 (INNCB), while the number of females with onset between 11 and 40 years were 174 (Duke) and 286 (INNCB).

However, the distribution of the onset of MG symptoms in AChR-ab-positive patients without thymoma followed the classic pattern in both

Table 2. Clinical manifestations of disease at the initial visit to the Duke and INNCB MG clinics, grouped by the MGFA classification

	MG classification	Duke N° (%)	INNCB N° (%)
	MGFA-I	239 (26.5%)	145 (14.4%)
Mild	MGFA-IIA	262 (29.1%)	336 (33.4%)
	MGFA-IIB	43 (4.8%)	298 (29.7%)
Moderate	MGFA-IIIA	21(2.3%)	80 (8.0%)
	MGFA-IIIB	199 (22.1%)	25 (2.5%)
Severe	MGFA-IVA	68 (7.5%)	9 (0.9%)
	MGFA-IVB	20 (2.2%)	10 (1.0%)
	MGFA-V	14 (1.6%)	32 (3.2%)
	PR-CSR	35 (3.9%)	70 (7.0%)
		N = 901	N = 1005
Ocular signs (MGFA-I)		239 (26.5%)	145 (14.4%)
Limb or axial muscles (sum of MGFA IIA+IIIA+IVA)		351 (39.0%)	425 (42.3%)
Oropharyngeal or respiratory muscles (sum of MGFA IIB+IIIB+IVB)		262 (29.1%)	333 (33.1%)

populations, with most women developing MG in the third decade, and men in the sixth/seventh decades.

Figure 2 shows the mean age at onset of MG symptoms and the percentage of affected MG males, calculated for each decade in which symptoms began, from before 1960 to 2010, for the Duke and INNCB MG clinics. A progressive increase in the mean onset age can be seen in both cohorts, starting from a mean age of 20 years for patients that showed MG symptoms before 1960 and reaching a mean of 50 years in 2000–2010. The percentage of males in the Duke cohort (Fig. 2A) increased from 30% to 52% during the interval before 1960 until 1981–1990, and has remained relatively stable thereafter. On the contrary, in the INNCB the percentage of males was relatively stable at 30%–40% over the decades (Fig. 2B), except for an unexpected drop between 1971 and 1980. The mean onset age for males and females are shown in Figure 2C and D; mean onset age for males was almost always greater than that of females.

The clinical manifestations of disease at the initial MG Clinic visit are shown in Table 2, and the relative frequencies are depicted in Supporting Figure S1. MG was classified according to the MGFA recommendations;[2] these data were available for 901 Duke patients and 1,005 INNCB patients.

Major differences were observed in the percentages of patients with oropharyngeal or respiratory muscles involvement: patients with mild disease with predominant bulbar manifestations (MGFA-IIB) were 4.7% (Duke) compared with 29.7% (INNCB), while those with moderate disease with predominant bulbar manifestations (MGFA-IIIB) were 22.1% (Duke) compared with 2.5% (INNCB).

Similar differences were seen for patients with predominant limb or axial muscle involvement: 2.3% of patients were classified as MGFA-IIIA at Duke and 8.0% at INNCB, while 7.5% were classified as MGFA-IVA at Duke and 0.9% at INNCB.

However, the total number of patients classified as having predominant limb or axial muscle involvement (MGFAIIA + IIIA + IVA) and of patients having predominantly oropharyngeal or respiratory muscle weakness (MGFAIIB + IIIB + IVB) was similar in the two cohorts. This suggests that the severity distinctions within the A and B subcategories of the MGFA clinical classification are probably inherently too subjective to be precise, in that some evaluators would consider that even mild bulbar weakness would raise the numeric level (e.g., from IIB to IIIA).

As recently pointed out by the Myasthenia Gravis Task Force,[8] patient registries could significantly improve our knowledge of MG. Indeed, proper data mining and analysis of large MG registries currently in use in several centers should help to develop and validate outcome measures, obtain preliminary data to justify future clinical trials, and provide data for realistic sample size calculations during the planning stages of clinical trials on specific MG sub-populations.

In order to increase the efficiency of MG registries, a common language must be adopted in the design or reshape of existing databases, to assure collection of data in a standardized format that permits ready analysis. The multitude of data formats in use create barriers to data sharing, which would require extensive reformatting. The NINDS of the National Institute of Health has recently completed a project to identify common data elements (CDEs) for neuromuscular diseases, including MG. This project defines uniform formats by which data for different disorders will be collected, analyzed, and shared across the research community. The results and the MG specific CDEs are available on the NINDS web site: www.commondataelements.ninds.nih.gov.

The use of a common language in the Duke and the INNCB MG registries, even though on only a subset of the data elements in each database (72 out of 160), allowed us to perform the study presented in this report. The two MG registries are hospital based, and neither cohort fully represents the entire regional or even national MG population. The assessment of MG prevalence and incidence requires nation-wide epidemiological studies that can collect clinical data, via a multicentric collaboration, from the largest population of patients; these studies do not detect differences in the cohorts of patients coming from different MG referring centers.

The demographic analysis of the Duke and INNCB MG cohorts identified several differences with respect to the different MG subcategories. Among other factors, these differences might be related to referral patterns that are affected by geographical location and specific expertise that attracts patents to these centers.

The differences we observed in MG disease severity classification by the MGFA classification at first visit suggests that this classification system is limited by intrinsic subjective bias by MG evaluators, and hence may be inadequate to categorize MG subpopulations. Standardized quantitative scales and refined CDEs should be adopted in order to classify patients, and to allow consistent assessments and further comparison among MG cohorts.

In conclusion, although the comparison of MG registries might be hampered by several drawbacks

(language, MG classification and scoring systems, missing information, and quality and consistency of the collected data), it can provide basic epidemiological information highlighting distinctive and cohort-specific features that might affect future analyses, such as the disease severity at maximal worsening, at the last observation, or the postintervention status. Moreover, the comparison of two patient registries from different countries underlines the importance of further research on the use of common tools of clinical classification and evaluation in order to achieve the best possible agreement and accuracy in data collection.

Physician-derived patient registries have the advantage of incorporating diagnostic and treatment data that can be supplemented with patient self-reported data. Hopefully, the overall end value of MG Registries would be an easy and rapid comparison of outcomes in order to identify optimal treatment approaches for MG subgroups.

Acknowledgments

The authors thank Janice M. Massey, Vern C. Juel, Lisa Hobson-Webb, Edward C. Smith, and Jeffrey T. Guptill at Duke University, and Ferdinando Cornelio, Paolo Confalonieri, Lucia Morandi, Lorenzo Maggi, Giorgia Camera at Istituto Neurologico Carlo Besta, Milan, who have generously shared their patients' clinical information.

Supporting Information

Additional supporting information may be found in the online version of this article.

Figure S1. Distribution of MG findings at first visit, according to the MGFA clinical classifications[2] are shown for the Duke (left) and INNCB (right) patients. See also Table 2.

Conflicts of interest

The authors declare no conflicts of interest.

References

1. Gliklich, R.E. & N.A. Dreyer, eds. 2010. *Registries for Evaluating Patient Outcomes: A User's Guide.* 2nd ed. (Prepared by Outcome DEcIDE Center [Outcome Sciences, Inc. d/b/a Outcome] under Contract No. HHSA29020050035I TO3.) AHRQ Publication No.10-EHC049. Agency for Healthcare Research and Quality. Rockville, MD.

2. Jaretzki, A. 3rd *et al.* 2000. Myasthenia gravis: recommendations for clinical research standards. Task Force of the Medical

Scientific Advisory Board of the Myasthenia Gravis Foundation of America. *Neurology* **55:** 16–23.

3. Sanders, D.B., B. Tucker-Lipscomb & J.M. Massey. 2003. A simple manual muscle test for myasthenia gravis: validation and comparison with the QMG score. *Ann. N.Y. Acad. Sci.* **998:** 440–444.

4. Burns, T.M. *et al.* 2010. The MG composite: a valid and reliable outcome measure for myasthenia gravis. *Neurology* **74:** 1434–1440.

5. Osserman, K.E. & G. Genkins. 1971. Studies in myasthenia gravis: review of a twenty-year experience in over 1200 patients. *Mt. Sinai J. Med.* **38:** 497–537.

6. Mantegazza, R. *et al.* 1988. Azathioprine as a single drug or in combination with steroids in the treatment of myasthenia gravis. *J. Neurol.* **235:** 449–453.

7. Burns, T.M. *et al.* 2008. Construction of an efficient evaluative instrument for myasthenia gravis: the MG composite. *Muscle Nerve* **38:** 1553–1562.

8. Benatar, M. *et al.* 2012. Recommendations for myasthenia gravis clinical trials. *Muscle Nerve* **45:** 909–917.

Ann. N.Y. Acad. Sci. ISSN 0077-8923

ANNALS OF THE NEW YORK ACADEMY OF SCIENCES

Issue: *Myasthenia Gravis and Related Disorders*

The Myasthenia Gravis-Specific Activities of Daily Living Profile

Srikanth Muppidi

Department of Neurology and Neurotherapeutics, University of Texas Southwestern Medical Center, Dallas Texas

Address for correspondence: Srikanth Muppidi, M.D., UT Southwestern Medical Center, 5323 Harry Hines Blvd., Dallas, TX 75390-9036. Srikanth.muppidi@utsouthwestern.edu

The myasthenia gravis activities of daily living (MG-ADL) profile is an eight-item patient-reported scale developed to assess MG symptoms and their effects on daily activities. The MG-ADL profile correlated well with the Quantitative MG (QMG) score ($r = 0.58$, $P < 0.001$) in 254 consecutive patient visits. Further analysis during clinical trials confirmed the excellent correlation with the QMG test and provided additional evidence that the MG-ADL profile is responsive to clinical improvement. MG-ADL performance was further analyzed during a recent multicenter, prospective scale validation study for two new outcome measures. At the first visit, there was a strong positive correlation between the MG-ADL and the MG Composite ($r = 0.85$, $P < 0.0001$) and between the MG-ADL and the MG-Quality of life15 (MG-QOL15) ($r = 0.76$, $P < 0.0001$). Test–retest analysis demonstrated a high reliability coefficient. Sensitivity/specificity analysis revealed that a 2-point improvement has the best trade-off attributes to predict clinical improvement. The MG-ADL profile also performed well on Rasch analysis. The MG-ADL scoring system is useful as a secondary outcome measure and in routine clinical management.

Keywords: myasthenia gravis outcome measures; MG-ADL; MG Composite; MG QOL15

Introduction

Outcome measures when developed for various diseases are tested for multiple psychometric properties. Routine psychometric analysis of outcome measures includes validity (construct and concurrent), test–retest reliability, and responsiveness of the outcome measure to change, in addition to sensitivity and specificity analysis. Recently, advanced psychometric analysis such as Rasch analysis is also performed. Ideally, various psychometric properties of an outcome measure should be assessed before it is adopted into clinical practice or is used as an outcome measure in therapeutic trials since using a nonvalid or unreliable measure could potentially affect the outcome of the clinical trial or, in worst-case scenario, lead to incorrect conclusions about the drug or treatment effect. However, occasionally an outcome measure, in this case the myasthenia gravis-specific activities of daily living (MG-ADL) scoring system, might be adopted into clinical practice and research studies well before it is extensively studied and yet ultimately perform well on subsequent psychometric evaluation. In this review, we will address the initial creation of the MG-ADL profile, psychometric evaluation of the MG-ADL profile, and its use in research and clinical practice.

Over the last two decades, numerous MG outcome measures have been studied.[1] These vary in terms of time taken to complete, ease of use, and finally, whether a physician or patient completes them. Some outcome measures such as the Quantitative MG (QMG) score[2] will also require specialized equipment and training. The MG-ADL profile was developed in the late 1990s since there were no other outcome measures at that time that would reflect the effect of MG-related disability on patient's activities of daily living.[3] At that time, the QMG test was considered the gold standard and was routinely used as a primary outcome measure in MG clinical trials. The MG-ADL profile was partially derived from the QMG test, a 13-item linearly scored scale. The MG-ADL profile is an 8-item scale, with linear scoring from 0 to 3. The range of total MG-ADL score is

doi: 10.1111/j.1749-6632.2012.06817.x

Ann. N.Y. Acad. Sci. 1274 (2012) 114–119 © 2012 New York Academy of Sciences.

Table 1. MG activities of the daily living scale

Items	Grade 0	Grade 1	Grade 2	Grade 3	Score (0,1,2,3)
1. Talking	Normal	Intermittent slurring of nasal speech	Constant slurring or nasal, but can be understood	Difficult to understand speech	
2. Chewing	Normal	Fatigue with solid food	Fatigue with soft food	Gastric tube	
3. Swallowing	Normal	Rare episode of choking	Frequent choking necessitating changes in diet	Gastric Tube	
4. Breathing	Normal	Shortness of breath with exertion	Shortness of breath at rest	Ventilator dependence	
5. Impairment of ability to brush teeth or comb hair	None	Extra effort, but no rest periods needed	Rest periods needed	Cannot do one of these functions	
6. Impairment of ability to arise from a chair	None	Mild, sometimes uses arms	Moderate, always uses arms	Severe, requires assistance	
7. Double vision	None	Occurs, but not daily	Daily, but not constant	Constant	
8. Eyelid droop	None	Occurs, but not daily	Daily, but not constant	Constant	
				Total MG-ADL SCORE (items 1–8)	

0–24. Completing the MG-ADL usually takes less than five minutes and is entirely reported by the patient. The eight items of the MG-ADL aim to assess disability secondary to ocular (2 items), bulbar (3 items), respiratory (1 item), and limb (2 items)-related effects from myasthenia gravis. There are no items to assess the disability from pure axial weakness such as neck extension weakness (See Table 1).

Initial MG-ADL analysis

Initial analysis of the MG-ADL was conducted at a single center.[3] Patients with MG were prospectively evaluated for this study. The study included 254 unique evaluations (156 patients, 90 were women), in patients with confirmed diagnosis of myasthenia gravis irrespective of clinical severity of MG. A single examiner performed a QMG test and asked the patient to complete the MG-ADL questions. The mean MG-ADL score was 4.80 ($\pm$3.63) with a range of 0–18. The mean QMG score was 10.80 ($\pm$5.70) with a range of 0–27. The Pearson correlation coefficient was 0.583 ($P < 0.001$). Authors correctly concluded that the MG-ADL was an easy to administer outcome measure and that the MG-ADL profile correlates well with QMG scores. Based on the above findings, the authors suggested that the MG-ADL profile may be used as a secondary endpoint in clinical trials in MG and because it does not require any specialized equipment could be easily adopted into routine clinical practice.

Enthusiastic adoption of the MG-ADL profile

After the above initial analysis, because of the ease of use and lack of similar MG outcome measures, the MG-ADL profile was used as a tool in both routine patient care and as an outcome measure in research studies. In the early 2000s, the MG-ADL was used as a secondary outcome measure in multiple therapeutic clinical trials evaluating the benefit of etanercept,[4] IVIG,[5] and tacrolimus.[6–8] Improvements in MG-ADL scores in these studies mirrored improvements in QMG scores.

Further analysis of the MG-ADL profile

Even though the MG-ADL continued to be used in clinical practice and in various clinical trials as a secondary outcome measure, further psychometric testing was not performed until the mycophenolate mofetil (MMF) clinical trials.[9,10] One of these prospective randomized placebo-controlled studies completed by the Muscle Study Group[10] evaluated the effectiveness of MMF and prednisone as initial therapy in MG. The study was double blinded for the first 12 weeks followed by an open-label extension phase for 36 weeks. Eighty patients were randomized to either MMF or placebo in addition to 20 mg of prednisone. The primary outcome measure was the improvement in QMG scores at 12 weeks. The MG-ADL and MG manual muscle tests (MG-MMT) were secondary outcome measures. Importantly, MG-ADL and MG-MMT scores were not available to the QMG scorers and physicians who would assess global impression of change in patients and this allowed for unbiased evaluation of psychometric properties of the MG-ADL test. During the study period, patients in both groups improved, and there was no significant difference between the two treatment arms in this study, but a subset of patients had significant improvement. This provided an opportunity to assess one of the key psychometric properties: the responsiveness of the MG-ADL to clinically significant improvement in MG status.[11]

Similar to initial analysis, MG-ADL scores correlated well with QMG scores at baseline and throughout the double blind study period of 12 weeks. The correlation coefficients ranged from 0.51 to 0.65 ($P < 0.0001$). Correlation of the change in QMG and MG-ADL scores was also good, 0.55 at 12 weeks and 0.44 at 36 weeks ($P < 0.001$). Since a subset of patients improved significantly, responsiveness of the MG-ADL to change in clinical status was analyzed. This revealed a mean change of 3.66 points at 12 weeks and 5.48 at 36 weeks. The effect size was 1.16 at 12 weeks and 1.59 at 36 weeks. Interestingly, in this study MG-ADL scores were more sensitive to change in clinical status than were QMG scores.[11] Finally, the most important finding was that im-

provement in MG-ADL score was incremental. Patients with significant improvement had greater decrease in their MG-ADL score than those with mild improvement or no improvement. There was no significant change in MG-ADL scores in patients who did not improve at 12 weeks. MG-ADL scores improved by 3.29 at 12 weeks in patients with improvement on global assessment of MG and by 4.83 in patients with marked improvement on global assessment of MG. This analysis provided clear evidence that the MG-ADL test was sensitive to clinical change in MG status and reinforced continued usage of the MG-ADL profile in clinical practice and in research studies.

The final assessment of MG-ADL came with a multicenter study of two new MG outcome scales, the MG Composite (MGC)[12] and the MG-Quality of life15 (MG-QOL15).[13] Eleven centers participated in the multicenter validation studies for the MGC and the MG-QOL15, and out of these five centers also simultaneously assessed the MG-ADL. This provided a unique opportunity to perform validity and reliability testing of the MG-ADL profile. Unlike previous therapeutic trials with narrow inclusion criteria, all patients with confirmed MG seen in routine clinical practice were recruited and this allowed us to assess the MG-ADL as an outcome measure in clinical practice. Patients with MG seen in clinics or hospitals had baseline evaluation of MGC, MG-QOL15, and MG-ADL scores at the first visit and again within six months. Eighty-seven patients completed the MG-ADL profile on the first visit and 76 returned for second visit.[14] Most patients had some improvement in MG-ADL scores between visits. Correlation of MG-ADL and MGC scores was robust during the first ($r = 0.846$, $P < 0.0001$) and second ($r = 0.869$, $P < 0.0001$) visits. Since the MGC shares a number of items with the MG-ADL profile, concerns about inflated correlation were raised, but a similar degree of correlation was seen with the MG-QOL15 ($r = 0.763$, $P < 0.0001$). Correlation of the delta in the MG-ADL score and physician impression of change in MG status between the two visits was also strong ($r = 0.70$, $P < 0.0001$).[14]

Sensitivity and specificity analysis

Since previous analysis did not provide an opportunity to perform sensitivity and specificity testing, during this new MG scale validation study we

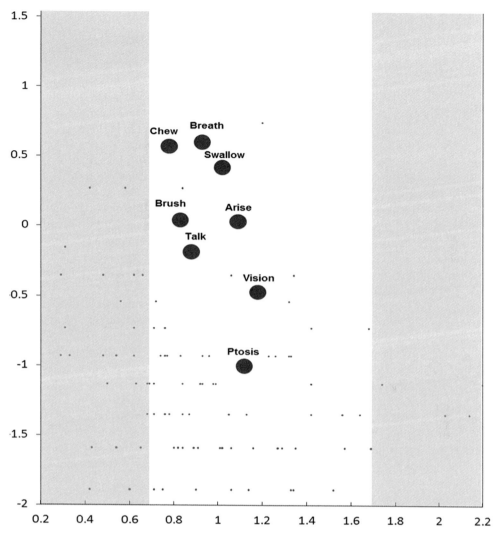

Figure 1. This figure depicts item difficulty and person ability measures (on the vertical logarithmic axis) and item fitting (on the horizontal logarithmic axis) for the MG-ADL profile. Each dot represents a subject and each circle represents an item. The vertical spacing approximates the items' placement on the linear probabilistic Rasch model. None of the items in the MG-ADL are misfitting, as they do not fall outside into the gray zone.

compared the changes in MG-ADL scores with the presumed gold standard, that is, physician impression of change plus improvement in MG-QOL15 for improvement in MG status. An MG-ADL score change of 2 points seemed to have the best balance between sensitivity and specificity. A 2-point change had a sensitivity of 77 and specificity of 82.[14] A 3-point improvement had much higher specificity of 90, but the sensitivity was diminished to 62. A receiver operating curve analysis was also performed. This revealed an area under the curve of 0.90, suggestive of high accuracy of the MG-ADL test to assess clinical improvement.[14]

Test and retest reliability analysis

After the above study, at a single center, test–retest reliability for the MG-ADL profile was performed. Twenty-six patients completed MG-ADL in clinic and were asked to repeat this again at home after one week. Twenty out of the 26 patients completed the second MG-ADL at home and mailed it back to the physician. A one-week interval was chosen to complete the MG-ADL profile again as it was considered too short a period to be affected by therapeutic changes made during the clinic visit but long enough that patients might not remember their individual item score. Patients who were on plasma exchange were excluded. Reliability coefficient was 93.7, suggesting excellent test–retest reliability,[14] and the repeat MG-ADL scores did not differ by more than 2 points 85% of the time.

Rasch analysis

Psychometric testing of outcome measures usually includes tests to evaluate reliability, validity, sensitivity and specificity analysis, and responsiveness to change. By these measures, the MG-ADL profile performed well. However, these traditional methods do not measure the overall estimate of an individual item (or question) score to the total score and do not measure the behavior of an item in relation to others in an outcome measure. To understand these properties, item response theory (IRT) models are used. Among the types of IRT models, Rasch analysis is commonly used. In Rasch analysis, the two important features of item measures tested are item difficulty and person ability. *Item difficulty* refers to ability of an item to differentiate patients with worse MG manifestations from those who are not as affected, whereas *person ability* refers to how difficult it is for a person to respond to an item in an outcome measure. Rasch analysis can assess the item difficulty and person ability, identify any misfitting items and effects of these items on the unidimensionality of the outcome measure, and assess category response functioning. Questions related to ptosis and vision were easy items, and questions about chewing and breathing were difficult items. Category probability functioning testing revealed that the empirical category response probability ascends for all items in MG-ADL except for the vision item. Developmental pathway analysis revealed that none of the items in MG-ADL fall into the misfitting category (see Fig. 1). These findings suggest that MG-ADL performed well on Rasch analysis without any misfitting items and does not require any major revisions.

Discussion

Since development of the MG-ADL numerous other outcome measures have been created and are being used in clinical care of patients with MG and in research trials. Recently the task force of the Medical Scientific Advisory Board (MSAB) of the Myasthenia Gravis Foundation of America (MGFA) suggested that the MGC be used as a primary outcome measure in clinical trials. Going forward, the MG-ADL profile may still be used a secondary outcome measure and it is currently used in the MGTX study[15] and the study to assess the efficacy of Methotrexate in MG (http://clinicaltrials.gov/show/NCT00814138). The MG-ADL test has one unique feature that differentiates it from the other MG outcome scales: it is completed solely by the patient. Since it does not require a physician or nurse to administer this test, the MG-ADL test could potentially be used as an outcome measure in long-term MG studies. In addition, with the advent of electronic records and electronic communication with patients, the MG-ADL test could potentially be completed by the patient between and during the clinic visits. For example, many patients are now receiving maintenance intravenous immunoglobulin therapy at home for myasthenia gravis and a test like the MG-ADL profile might provide information about their ongoing MG clinical state. One could also foresee the MG-ADL test as a valuable tool in observational studies or clinical trials with long-term follow-up of years where it is not feasible to have frequent clinic visits, since patients can provide their MG-ADL score in-between clinic visits.

For all its positive attributes, the MG-ADL test has two important deficiencies as an outcome measure. One, there is no item to measure the effect of axial weakness (such as neck extension weakness). This is important because neck extension weakness when significant can cause head drop, a very disabling manifestation, and yet the MG-ADL score will not reflect this limitation on a patient's activity level. Secondly, items in the MG-ADL test are linearly scored and are not weighted. Linear scoring would suggest that degree of disability or effect on daily living activities of various individual items is the same. For example, if a patient has constant double vision, he would score 3 for diplopia item, but at the same time, being on ventilator for respiratory assistance would also score 3 for breathing item. Even though the contribution to the final MG-ADL score is the same, the degree of disability experienced by the patient on ventilator is many times higher than the disability of the patient with constant double vision. Newer MG scales such as MGC are weighted to correct for this limitation. Despite the above deficiencies, the MG-ADL self-test profile continues to be a useful tool and will probably have a role as an outcome measure going forward in clinical trials and patient care, in myasthenia gravis.

Acknowledgments

The author would like to thank Dr. Reza Sadjadi and Dr. Ted Burns for providing Figure 1 and information on the Rasch analysis of the MG-ADL. Rasch analysis data were presented at the 12th International Conference on Myasthenia Gravis and Related Disorders, May 21–23, 2012 at the New York Academy of Sciences in New York City.

Conflicts of interest

The author declares no conflicts of interest.

References

1. Burns, T.M. 2010. History of outcome measures for myasthenia gravis. *Muscle Nerve* **42:** 5–13.
2. Barohn, R.J. *et al.* 1998. Reliability testing of the quantitative myasthenia gravis score. *Ann. N.Y. Acad. Sci.* **841:** 769–772.
3. Wolfe, G.I. *et al.* 1999. Myasthenia gravis activities of daily living profile. *Neurology* **52:** 1487–1489.
4. Rowin, J. *et al.* 2004. Etanercept treatment in corticosteroid-dependent myasthenia gravis. *Neurology* **63:** 2390–2392.
5. Wolfe, G.I. *et al.* 2002. Randomized, controlled trial of intravenous immunoglobulin in myasthenia gravis. *Muscle Nerve* **26:** 549–552.
6. Kawaguchi, N. *et al.* 2004. Low-dose tacrolimus treatment in thymectomised and steroid-dependent myasthenia gravis. *Curr. Med. Res. Opin.* **20:** 1269–1273.
7. Konishi, T. *et al.* 2003. Clinical study of FK506 in patients with myasthenia gravis. *Muscle Nerve* **28:** 570–574.
8. Nagaishi, A., M. Yukitake & Y. Kuroda. 2008. Long-term treatment of steroid-dependent myasthenia gravis patients with low-dose tacrolimus. *Intern. Med.* **47:** 731–736.
9. Sanders, D.B. *et al.* 2008. An international, phase III, randomized trial of mycophenolate mofetil in myasthenia gravis. *Neurology* **71:** 400–406.
10. Muscle Study, G. 2008. A trial of mycophenolate mofetil with prednisone as initial immunotherapy in myasthenia gravis. *Neurology* **71:** 394–399.
11. Wolfe, G.I. *et al.* 2008. Comparison of outcome measures from a trial of mycophenolate mofetil in myasthenia gravis. *Muscle Nerve* **38:** 1429–1433.
12. Burns, T.M. *et al.* 2010. The MG composite: a valid and reliable outcome measure for myasthenia gravis. *Neurology* **74:** 1434–1440.
13. Burns, T.M. *et al.* 2011. The MG-QOL15 for following the health-related quality of life of patients with myasthenia gravis. *Muscle Nerve* **43:** 14–18.
14. Muppidi, S. *et al.* 2011. MG-ADL: still a relevant outcome measure. *Muscle Nerve* **44:** 727–731.
15. Wolfe, G.I. *et al.* 2003. Development of a thymectomy trial in nonthymomatous myasthenia gravis patients receiving immunosuppressive therapy. *Ann. N.Y. Acad. Sci.* **998:** 473–480.

Ann. N.Y. Acad. Sci. ISSN 0077-8923

Regulatory T cell–based immunotherapies in experimental autoimmune myasthenia gravis

Miriam C. Souroujon,[1,2] Revital Aricha,[1] Tali Feferman,[1] Keren Mizrachi,[1,3] Debby Reuveni,[1,2] and Sara Fuchs[1]

[1]Department of Immunology, The Weizmann Institute of Science, Rehovot, Israel. [2]Department of Natural Sciences, The Open University of Israel, Raanana, Israel. [3]The Leslie and Susan Gonda (Goldschmidt) Multidisciplinary Brain Research Center, Bar-Ilan University, Israel.

Address for correspondence: Miriam C. Souroujon, Department of Natural Sciences, The Open University. 1 University Rd, Raanana 43107, Israel. miriso@openu.ac.il

Establishment of tolerance in myasthenia gravis (MG) involves regulatory T (T_{reg}) cells. Experimental autoimmune MG (EAMG) in rats is a suitable model for assessing the contribution of T_{reg} cells to the immunopathology of the disease and for testing novel T_{reg} cell–based treatment modalities. We have studied two immunotherapeutic approaches for targeting of T_{reg} cells in myasthenia. By one approach we demonstrated that treatment of sick rats by *ex vivo*–generated exogenous T_{reg} cells derived from healthy donors suppressed EAMG. By a different approach, we aimed at affecting the endogenous T_{reg} /Th17 cell balance by targeting IL-6, which has a key role in controlling the equilibrium between pathogenic Th17 and suppressive T_{reg} cells. We found that treatment of myasthenic rats by neutralizing anti-IL-6 antibodies shifted this equilibrium in favor of T_{reg} cells and led to suppression of EAMG. Our results show that T_{reg} cells could serve as potential targets in treating MG patients.

Keywords: T_{reg} cells; experimental autoimmune myasthenia gravis; Th17 cells; IL-6

Introduction

The involvement of regulatory T (T_{reg}) cells in autoimmunity was demonstrated in various autoimmune diseases and in their respective experimental models. These include type 1 diabetes, multiple sclerosis, systemic lupus erythematosus (SLE), rheumatoid arthritis, inflammatory bowel disease, and psoriasis, some of which are antibody-dependent autoimmune disorders.[1–10] Functional defects in T_{reg} cells and a decreased expression of Foxp3 (Forkhead box P3), a key transcription factor in the development and function of T_{reg}, have also been demonstrated in the thymus of MG patients,[4] and some reports also describe lower numbers of $CD4^+$ $CD25^+$ $GITR^+$ T regulatory cells in PBL of MG patients.[5] It was also reported that after thymectomy or effective immunosuppression in MG patients, $CD4^+$ $CD25^{high}$ cell numbers increased and reached normal or elevated values compared to healthy controls.[6,7]

These observations have triggered the attempts to target T_{reg} cells for the treatment of MG. Reconstitution of the T_{reg} cell compartment in myasthenia can be approached either by treatments that affect the endogenous T_{reg} cell population or by the adaptive transfer of compatible exogenous and possibly autologous functional T_{reg} cells. We have used the experimental model disease EAMG in rats, in which the disease is induced by immunization with acetylcholine receptor (AChR), to assess the feasibility of both approaches.[11–13] This experimental disease mimics well the human disease, especially during its chronic phase and therefore serves as a suitable model for studying the immunopathogenesis of myasthenia and for testing novel therapeutic approaches.

Adoptive transfer of exogenous functional T_{reg} cells

The impairments of T_{reg} cells reported in MG patients seem to be present also in the experimental

doi: 10.1111/j.1749-6632.2012.06844.x

model EAMG. We found that the frequency of $CD4^+$ $CD25^+$ cells is lower in EAMG (AChR-immunized) rats compared to naive rats and to CFA-immunized rat controls. Moreover, the percentage of $CD4^+$ $CD25^{high}$ cells is also lower in myasthenic rats compared to healthy controls,[11] and since high CD25 expression has been associated with regulatory activity of T_{reg} cells in peripheral blood, these observations suggest an impaired suppressive activity of T_{reg} cells in EAMG. Thus, adoptive transfer of functional T_{reg} cells could reconstitute the T_{reg} cell compartments in myasthenia.

The natural frequency of $CD4^+CD25^+$ T_{reg} cells in lymphoid organs or in peripheral blood is very low.

We had therefore to design an effective method to produce the large numbers of T_{reg} cells required for administration into myasthenic rats. $CD4^+$ splenic lymphocytes were isolated from healthy rats and cultured for three days in the presence of TGF-β (50 ng) and IL-2 (5 ng) in tissue culture plates coated by anti-CD28 and anti-CD3 antibodies. While the prevalence of $CD4^+$ $CD25^+$ cells was 5% on day 0 it increased three days later to 94–96% (Fig. 1A). The *ex vivo*–generated $CD4^+$ $CD25^+$ ($evCD4^+CD25^+$) had significantly upregulated mRNA levels of CTLA-4 and Foxp3 compared to naturally occurring CD4+ $CD25^-$ ($nCD4^+CD25^-$) (Fig. 1B). To determine the *in vitro* suppressive function of the

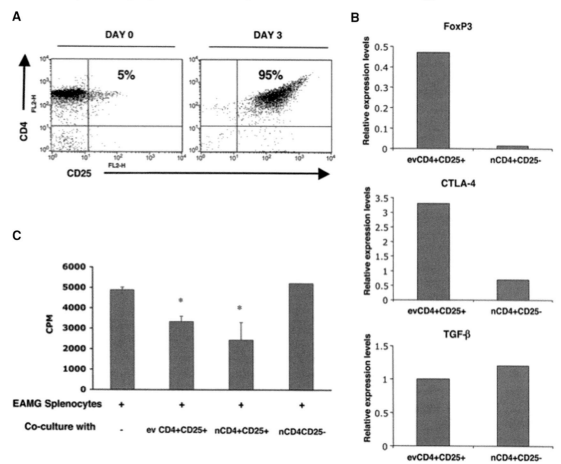

Figure 1. Characterization of *ex vivo*–generated $CD4^+$ $CD25^+$ T_{reg} cells. (A) FACS analysis monitoring the prevalence of $CD4^+$ $CD25^+$ cells among freshly isolated $CD4^+$ splenic lymphocytes (day 0) and following a three-day culture in the presence of anti-CD3, anti-CD28, IL-2 and TGF-β. (B) mRNA expression levels of Foxp3, CTLA-4, and TGF-β in *ex vivo*–generated $CD4^+CD25^+$ ($evCD4^+CD25^+$) and in freshly isolated naturally occurring $CD4^+CD25^-$ cells ($nCD4^+CD25^-$). mRNA levels were determined by quantitative real time RT-PCR using β-actin as an inner control for normalization, and are representative of two independent experiments. (C) Effect of *ex vivo*–generated $CD4^+CD25^+$ cells ($evCD4^+CD25^+$) and of freshly isolated naturally occurring $CD4^+CD25^+$ ($nCD4^+CD25^+$) or $CD4^+CD25^-$ ($nCD4^+CD25^-$) on the proliferation of splenocytes from myasthenic rats in response to AChR (0.125 μg/ml). Error bars indicate SEM value ($n = 6$). *$P < 0.05$. Data from Ref. 11.

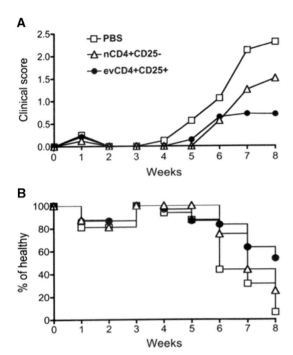

Figure 2. Suppression of EAMG by *ex vivo*–generated T$_{reg}$ cells from healthy donors. Rats were administered i.p. with *ex vivo*–generated CD4$^+$CD25$^+$ cells (evCD4$^+$CD25$^+$; 4 × 10^6/rat), freshly isolated CD4$^+$CD25$^-$ cells (nCD4$^+$CD25$^+$; 4 × 10^6/rat), or with PBS starting four days after EAMG induction and every two weeks thereafter. (A) Mean clinical scores of the different groups (*n* = 8 for each group). Representative of three independent experiments. (B) Cumulative data presenting percent of healthy rats at different time points in three independent experiments. *P* < 0.02. Analyzed by the two-way ANOVA test. Data from Ref. 11.

ex vivo–generated T$_{reg}$ cells, they were added to spleen cells from AChR-immunized rats that were cultured in the presence of AChR. The freshly isolated nCD4$^+$CD25$^+$ T$_{reg}$ cells and the evCD4$^+$CD25$^+$ significantly suppressed the proliferation in response to AChR, whereas freshly isolated nCD4$^+$CD25$^-$ cells were not suppressive (Fig. 1C).

We next tested the potential of the *ex vivo*–generated CD4$^+$ CD25$^+$ cells to modulate EAMG. These cells were administered intraperitoneally four times (4 × 10^6 cells per treatment per rat), at two-week intervals to myasthenic rats. For control, rats were treated by either PBS or by nCD4$^+$CD25$^-$ cells isolated from naive rats. As can be seen in Figure 2, *ex vivo*–generated T$_{reg}$ cells suppressed EAMG. The recipient rats were followed for eight weeks starting from disease induction. At the end of the experiments, 53% of the rats treated by *ex vivo*–generated

CD4$^+$ CD25$^+$ cells remained healthy (Fig. 2B), whereas only 6.25% of PBS-treated rats and 25% of rats treated by nCD4$^+$CD25$^-$ did not show clinical signs of disease (Fig. 2B).[11] The evCD4$^+$CD25$^+$ treated rats had a decreased total anti-rat AChR antibody titer and decreased IgG1, IgG2a, and IgG2b anti-AChR antibody titers compared with PBS-treated control rats. In the rat, IgG1 and IgG2a represent respectively Th2 and Th1-regulated responses, suggesting that the treatment by the evCD4$^+$CD25$^+$ cells affected both these types of AChR-specific responses.[11] This may be of importance in MG that is known to be a mixed Th1/Th2 disease. In order to test whether this is indeed the case, we used real time RT-PCR to determine mRNA levels of selected cytokines in lymph node cells of rats that received the different treatments. Administration of *ex vivo*–generated T$_{reg}$ cells to EAMG rats led to downregulation of Th2 as well as Th1 type cytokines. This is in agreement with previous reports on the effect of T$_{reg}$ cells on Th1 and Th2 cytokine production.[14–16]

Interestingly administration of *ex vivo*–generated CD4$^+$ CD25$^+$ affected the endogenous T$_{reg}$ cell compartment in the recipients. This was shown by FACS analysis performed on splenic lymphocytes derived from the treated rats 10 days after the last treatment. Rats treated by *ex vivo*–generated CD4$^+$ CD25$^+$ cells had significantly higher numbers of CD4$^+$ CD25$^+$ Foxp3$^+$ cells compared to PBS-treated rats and to rats treated by *ex vivo*–generated CD4$^+$ CD25$^-$ cells. It has been shown that following the administration of T$_{reg}$ only 20% of these cells are located in the spleen of the recipients.[17] Moreover, we administered exogenous CD4$^+$ CD25$^+$ cells, but only a specific subpopulation of CD4$^+$ CD25$^+$ Foxp3$^+$ cells was elevated in the spleens of the recipients eight weeks following disease induction. These observations lead us to believe that the increase in CD4$^+$ CD25$^+$ Foxp3$^+$ cells represents a *de novo* induction of T$_{reg}$ cells and that these cells are not of donor origin. This is in agreement with findings of Zheng *et al.*,[18] who showed that transferred graft rejection can be controlled by administration of regulatory T cells that induce in the recipient *de novo* tolerogenic CD4$^+$ CD25$^+$ cells.

The suppressive effects on EAMG that we obtained by administration of T$_{reg}$ cells from healthy donors encouraged us to test whether T$_{reg}$ cells generated from CD4$^+$ cells of myasthenic rats would have similar effects on EAMG. If indeed MG patients

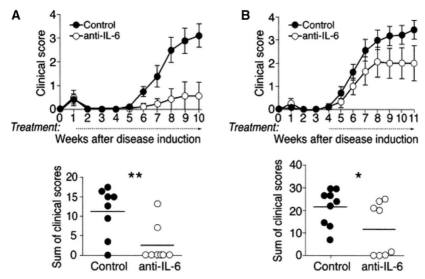

Figure 3. Suppression of EAMG by anti-IL-6 treatment. Mean clinical scores (upper panel) and sums of cumulative weekly clinical score values for individual rats (lower panel), or rats treated by anti-IL-6 or normal goat IgG starting at the acute (A) or at the chronic phase (B) of EAMG; $n = 8$ for each group. Data represent one out of two or three independent experiments. $P < 0.0001$ in A and $P < 0.001$ in B. Analyzed by the two-way ANOVA test. Data from Ref. 12.

could be treated by T$_{reg}$ cells derived from autologous CD4$^+$ cells, this would have a clear advantage in clinical terms. For that, CD4$^+$ CD25$^+$ T$_{reg}$ cells were generated from CD4$^+$ cells of AChR-immunized rats in a similar procedure to the *ex vivo* generation of T$_{reg}$ cells from healthy donors. After three days in culture over 90% of the cells expressed CD4 and CD25, but their expression of Foxp3 and CD25^{high} was lower compared to cells generated from CD4$^+$ cells of healthy donors. When tested *in vivo*, CD4$^+$ CD25$^+$ cells generated from myasthenic donors were not as effective as evCD4$^+$CD25$^+$ from healthy donors in modulating EAMG and in some cases even led to disease exacerbation.[11] The latter observations imply that the future clinical application of this approach would require effective methods for generating functional and effective autologous T$_{reg}$ cells from CD4$^+$ cells of MG patients.

Affecting the equilibrium between endogenous T$_{reg}$ and Th17 cells

The differentiation of naive T cells into specific subsets is controlled by cytokines in the local milieu. The differentiation of naive T cells into T$_{reg}$ cells requires TGF-β and IL-2, whereas TGF-β and IL-6 synergistically induce their differentiation into Th17 cells. The equilibrium between these two T cell sub-

sets thus determines the critical balance between inflammatory and autoimmune responses[19–21] and IL-6 has a key role in determining whether suppressive T$_{reg}$ or proinflammatory Th17 cells will be formed. IL-6 is a pleiotropic cytokine that was shown to be involved in the pathogenesis of MG. It promotes B cell differentiation and proliferation and induces their maturation into plasma cells.[22–24] IL-6 knockout mice are resistant to the induction of EAMG by immunization with Torpedo AChR and their CD4$^+$ cells do not produce IL-17 in response to AChR *in vitro*.[25,26] IL-6 is also known to act as a myokine and may be involved in myasthenia via its direct effects on the target organ—the muscle. Since IL-6 governs the balance between T$_{reg}$ and Th17 cells, it could serve as a potential target for blocking the differentiation of Th17 *in vivo*, thereby shifting the balance between T$_{reg}$ and Th17 cells.

In order to test the potential efficacy of IL-6 blockade in the treatment of EAMG we have first addressed the question whether the balance between T$_{reg}$ and Th17 is perturbed in EAMG.[12] Since the balance between regulatory and effector cells is governed by cytokines we tested the mRNA levels of IL-17 that is produced by Th17 cells as well as of IL-23, a proinflammatory cytokine that is involved in the maintenance, expansion, and further

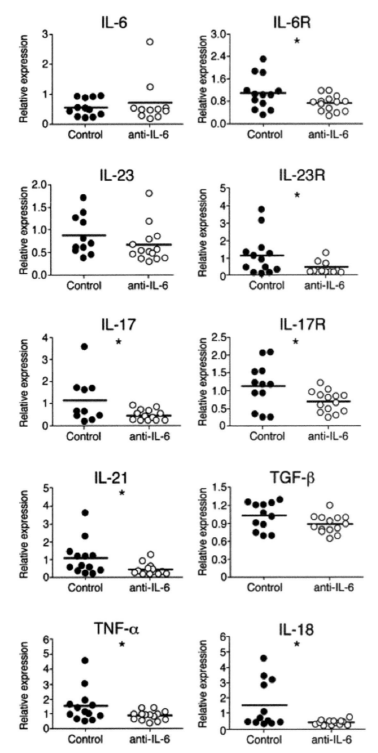

Figure 4. Effect of anti-IL-6 treatment on the expression of Th-17 related genes. mRNA expression levels of cytokines and Th-17–related genes in lymph node cells from EAMG rats treated by anti-IL-6 ($n = 14$) or from the control group treated by normal IgG ($n = 13$) starting at the acute phase of EAMG were determined by quantitative real-time RT-PCR eight weeks after disease induction. β-Actin was used as an inner control for normalization for each gene. Horizontal bars represent the mean value of each group, $^{*}P \leq 0.05$. Data from Ref. 12.

differentiation of committed Th17 cells. We found that the mRNA expression levels of IL-6 and its receptor, IL-6R as well as IL-17, IL-17R, IL-23, and IL-23R were upregulated at different phases of EAMG, whereas TGF-β mRNA was downregulated at early stages of EAMG, compared to CFA-immunized healthy controls, suggesting that the balance between T$_{reg}$ and Th17 cells is perturbed in EAMG.

We next tested the effect of IL-6 blockade on this perturbed balance. Neutralizing anti-IL-6 antibodies (1 μg/rat/day) were injected i.p. to AChR-immunized rats on alternate days starting either at the acute or the chronic phase of EAMG. For control, rats received either PBS or control goat IgG. As seen in Figure 3, administration of anti-IL-6 antibodies had a suppressive effect on EAMG when treatment was initiated either at the acute phase of disease (Fig. 3A) or at the chronic phase of EAMG (Fig. 3B), with a more pronounced effect when treatment started earlier. At the end of the experiment (10 weeks after disease induction) the meant clinical scores of the rats treated by anti-IL-6 antibodies were significantly lower than those of control treated rats: 0.68 compared to 3.1 when treatment started at the acute phase and 2.0 compared to 3.5 when treatment was initiated at the chronic phase of disease.

Administration of anti-IL-6 antibodies led to a reduction in the percentage of B cells in lymph node cells derived from the treated rats and to lower anti-rat AChR IgG levels, in particular anti-rat AChR IgG2a titers.[12] These observations are in line with the role of IL-6 as a promoter of B cell development and plasma cell maturation.[24] Since IL-6 is known to inhibit the conversion of conventional T cells into Foxp3$^+$ regulatory T cells,[27] we expected to see an elevated number of T$_{reg}$ cells in rats treated by anti-IL-6 antibodies. However, the mRNA expression level of Foxp3, as well as the frequency of CD4$^+$ CD25$^+$ Foxp3$^+$ cells, was similar in lymph node cells from anti-IL-6 treated rats and control treated rats.[12] In order to assess the effects of IL-6 blockade of the Th17 subset, we determined the mRNA expression levels of IL-17 related cytokines and their respective receptors. Treatment by anti-IL-6 antibodies led to a significant decrease in the mRNA levels of IL-17–related cytokines (Fig. 4) and to lower serum levels of IL-17 in the treated rats. In addition to the effect on the Th17 cell subset, treatment by anti-IL-6 antibodies also led to downregulated mRNA levels of the Th1 cytokines TNF-α and IL-18.[12]

Our results indicate that blockade of IL-6, a key regulator of the balance between T$_{reg}$ and Th17 cells, suppresses EAMG. This suppression was accompanied by a lower humoral response to AChR and a decreased Th1 response. Moreover, blockade of IL-6 signaling led to a shift in the T$_{reg}$ /Th17 cell balance in favor of T$_{reg}$ cells and should therefore be considered as a potential treatment for myasthenia gravis and possibly other noninflammatory autoimmune diseases.

Summary

The involvement of CD4$^+$ CD25$^+$ T$_{reg}$ cells in the pathogenesis of EAMG renders these cells potential targets for therapeutic intervention. This may be achieved either by administration of exogenous functional T$_{reg}$ cells or by shifting the endogenous T$_{reg}$ /Th17 cell balance in favor of T$_{reg}$ cells. Studies in the rat experimental model indicate that both these approaches may be feasible and effective for the treatment of myasthenia gravis. Our results suggest that autologous T$_{reg}$ cells derived from myasthenic patients would have to be manipulated *ex vivo* in order to reconstitute their suppressive activity before they can be applied for clinical use in these patients.

Achnowledgments

The work from our lab described in this article was supported by grants from the Muscular Dystrophy Association of America (MDA), the Association Francaise Contre les Myopathies (AFM), the European Commission (FIGHT-MG, contract #FP7 HEALTH-2009-242-210), and the Open University of Israel Research Fund.

Conflicts of interest

The authors declare no conflicts of interest.

References

1. Brunkow, M.E. *et al.* 2001. Disruption of a new forkhead/winged-helix protein, scurfin, results in the fatal lymphoproliferative disorder of the scurfy mouse. *Nat. Genet.* **27:** 68–73.
2. Sakaguchi, S. *et al.* 2006. Foxp3$^+$ CD25$^+$ CD4$^+$ natural regulatory T cells in dominant self-tolerance and autoimmune disease. *Immunol. Rev.* **212:** 8–27.
3. Buckner, J.H. 2010. Mechanisms of impaired regulation by CD4(+)CD25(+)FOXP3(+) regulatory T cells in human autoimmune diseases. *Nat. Rev. Immunol.* **10:** 849–859.
4. Balandina, A. *et al.* 2005. Functional defect of regulatory CD4(+)CD25+ T cells in the thymus of patients with autoimmune myasthenia gravis. *Blood* **105:** 735–741.

5. Masuda, M. *et al.* 2010. Clinical implication of peripheral CD4$^+$CD25$^+$ regulatory T cells and Th17 cells in myasthenia gravis patients. *J. Neuroimmunol.* **225:** 123–131.

6. Fattorossi, A., Battaglia, A., Buzzonetti, A., *et al.* 2005. Circulating and thymic CD4 CD25 T regulatory cells in myasthenia gravis: effect of immunosuppressive treatment. *Immunology* **116:** 134–141.

7. Sun, Y., Qiao, J., Lu, C.Z., *et al.* 2004. Increase of circulating CD4+CD25+ T cells in myasthenia gravis patients with stability and thymectomy. *Clin. Immunol.* **112:** 284–289.

8. Sakaguchi, S. *et al.* 2012. Re-establishing immunological self-tolerance in autoimmune disease. *Nat. Med.* **18:** 54–58.

9. Hsu, W.T. *et al.* 2006. The role of CD4 CD25 T cells in autoantibody production in murine lupus. *Clin. Exp. Immunol.* **145:** 513–519.

10. Iikuni, N. *et al.* 2009. Cutting edge: regulatory T cells directly suppress B cells in systemic lupus erythematosus. *J. Immunol.* **183:** 1518–1522.

11. Aricha, R. *et al.* 2008. Ex vivo generated regulatory T cells modulate experimental autoimmune myasthenia gravis. *J. Immunol.* **180:** 2132–2139.

12. Aricha, R. *et al.* 2011. Blocking of IL-6 suppresses experimental autoimmune myasthenia gravis. *J. Autoimmunity* **36:** 135–141.

13. Souroujon, M.C. *et al.* 2010. Development of novel therapies for MG. *Autoimmunity* **43:** 446–460.

14. Shevach, E.M. 2002. CD4$^+$ CD25$^+$ suppressor T cells: more questions than answers. *Nat. Rev. Immunol.* **2:** 389–400.

15. Piccirillo, C.A. & E.M. Shevach. 2004. Naturally-occurring CD4$^+$ CD25$^+$ immunoregulatory T cells: central players in the arena of peripheral tolerance. *Semin. Immunol.* **16:** 81–88.

16. Nolte-'t Hoen, E.N. *et al.* 2004. Identification of a CD4$^+$ CD25$^+$ T cell subset committed in vivo to suppress antigen-specific T cell responses without additional stimulation. *Eur. J. Immunol.* **34:** 3016–3027.

17. Feng, N.H. *et al.* 2004. Transplantation tolerance mediated by regulatory T cells in mice. *Chin. Med. J.* **117:** 1184–1189.

18. Zheng, S.G. *et al.* 2006. Transfer of regulatory T cells generated ex vivo modifies graft rejection through induction of tolerogenic CD4$^+$ CD25$^+$ cells in the recipient. *Int. Immunol.* **18:** 279–289.

19. Weaver, C.T. & K.M. Murphy. 2007. The central role of the Th17 lineage in regulating the inflammatory/autoimmune axis. *Semin. Immunol.* **19:** 351–352.

20. Korn, T. *et al.* 2007. Th17 cells: effector T cells with inflammatory properties. *Semin. Immunol.* **9:** 362–371.

21. Ishihara, K. & T. Hirano. 2002. IL-6 in autoimmune disease and chronic inflammatory proliferative disease. *Cytokine Growth Factor Rev.* **13:** 357–368.

22. Cohen-Kaminsky, S. *et al.* 1993. High IL-6 gene expression and production by cultured human thymic epithelial cells from patients with myasthenia gravis. *Ann. N. Y. Acad. Sci.* **681:** 97–99.

23. Endo, S. *et al.* 2005. Inhibition of IL-6 overproduction by steroid treatment before transsternal thymectomy for myasthenia gravis: does it help stabilize perioperative condition? *Eur. J. Neurol.* **12:** 768–773.

24. Van Snick, J. 1990. Interleukin-6: an overview. *Annu. Rev. Immunol.* **8:** 253–278.

25. Chen-Kiang, S. 1995. Regulation of terminal differentiation of human B-cells by IL-6. *Curr. Top Microbiol. Immunol.* **194:** 189–198.

26. Takatsu, K. 1997. Cytokines involved in B-cell differentiation and their sites of action. *Proc. Soc. Exp. Biol. Med.* **215:** 121–133.

27. Korn, T. *et al.* 2008. IL-6 controls Th17 immunity in vivo by inhibiting the conversion of conventional T cells into Foxp3$^+$ regulatory T cells. *Proc. Natl. Acad. Sci. USA* **105:** 18460–18465.

Ann. N.Y. Acad. Sci. ISSN 0077-8923

ANNALS OF THE NEW YORK ACADEMY OF SCIENCES
Issue: *Myasthenia Gravis and Related Disorders*

The role of complement in experimental autoimmune myasthenia gravis

Linda L. Kusner[1] and Henry J. Kaminski[2]

[1]Department of Pharmacology and Physiology, [2]Department of Neurology, The George Washington University, Washington, DC

Address for correspondence: Linda L. Kusner, The George Washington University, Pharmacology and Physiology, Ross Hall, 2300 I St NW, Washington, DC 20037. lkusner@gwu.edu

Complement plays an important role in the pathophysiology of experimental autoimmune myasthenia gravis (EAMG). The deposition of IgG at the neuromuscular junction, followed by the activation and observance of C3 at the site, and finally the insertion of the membrane attack complex results in the destruction of the plasma membrane at the neuromuscular junction. Animal models of complement-deficient components show the importance of the mediated lysis in EAMG. These events have regulators that allow for the limitation in the cascade and the ability of the cell to inhibit complement at many places along the pathway. The complement regulatory proteins have many roles in reducing the activation of the complement cascade and the inflammatory pathways. Mice deficient in complement regulatory proteins, decay accelerating factor, and CD59 demonstrate a significant increase in the destruction at the neuromuscular junction. Inhibition of complement-mediated lysis is an attractive therapeutic in MG.

Keywords: complement; complement regulators; myasthenia gravis; C5; autoimmunity

Introduction

Myasthenia gravis (MG) is an antibody-mediated autoimmune disease that targets the neuromuscular junction (NMJ). The preponderance of experimental data indicates that the deleterious effects of AChR autoantibody are mediated through activation of complement in animal models. Among this evidence, it has been observed that C3 activation fragments, C9, and other components of the membrane attack complex (MAC) are readily detectable at motor endplates in animals with EAMG;[1–3] depletion of C3 by cobra venom factor protects rats against induction of EAMG;[4,5] and administration of complement inhibitors (anti-C6, anti-C5, soluble CR1, or rEV576)[6–9] protects in passively induced and active EAMG. The data, taken together, strongly support the notion that complement activation in particular assembly of the MAC at the NMJ leads to destruction of postsynaptic structure, compromising neuromuscular transmission.

In human MG, there is strong evidence for complement as the primary pathogenic mechanism.
This derives from identification of C3 and MAC deposition at NMJ of patients.[2,3,10] NMJ consistently demonstrates a simplified structure consistent with complement injury.[11] Depletion of serum complement components, C3 and C4, is observed in patients,[12] terminal components of complement are present in MG patient sera,[13] and sera induces complement-mediated lysis of cultured myotubes.[14] The role of complement in MG associated with antibodies directed toward the muscle specific kinase or LRP-4 has not been fully defined and is not discussed in this review.

Complement

Complement is a major defense in the innate immune system and is recognized as augmenting the adaptive immune response. The complement system is made up of over 30 proteins with the function to eliminate invading pathogens, prevent infection, and clear altered host cells. The initiation of complement can occur by three separate mechanisms: classical, alternative, and lectin pathways. Although

doi: 10.1111/j.1749-6632.2012.06783.x

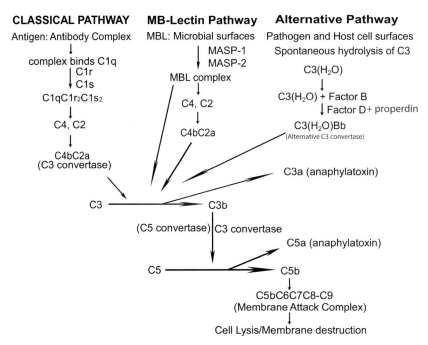

CLASSICAL PATHWAY   **MB-Lectin Pathway**   **Alternative Pathway**

Figure 1. Complement cascade. The three pathways of complement are initiated by different mechanisms and intersect at the C3 level. The classical pathway is involved in the pathology of EAMG, initiated by the antibody–antigen complex. The final steps in the cascade are focused on the formation of the membrane attack complex, with C5b-C8 accumulation on the plasma membrane and C9 recruitment to form the pore, which causes the destruction of the nerve–muscle communication.

the activation of the pathways differs, all intersect at the C3 level, and progress to the membrane attack complex (Fig. 1). In MG, the classical pathway is involved by the initiation of the antigen–antibody complex being recognized by C1q. The process progresses to the membrane attack complex (MAC) insertion into the postsynaptic membrane of the NMJ.

The initiation of the classical pathway by the binding of the antibody (IgG or IgM) to the antigen (AChR) is recognized by C1q (Fig. 1). The C1q forms a pentameric complex with the C1r2C1s2 serine protease tetramer. The conformational change of C1q binding to the cell surface allows C1r to activate through autocleavage.[15] Active C1r can then cleave C1s. The zymogen reaction continues by C1s proteolytic activation of C4 to C4a (peptide analphylatoxin), and C4b, which attaches to the cell surface and binds C2. C2 also becomes cleaved by C1s to form the C3 convertase (C4b2a). The C3 convertase cleaves C3 forming C3a (peptide analphylatoxin) and C3b, which binds the C3 convertase to become the C5 convertase (C4b2a3b). The activation of C5 by C5 convertase to form C5a and C5b

initiates formation of the membrane attack complex by recruitment of C6, C7, C8, and C9.

Complement-deficient EAMG models

Animal models are efficient means of analyzing the effect of the complement system in MG. Animals can be induced in a passive form of EAMG with an antibody to the AChR or actively by administering the antigen. By these methods, the roles of the particular components of the complement system can be discriminated by producing NMJ damage and resultant weakness. Components to the complement system have been genetically deleted from mice and rats to discern the nature of the classical pathway and the relevance to the NMJ injury and antibody production.

Studies of complement depletion were the first approaches to assess the necessity of complement to the pathology of EAMG. Cobra venom was injected during the acute phase of the active EAMG in rats and before the passive transfer of antibodies to the AChR. In each experimental design, the lack of complement resolved the NMJ pathology that was seen in the complement-sufficient groups.[4] Direct evidence for the involvement of the classical complement pathway in EAMG derives from the identification of IgG, C3, and MAC deposition at the neuromuscular junctions of both EAMG animals and MG patients.[2,3,10,16,17]

Mice deficient in C3 and C4 demonstrate reduced clinical scores compared to their wild-type littermates during the course of active EAMG, with C3-knockout mice showing no signs of weakness.[18] The total IgG- and AChR-specific IgG levels were equivalent in the C4-deficient animals compared to their wild-type littermates, whereas C3-deficient animals showed a reduction in total IgG and AChR-specific IgG. Both C3- and C4-deficient animals demonstrate reduced AChR IgG2b levels. Reduced B cell expression was also seen in nonimmunized C3- and C4-deficient mice, which remained low in the EAMG state. Therefore, the state of the immune system is altered in the complement-deficient animals. Despite the presence of AChR-specific antibodies neuromuscular junctions show an absence of C3 or MAC deposits when EAMG was induced in C3-deficient mice. Complement-deficient EAMG animals showed a preservation of AChR density at the neuromuscular junction.

A later component of the complement cascade, C5, also is involved in the development of EAMG. C5 cleavage by the C5 convertase results in C5a, a potent anaphylatoxin, and C5b, an initiator of MAC assembly. The influence of the C5 on EAMG susceptibility was analyzed in C5-sufficient and C5-deficient mice in an active model.[19] During the time course of EAMG, both strains had comparable levels of serum AChR-specific antibodies. C5-deficient mice demonstrated reduced incidence of disease compared to the C5-sufficient mice. Therefore, C5 appeared to be critical in EAMG pathogenesis, likely through activation of the terminal C5b-C9 sequence required for neuromuscular junction destruction. As a potential for therapeutic target, blocking of C5 does not impair function of early activated complement components.[7]

The final components of the MAC involve C5b recruiting C6–C7–C8, which then accumulates C9, which forms the pose of the complex. A study of C6-deficient rats demonstrated that the lack of one of these components to the MAC causes resistance to passively induced EAMG.[17] The study also looked at the ability to restore the MAC complex and its destruction to the NMJ resulting in weakness by addition of C6 to a C6-deficient EAMG animal. Therefore, all components in the classical pathway must be in place for MAC deposition.

Therapeutic targets in EAMG

Since complement-deficient animals demonstrated a resistance to EAMG, therapeutic agents that target the classical pathway of the complement system may allow improved outcome in MG. The classical pathway has many components that could be potential targets for inhibition of MAC and the reduction in the damage done to the NMJ in EAMG.

The target for the therapeutic effect has focused on the C5 component. An antibody to C5 was used in a passive study on rats.[7] The rats were given injections of anti-C5 or a control IgG four hours before being induced by AChR-specific antibody. The IgG control and untreated rats showed weakness in 24 hours with untreated decreasing in strength over the time course. The rats treated with anti-C5 demonstrated only mild weakness on day 3, which resolved by day 5. Complement deposition at the NMJ was assessed by immunohistochemistry to C9. The C9 is relatively absent at the NMJ of the anti-C5–treated group compared to the untreated and control IgG treated animals. The anti-C5–treated animal showed preserved synaptic folds of the NMJ, whereas the untreated animals demonstrated reduced synaptic folds of the neuromuscular junction and increase in cell membrane debris.

A complement inhibitor has been discovered in the saliva of the soft tick. The compound was found to bind and modify C5, inhibiting its interaction with C5 convertase.[20] To determine the effect of the complement inhibitor, labeled rEV576, a passive model of EAMG was employed in rats.[6] Treatment with rEV576 demonstrated significantly less weakness compared to the untreated group. As part of the same study, the active model of EAMG was produced in Lewis rats. After weakness was observed, treatment was initiated with rEV576 or vehicle. The rats in the control group declined rapidly over the course of 12 days, whereas, the treated group improved. C9 deposition at the NMJ of the treated group was significantly less than the vehicle-treated group.

Cell surface complement regulators

The complement cascade has regulators that are responsible for limiting damage of spontaneously activated complement. For the classical pathway of the complement cascade, decay accelerating protein (Daf, CD55), membrane cofactor protein (MCP, CD46), CR1-related gene/protein Y (Crry), and CD59 are critical inhibitors of activation. These regulators have been found on the surface of most myofibers and concentrated at the NMJ.[21,22] The CD59 inhibits the membrane attack complex formation and decay accelerating factor accelerates the decay of C3 convertase and C5 convertase. Both have been investigated in EAMG (see below).

Levels of complement regulators vary among muscles

The levels of complement regulators have been evaluated in diaphragm and extraocular muscle and found to change in response to passive EAMG induction.[22] The transcript levels of *Daf1*, *Crry*, and *CD59* were determined in the extraocular muscle and the diaphragm of C57BL/6 mice under normal and passive EAMG conditions. Under the normal condition, all three complement regulators' transcripts were lower in extraocular muscle compared to diaphragm. When comparing normal muscle to passive EAMG-induced muscle, extraocular muscle had a reduction of the level of transcripts of the complement regulators during disease state. However, the diaphragm did not show any changes in complement regulators due to EAMG. In assessing the protein level, immunohistochemistry showed an increase in *Daf1* expression at the NMJ of extraocular under EAMG conditions, whereas, EAMG induced showed an increase in *Crry* at the NMJ of the diaphragm. The study demonstrates a dynamic expression of complement regulators and the decrease expression may affect the susceptibility of muscles to complement-mediated diseases.

The complement regulators have been assessed in the background of genetic modification of specific complement regulator expression.[23] The transcript levels of *Daf*, *CD59a*, and *CD59b* did not show any increases to compensate for the loss of the other complement regulator in genetically modified mice. However, the genetic knockout of both the *Daf* and *CD59ab* showed an increase in the *Crry* transcript levels. These results suggest that the modification of one of the complement regulators can affect the expression of other complement regulators. Also, disease and tissue type influence complement regulator levels.

C9 deposition increases in complement regulator knockout mice with passive EAMG

To determine the effect of EAMG on complement regulator knockouts, wild-type mice and mice deficient in Daf1, CD59ab, or both Daf1and CD59ab were induced by McAb3 (gift of Dr. Vanda Lennon).[23] After 24 h, the Daf1$^{-/-}$CD59ab$^{-/-}$ mice required euthanasia due to the severity of weakness. The level of MAC deposition was much greater in CD59ab-deficient mice compared to wild-type and Daf1$^{-/-}$ mice. The nature of MAC deposits differed among the Daf1$^{-/-}$CD59ab$^{-/-}$ mice, with deposits internalized in the myofiber. Ultrastructural analysis of the NMJ of the Daf1$^{-/-}$CD59ab$^{-/-}$ animals demonstrated extensive damage at the NMJ, as well as myofibers that were necrotic. Comparing only CD59ab-deficient mice to the Daf1$^{-/-}$ mice, MAC deposition was much greater at the NMJ of the CD59ab$^{-/-}$ mice at 24 and 60 h of EAMG induction. However, the Daf1$^{-/-}$ mice appeared weaker. Both complement regulator knockout animals had much more severe weakness and MAC deposition than did the wild-type mice. These and other studies[24–26] signal the critical importance of complement regulation confined to the NMJ and point to the possibility that enhancing complement inhibition at the NMJ may be a successful form of therapy.

Increasing complement inhibitors to the NMJ as a therapeutic

In light of the complement regulator studies, we have developed a therapeutic approach to concentrate complement inhibitors to the NMJ. In a preliminary study, we produced a compound consisting of the Daf regulatory region conjugated to a single chain antibody that binds the acetylcholine receptor. The construct was found to bind the AChR and demonstrated *in vivo* complement inhibitory function.[27] In unpublished studies, we have demonstrated *in vitro* efficacy and importantly have not found evidence of compromise of neuromuscular transmission by the compound.

Conclusion

We have briefly summarized work performed in rodents that support a therapeutic benefit for EAMG produced by complement inhibition. The extensive studies of complement and its regulators in EAMG have led to consideration that therapies could be targeted against the complement system for human MG, and in fact, for generalized MG, a phase 2 trial of eculizumab, which targets the C5 component, was recently completed. It is clear that complement inhibition is a fruitful path for therapeutic evaluation; however, greater elucidation of the complement-mediated pathology of MG is required. The differential susceptibility and response of muscle groups will be critical to define further in order to determine whether complement inhibition may be of greater benefit to patients with ocular myasthenia compared to generalized MG. Thus far, the C5 step of complement activation has been a focus for inhibition, but MAC assembly may be more important. Finally, limiting the adverse effects of chronic complement inhibition will be critical to enhance the treatment benefit; one approach would be to develop agents that specifically concentrate to the NMJ.

Acknowledgments

Work contained in this review was supported by Grants from the National Institutes of Health, (R24EY014837and R01EY013238 to HJK) and the Myasthenia Gravis Foundation of America (LLK).

Conflicts of interest

The authors declare no conflicts of interest.

References

1. Sahashi, K. *et al*. 1978. Ultrastructural localization of immune complexes (IgG and C3) at the end-plate in experimental autoimmune myasthenia gravis. *J. Neuropathol. Exp. Neurol.* 37: 212–223.

2. Sahashi, K. *et al*. 1980. Ultrastructural localization of the terminal and lytic ninth complement component (C9) at the motor end-plate in myasthenia gravis. *J. Neuropathol. Exp. Neurol.* 39: 160–172.

3. Nakano, S. & A.G. Engel. 1993. Myasthenia gravis: quantitative immunocytochemical analysis of inflammatory cells and detection of complement membrane attack complex at the end-plate in 30 patients. *Neurology* 43: 1167–1172.

4. Lennon, V.A. *et al*. 1978. Role of complement in the pathogenesis of experimental autoimmune myasthenia gravis. *J. Exp. Med.* 147: 973–983.

5. Tsujihata, M. *et al*. 2003. Effect of myasthenic immunoglobulin G on motor end-plate morphology. *J. Neurol.* 250: 75–82.

6. Soltys, J. *et al*. 2009. Novel complement inhibitor limits severity of experimentally myasthenia gravis. *Ann. Neurol.* 65: 67–75.

7. Zhou, Y. *et al*. 2007. Anti-C5 antibody treatment ameliorates weakness in experimentally acquired myasthenia gravis. *J. Immunol.* 179: 8562–8567.

8. Biesecker, G. & C.M. Gomez. 1989. Inhibition of acute passive transfer experimental autoimmune myasthenia gravis with Fab antibody to complement C6. *J. Immunol.* 142: 2654–2659.

9. Piddlesden, S.J. *et al*. 1996. Soluble complement receptor 1 (sCR1) protects against experimental autoimmune myasthenia gravis. *J. Neuroimmunol.* 71: 173–177.

10. Engel, A.G. *et al*. 1977. Immune complexes (IgG and C3) at the motor end-plate in myasthenia gravis: ultrastructural and light microscopic localization and electrophysiologic correlations. *Mayo Clin. Proc.* 52: 267–280.

11. Selcen, D. *et al*. 2004. Are MuSK antibodies the primary cause of myasthenic symptoms? *Neurology* 62: 1945–1950.

12. Romi, F. *et al*. 2005. The role of complement in myasthenia gravis: serological evidence of complement consumption in vivo. *J. Neuroimmunol.* 158: 191–194.

13. Barohn, R.J. & R.L. Brey. 1993. Soluble terminal complement components in human myasthenia gravis. *Clin. Neurol. Neurosurg.* 95: 285–290.

14. Ashizawa, T. & S.H. Appel. 1985. Immunopathologic events at the endplate in myasthenia gravis. *Springer Semin. Immunopathol.* 8: 177–196.

15. Wallis, R. *et al*. 2010. Paths reunited: initiation of the classical and lectin pathways of complement activation. *Immunobiology* 215: 1–11.

16. Engel, A.G. *et al*. 1979. Passively transferred experimental autoimmune myasthenia gravis. Sequential and quantitative study of the motor end-plate fine structure and ultrastructural localization of immune complexes (IgG and C3), and of the acetylcholine receptor. *Neurology* 29: 179–188.

17. Chamberlain-Banoub, J. *et al*. 2006. Complement membrane attack is required for endplate damage and clinical disease in passive experimental myasthenia gravis in Lewis rats. *Clin. Exp. Immunol.* 146: 278–286.

18. Tuzun, E. *et al*. 2003. Genetic evidence for involvement of classical complement pathway in induction of experimental autoimmune myasthenia gravis. *J. Immunol.* 171: 3847–3854.

19. Christadoss, P. 1988. C5 gene influences the development of murine myasthenia gravis. *J. Immunol.* 140: 2589–2592.

20. Roversi, P. *et al*. 2007. The structure of OMCI, a novel lipocalin inhibitor of the complement system. *J. Mol. Biol.* 369: 784–793.

21. Navenot, J.M. *et al*. 1997. Expression of CD59, a regulator of the membrane attack complex of complement, on human skeletal muscle fibers. *Muscle Nerve* 20: 92–96.

22. Kaminski, H.J. *et al*. 2004. Complement regulators in extraocular muscle and experimental autoimmune myasthenia gravis. *Exp. Neurol.* 189: 333–342.

23. Kusner, L.L. *et al.* 2012. Cell surface complement regulators moderate experimental myasthenia gravis pathology. *Muscle Nerve* DOI: 10.1002/mus.23448

24. Tuzun, E. *et al.* 2006. Complement regulator CD59 deficiency fails to augment susceptibility to actively induced experimental autoimmune myasthenia gravis. *J. Neuroimmunol.* **181:** 29–33.

25. Morgan, B.P. *et al.* 2006. The membrane attack pathway of complement drives pathology in passively induced experimental autoimmune myasthenia gravis in mice. *Clin. Exp. Immunol.* **146:** 294–302.

26. Kaminski, H.J. *et al.* 2006. Deficiency of decay accelerating factor and CD59 leads to crisis in experimental myasthenia. *Exp. Neurol.* **202:** 287–293.

27. Song, C. *et al.* 2012. Protective effect of scFv-DAF fusion protein on the complement attack to acetylcholine receptor: a possible option for treatment of myasthenia gravis. *Muscle Nerve* **45:** 668–675.

Ann. N.Y. Acad. Sci. ISSN 0077-8923

ANNALS OF THE NEW YORK ACADEMY OF SCIENCES

Issue: *Myasthenia Gravis and Related Disorders*

Novel animal models of acetylcholine receptor antibody–related myasthenia gravis

Erdem Tüzün,[1,2] Windy Allman,[1] Canan Ulusoy,[2] Huan Yang,[3] and Premkumar Christadoss[1]

[1]Department of Microbiology and Immunology, The University of Texas Medical Branch, Galveston, Texas. [2]Department of Neuroscience, Institute of Experimental Medicine and Research, Istanbul University, Istanbul, Turkey. [3]Department of Neurology, Xiang Ya Hospital of Central South University, Changsha, China

Address for correspondence: Premkumar Christadoss, M.D., Department of Microbiology and Immunology, The University of Texas Medical Branch, 301 University Blvd., Galveston, TX 77555-1070. pchrista@utmb.edu

Experimental autoimmune myasthenia gravis (EAMG) in mice has been used to unravel the pathogenic mechanisms and to be used as a preclinical model of myasthenia gravis (MG). Induction of predominantly ocular EAMG in HLA-DQ8 transgenic mice immunized with acetylcholine receptor (AChR) subunits demonstrated the importance of nonconformationally expressed AChR subunits in extraocular muscle involvement. Wild-type (WT) and CD4+ T cell knockout (KO) C57BL/6 mice developed EAMG upon immunization with AChR in incomplete Freund's adjuvant plus lipopolysaccharide. AChR-specific IgG2+ B cell frequencies, estimated by Alexa-conjugated AChR, and AChR-reactive IgG2b levels significantly correlated with the clinical grades of EAMG in WT mice. CD4+ T cell–deficient EAMG mice exhibited AChR antibodies mainly of the IgG2b isotype, emphasizing T helper–independent B cell activation pathways in EAMG induction. These novel EAMG models have suggested that diverse immunopathological mechanisms might contribute to EAMG or MG pathogenesis.

Keywords: myasthenia gravis; experimental autoimmune myasthenia gravis; autoimmunity; lipopolysaccharide; CD4+ T cell

Introduction

Myasthenia gravis (MG) is an acquired autoimmune disorder in which autoantibodies to the postsynaptic acetylcholine receptors (AChRs) are reduced in number or function, leading to muscle fatigue and weakness.[1,2] One of the most commonly used animal models of MG is induced by immunization of mice or rats with AChR in complete Freund's adjuvant (CFA). This experimental autoimmune myasthenia gravis (EAMG) model is induced by an immune response against foreign antigens with cross-reactivity to mouse/rat AChR. By contrast, the autoimmunity in human MG is triggered and maintained by as yet unknown mechanisms. Although EAMG animals do not display thymic pathology, MG patients often present with thymoma and thymic hyperplasia. The thymus gland probably serves as the site of initial autoimmunization and subsequent maintenance of autoimmunity in at least MG patients with thymic pathology.

Therefore, EAMG induced by AChR immunization is not an entirely ideal model for the spontaneous autoimmunity that occurs in humans. Nevertheless, EAMG imitates the clinical, pathological, and electrophysiological features of human MG as closely as possible and thus has been extensively used to unravel the pathogenic mechanisms of MG and explore potential treatment methods for MG.[1–5]

Data from AChR-CFA–induced EAMG suggest that MG is a T cell–dependent B cell–mediated autoimmune disease.[4] Activation of AChR-reactive B cells by T helper (Th) cells culminates in production of complement-fixing anti-AChR IgG isotypes, ultimately leading to membrane attack complex (MAC) formation and subsequent neuromuscular junction (NMJ) destruction.[3–10] Although AChR-antibodies are detected in around 80–90% of MG patients, autoantibodies to muscle-specific receptor tyrosine kinase (MuSK) and lipoprotein-related protein 4 (LRP4) have been identified in

doi: 10.1111/j.1749-6632.2012.06773.x

Table 1. Comparison of conventional and novel acetylcholine receptor–related experimental autoimmune myasthenia gravis models

Method of immunization	Mouse strains	Generalized weakness	Ocular weakness	MHC Class II or CD4 requirement	AChR-antibodies	NMJ deposits
Native whole *Torpedo* AChR in CFA[a]	B6	Mild to severe	None	Required	Present	Present
E. coli plasmid expressing recombinant human AChR α-subunit in CFA	HLA-DQ8 transgenic B10 B6 B10	None or mild	Mild to severe	Not essential	Present	Present
E. coli plasmid expressing recombinant human AChR γ-subunit in CFA	HLA-DQ8 transgenic B10	None or mild	Mild to severe	Unknown	Present	Present
Native whole *Torpedo* AChR in LPS	B6	Mild to severe	None	Not essential	Present	Present

MHC, major histocompatibility complex; HLA, human leukocyte antigen; NMJ, neuromuscular junction; AChR, acetylcholine receptor; C57BL/6, B6; C57BL/10, B10; CFA, complete Freund's adjuvant; LPS, lipopolysaccharide.
[a]The conventional immunization method commonly used to induce EAMG.

some MG patients previously considered to be seronegative.[11,12] Although, in general, MuSK antibody–related MG has similar features as AChR antibody–related MG, MuSK antibody–related MG patients are more likely to present with severe weakness that requires assisted ventilation and higher doses of immunosuppressive agents. Also, in contrast with AChR-antibody–positive MG, some MuSK-antibody–positive patients exhibit particularly severe facial and tongue muscle atrophy.[12] Notably, the animal model of MuSK-MG, induced by immunization of mice and rats with MuSK in CFA, also appears to have a more severe and debilitating course and is characterized with more significant weight loss than that observed in EAMG induced with AChR immunization.[13]

Our recent studies based on immunization of wild-type (WT), human leukocyte antigen (HLA)–DQ8 transgenic, or major histocompatibility complex (MHC) class II knockout (KO) C57BL/6 (B6)

mice using different AChR-subunit antigens or novel adjuvants have introduced novel EAMG models with different clinical and/or immunopathological features (Table 1). These studies have thus provided new insights into the current knowledge of MG pathogenesis.[14–17]

Ocular EAMG induced by AChR subunit immunization

EAMG has so far been conventionally induced by immunization with the purified whole native AChR molecule, generally obtained from electric ray *Torpedo californica*.[4] The absence of ocular symptoms is a major difference of this active AChR-EAMG model compared to human MG.[4,5] Ocular symptoms are the initial complaints in most MG patients and around 10% of MG patients present with only extraocular muscle involvement. The reason(s) behind this difference between EAMG and MG are not known.

EAMG induction does not necessarily require immunization with the native AChR heteromer. Immunization of rats with recombinant human AChR-α subunit and immunization of mice and rats with small AChR peptides obtained from human, mouse, or rat AChR leads to an EAMG-like disease that closely mimics the disease induced by whole AChR.[18–21] Notably, rats immunized with the immunodominant peptide (α97–116) of the rat AChR-α subunit develop the clinical and electrophysiological aspects of MG, suggesting that EAMG in rats can be induced by a single peptide of the self AChR.[19]

In contrast with the previous immunization methods, HLA-DQ8 transgenic and mouse MHC class II-deficient C57BL/10 (B10) mice immunized with an *Escherichia coli* plasmid expressing the recombinant human AChR-α or -γ subunit developed predominantly ocular symptoms (partial or full ptosis).[13,14] The same immunogen also induced ocular myasthenic symptoms in WT B6 and B10 mice, whereas HLA-DR3 transgenic mice were highly ocular EAMG resistant. In a similar fashion to human MG, mice first developed ptosis, followed by mild to moderate generalized muscle weakness. Some mice (around 20–40% in different experiments) never developed limb weakness and remained with purely ocular symptoms.[14,15] By contrast, HLA-DQ8 transgenic or WT mice immunized with the whole human AChR (derived from the TE671 cell line) only developed generalized muscle weakness.[22]

Mice with ocular symptoms displayed serum antibodies not only to human AChR-subunits but also to crude extraocular and limb muscle homogenates. Extraocular and limb muscles of the same mice showed C3, MAC, and IgG deposits in many NMJs, suggesting antibody- and complement-mediated AChR loss. In resemblance to clinical EAMG findings, antibody and complement accumulation was more frequently observed in the extraocular muscles (12–20% of NMJs) than limb muscles (5–15% of NMJs).[14,15] Notably, some mice with no generalized weakness also showed deposits at the limb NMJs, suggesting that some of the immunized mice develop subclinical EAMG with minimal NMJ dysfunction and no notable muscle weakness despite NMJ deposits. Similar MG patients with purely ocular MG, no limb muscle weakness, and limb NMJ deposits have also been reported.[23] In addition, in resemblance to conventional generalized EAMG in-

duced by the whole native AChR molecule, following immunization with the human AChR subunits, the extraocular and limb muscle samples demonstrated significantly increased mRNA levels for α, γ, and ε subunits, suggesting the existence of a compensating mechanism to attenuate the AChR loss induced by AChR subunit immunization.[15,24]

Immunization with the *E. coli* extract without the human AChR subunits failed to induce any clinical or immunohistochemical findings in HLA-transgenic or WT mice, suggesting that an AChR insert is required for development of pathologic deposits of IgG, C3, and MAC and subsequently myasthenic symptoms. Nevertheless, *E. coli*-immunized HLA-DQ8 transgenic mice had very low levels of serum anti-AChR antibodies and NMJ deposits, suggesting that miniscule amounts of *E. coli* proteins remaining in the immunogen might have acted as an adjuvant or molecular mimic and contributed to the induction of myasthenic pathology.[14,15] This assumption needs to be further scrutinized by future experiments.

Generation of ocular symptoms by human AChR-γ subunit immunization might be explained by abundant presence of this subunit in extraocular muscles. However, absence of the γ subunit in the upper eyelid elevator levator palpebrae muscle,[25] which is most profoundly affected in this new model, and induction of ptosis in mice immunized with the α subunit,[14] which is expressed in all striated muscles, contradict this assumption.

Obvious EAMG susceptibility of HLA-DQ8 transgenic mice and significant EAMG resistance of HLA-DR3 transgenic mice suggest that the intensity and location (ocular versus generalized) of myasthenic symptoms might depend on the autoimmune response induced by specific interactions between the individual MHC molecules and AChR subunits. The significance of these interactions has already been epitomized by the mutant mouse strain bm12, which differs from its parental strain B6 at the I-Aβ locus and in this way exhibits an immune response profile markedly different from that of B6. Only three nucleotide differences in the I-Aβ gene render bm12 mice highly resistant to EAMG.[26] Moreover, induction of ocular symptoms by nonconformational AChR subunits rather than the whole AChR molecule with the native conformation raises the question whether certain thymic cells expressing nonconformational epitopes of AChR might be the initial driving force behind the autoimmune response against extraocular muscles.[27] In this hypothetical setting, exposure to a nonconformational molecular mimic of the AChR subunit (of thymic or extrinsic origin) in a susceptible person could trigger T and B cell autoimmune responses to AChR subunit pathogenic epitopes and could culminate in ocular symptoms at an earlier phase of MG. As the immune system gains access to NMJ AChR molecules, which have the native conformation, generalized muscle weakness might ensue.

Interestingly, MHC class-II deficient ($A\beta^0$) mice in the B6 background developed extraocular muscle weakness, when immunized with the *E. coli* plasmid expressing the recombinant human AChR-α subunit. The clinical incidence and severity and levels of anti-AChR antibodies and NMJ deposits are much lower in AChR subunit-immunized $A\beta^0$ mice than those observed in WT and HLA-transgenic mice immunized with the same antigen.[14] Nevertheless, this finding suggests that, in contrast to the conventional view, myasthenic muscle weakness might be induced by non-MHC class II–restricted, Th-mediated, and purely B cell–dependent mechanisms.

Lipopolysaccharide-enhanced model of EAMG

Another EAMG model that appears to be induced predominantly by B cell–dependent mechanisms is generated by immunization with lipopolysaccharide (LPS) and incomplete Freund's adjuvant (IFA). CFA has long been the principal and standard adjuvant used for induction of EAMG, as well as many other autoimmune disease models. However, CFA, which contains inactivated mycobacteria, is a major promoter of both Th1- and Th2-type immunities.[28] This effect might blur the results obtained by CFA immunization and make it difficult to interpret whether the immunological profile of the immunized animals is genuinely modulated by the immunogen or CFA, even when only CFA-immunized mice are used as controls. Especially, when CFA is used to generate the animal model of a Th2-dominated disease, the resultant immunological and clinical phenotype might not be a perfect equivalent of the human disease. For example, in MG patients, MuSK antibodies are predominantly of noncomplement fixing IgG4 isotype, which is stimulated by Th2-immunity.[29,30] By contrast, mice immunized with a MuSK plus CFA emulsion develop MuSK antibodies of both noncomplement-fixing IgG1 (human IgG4 equivalent) and complement-fixing IgG2 (human IgG1 equivalent) isotypes, which are stimulated by Th2 and Th1 immunities, respectively.[31] This raises the question whether the AChR-EAMG model obtained by utilization of CFA as an adjuvant indisputably reflects the immunopathogenic features of the human disease and whether using a different adjuvant could unmask the alternative immunological pathways that are capable of inducing EAMG and MG.

Until now, the adjuvant effect of LPS has been tested in only a few models of autoimmunity, including those for experimental autoimmune thyroiditis, experimental autoimmune arthritis and lupus-prone MRL/lpr mice[32,33] and the precise effects of this adjuvant on autoimmunity are vastly unknown. To delineate these issues, B6 mice were immunized with AChR in IFA mixed with LPS, which is a strong Th1 promoter.[34] LPS-AChR immunization induced EAMG in B6 mice like that seen following CFA-AChR immunization. The clinical severity, EAMG incidence and grip strengths of mice immunized with LPS-AChR and CFA-AChR were exactly identical.[17] The CFA-AChR induced–EAMG has been shown to be strictly dependent upon the activation of AChR-specific CD4+ T cells.[8–10] By contrast, CD4+ T cell KO mice immunized with LPS-AChR were as susceptible to EAMG as WT mice immunized with LPS-AChR or CFA-AChR, whereas CD4+ T cell KO mice immunized with CFA-AChR were highly EAMG resistant. Both WT and CD4+ T cell KO mice immunized with LPS-AChR diplayed significantly reduced serum levels of anti-AChR IgG1 and increased levels of anti-AChR IgG2b, as compared to WT mice immunized with CFA-AChR, consistent with the Th1-promoting effect of LPS.[10,17] Moreover, CD4 KO mice immunized with LPS-AChR, but not CFA-AChR, showed an abundance of NMJ IgG and complement deposits.[17]

To further characterize the distinguishing features of CFA versus LPS immunization, AChR-specific B cell populations in the peripheral blood of B6 mice immunized with AChR in combination with LPS or CFA were evaluated. For this purpose, a flow cytometric assay was developed. Alexa-conjugated AChR was used as a probe for AChR-specific B cells (B220+Ig+). Mice with EAMG showed significantly elevated frequencies of AChR-specific IgG2+ and

IgM$^+$ B cells. Moreover, the frequencies of IgG2$^+$ B cells and plasma anti-AChR IgG2 levels significantly correlated with the clinical grades of EAMG, further validating this novel assay.[16]

This method was applied to assess the AChR-reactive B cell frequencies in the circulation of LPS- and CFA-immunized mice. There were no significant differences in the total frequencies of B cells (B220$^+$ lymphocytes) present in blood samples of naive, WT CFA-AChR, WT LPS-AChR, CD4$^+$ T cell

KO CFA$^+$AChR, and CD4 KO LPS-AChR immunized mice. All mice immunized with AChR, regardless of genotype or the adjuvant used, had significantly elevated frequencies of AChR-binding B cells compared to naive mice. Of particular interest, both LPS-AChR and CFA-AChR–immunized CD4$^+$ T cell KO mice had increased mean frequencies of AChR-binding B cells than naive, WT CFA-AChR, and WT LPS-AChR immunized mice. However, the frequency of AChR$^+$ peripheral B cells was higher

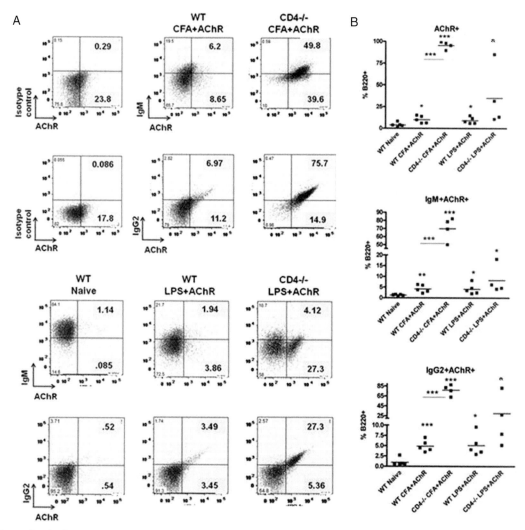

Figure 1. The frequencies of AChR-binding peripheral blood lymphocytes are elevated in CD4$^{-/-}$ mice. Representative flow cytometry analysis of peripheral blood lymphocytes from naive, LPS-AChR or CFA-AChR–immunized mice, 75 days postprimary immunization. Cells were first gated on B220$^+$ lymphocytes to characterize IgM or IgG2 expression and AChR binding (A). The numbers shown in bi-exponential plots indicate the relative percentage of cells in each quadrant. Mean frequency of total AChR-binding B cells (top row), IgM$^+$ AChR-binding B cells (middle row), and IgG2$^+$ AChR-binding B cells (bottom row) (B). $n = 4$–5, Student's t-test; $^*P < 0.05$, $^{***}P < 0.001$. Data are from Ref. 35.

in CD4$^+$ T cell KO CFA-AChR–immunized mice (Fig. 1).[35] Therefore, it is likely that AChR-specific B cells from CFA-AChR–immunized CD4$^+$ T cell KO mice are not deleted but may be either inhibited from differentiating into antibody- secreting plasma cells or perhaps preferentially shunted into the memory B cell repertoire and are anergic. The generation of different B cell subsets may be more dependent upon signals provided by adjuvant than CD4 costimulation, since LPS-AChR–immunized CD4$^+$ T cell KO mice are capable of producing high affinity secreted IgG.[17]

Overall, these results demonstrated that LPS can be used as an adjuvant to induce autoimmune NMJ destruction and EAMG can be induced via non-CD4$^+$ T helper cell-mediated mechanisms. The development of autoimmunity triggered by LPS or CFA occurs by activation of distinct B cell differentiation pathways. The CFA immunization requires the presence of CD4$^+$ T cell costimulation of B cells to induce anti-AChR IgG2 secretion, whereas LPS immunization does not require CD4$^+$ T cell costimulation to induce anti-AChR antibody production.

Conclusion

The recently introduced novel EAMG models have suggested that immunological mechanisms participating in EAMG and MG pathogenesis are far more complicated than once considered. The diversity of these mechanisms might also be the driving force behind the significant clinical heterogeneity of MG. Therefore, investigation of these mechanisms might generate novel diagnostic and therapeutic approaches for MG patients. Our results suggest that investigation of immunological phenotypes can be achieved by using specific and strategically selected adjuvants and antigens.

Acknowledgments

The studies reported in this review were supported by the Muscular Dystrophy Association (MDA) and the French Muscular Dystrophy Association (AFM).

Conflicts of interest

The authors declare no conflicts of interest.

References

1. Lang, B. & A. Vincent. 2009. Autoimmune disorders of the neuromuscular junction. *Curr. Opin. Pharmacol.* **9:** 336–340.
2. Vincent, A. & M.I. Leite. 2005. Neuromuscular junction autoimmune disease: muscle specific kinase antibodies and treatments for myasthenia gravis. *Curr. Opin. Neurol.* **18:** 519–525.
3. Tüzün, E., R. Huda & P. Christadoss. 2011. Complement and cytokine based therapeutic strategies in myasthenia gravis. *J. Autoimmun.* **37:** 136–143.
4. Christadoss, P., M. Poussin & C. Deng. 2000. Animal models of myasthenia gravis. *Clin. Immunol.* **94:** 75–87.
5. Wu, B. *et al.* 2011. Experimental autoimmune myasthenia gravis in the mouse. *Curr. Protoc. Immunol.* **15:** 15.23.1–15.23.26.
6. Tüzün, E. *et al.* 2008. Targeting classical complement pathway to treat complement mediated autoimmune diseases. *Adv. Exp. Med. Biol.* **632:** 265–272.
7. Christadoss, P. *et al.* 2008. Classical complement pathway in experimental autoimmune myasthenia gravis pathogenesis. *Ann. N.Y. Acad. Sci.* **1132:** 210–219.
8. Shenoy, M. *et al.* 1994. Effect of MHC class I and CD8 cell deficiency on experimental autoimmune myasthenia gravis pathogenesis. *J. Immunol.* **153:** 5330–5335.
9. Christadoss, P., J. Lindstrom & N. Talal. 1983. Cellular immune response to acetylcholine receptors in murine experimental autoimmune myasthenia gravis: inhibition with monoclonal anti-I-A antibodies. *Cell. Immunol.* **81:** 1–8.
10. Zhang, G.X. *et al.* Both CD4+ and CD8 +T cells are essential to induce experimental autoimmune myasthenia gravis. *J. Exp. Med.* **184:** 349–356.
11. Higuchi, O. *et al.* 2011. Autoantibodies to low-density lipoprotein receptor-related protein 4 in myasthenia gravis. *Ann. Neurol.* **69:** 418–422.
12. Farrugia, M.E. *et al.* 2006. MRI and clinical studies of facial and bulbar muscle involvement in MuSK antibody-associated myasthenia gravis. *Brain* **129:** 1481–1492.
13. Viegas, S. *et al.* 2012. Passive and active immunization models of MuSK-Ab positive myasthenia: electrophysiological evidence for pre and postsynaptic defects. *Exp. Neurol.* **234:** 506–512.
14. Yang, H. *et al.* 2007. A new mouse model of autoimmune ocular myasthenia gravis. *Invest. Ophthalmol. Vis. Sci.* **48:** 5101–5111.
15. Wu, X. *et al.* 2012. Ocular and generalized myasthenia gravis induced by human acetylcholine receptor γ subunit immunization. *Muscle Nerve* **45:** 209–216.
16. Allman, W. *et al.* 2011. Characterization of peripheral blood acetylcholine receptor-binding B cells in experimental myasthenia gravis. *Cell. Immunol.* **271:** 292–298.
17. Allman, W. *et al.* 2012. CD4 costimulation is not required in a novel LPS-enhanced model of myasthenia gravis. *J. Neuroimmunol.* **249:** 1–7.
18. Lennon, V.A. *et al.* 1991. Recombinant human acetylcholine receptor alpha-subunit induces chronic experimental autoimmune myasthenia gravis. *J. Immunol.* **146:** 2245–2248.
19. Baggi, F. *et al.* 2004. Breakdown of tolerance to a self-peptide of acetylcholine receptor alpha-subunit induces experimental myasthenia gravis in rats. *J. Immunol.* **172:** 2697–2703.
20. Oshima, M. *et al.* 1998. T cell responses in EAMG-susceptible and non-susceptible mouse strains after immunization with overlapping peptides encompassing the extracellular part of Torpedo californica acetylcholine receptor alpha chain. Implication to role in myasthenia gravis

of autoimmune T-cell responses against receptor degradation products. *Autoimmunity* **27**: 79–90.

21. Wang, H.B. *et al.* 2001. Anti-CTLA-4 antibody treatment triggers determinant spreading and enhances murine myasthenia gravis. *J. Immunol.* **166**: 6430–6436.

22. Yang, H. *et al.* 2002. Mapping myasthenia gravis-associated T cell epitopes on human acetylcholine receptors in HLA transgenic mice. *J. Clin. Invest.* **109**: 1111–1120.

23. Tsujihata, M. *et al.* 1989. Diagnostic significance of IgG, C3, and C9 at the limb muscle motor end-plate in minimal myasthenia gravis. *Neurology* **39**: 1359–1363.

24. Sheng, J.R. *et al.* 2009. Acetylcholine receptor-alpha subunit expression in myasthenia gravis: a role for the autoantigen in pathogenesis? *Muscle Nerve* **40**: 279–286.

25. Kaminski, H.J. *et al.* 1995. The gamma-subunit of the acetylcholine receptor is not expressed in the levator palpebrae superioris. *Neurology* **45**: 516–518.

26. Yang, B., K.R. McIntosh & D.B. Drachman. 1998. How subtle differences in MHC class II affect the severity of experimental myasthenia gravis. *Clin. Immunol. Immunopathol.* **86**: 45–58.

27. Vincent, A. *et al.* 1998. Determinant spreading and immune responses to acetylcholine receptors in myasthenia gravis. *Immunol. Rev.* **164**: 157–168.

28. Zhang, G.X. *et al.* 1997. Linomide suppresses both Th1 and Th2 cytokines in experimental autoimmune myasthenia gravis. *J. Neuroimmunol.* **73**: 175–182.

29. Basile, E. *et al.* 2006. During 3 years treatment of primary progressive multiple sclerosis with glatiramer acetate, specific antibodies switch from IgG1 to IgG4. *J. Neuroimmunol.* **177**: 161–166.

30. Füchtenbusch, M. *et al.* 2000. Exposure to exogenous insulin promotes IgG1 and the T-helper 2-associated IgG4 responses to insulin but not to other islet autoantigens. *Diabetes* **49**: 918–925.

31. Hussain, R. *et al.* 1995. Selective increases in antibody isotypes and immunoglobulin G subclass responses to secreted antigens in tuberculosis patients and healthy household contacts of the patients. *Clin. Diagn. Lab. Immunol.* **2**: 726–732.

32. Granholm, N.A. & T. Cavallo. 1994. Long-lasting effects of bacterial lipopolysaccharide promote progression of lupus nephritis in NZB/W mice. *Lupus* **3**: 507–514.

33. Yoshino, S., E. Sasatomi & M. Ohsawa. 2000. Bacterial lipopolysaccharide acts as an adjuvant to induce autoimmune arthritis in mice. *Immunology* **99**: 607–614.

34. Jamalan, M. *et al.* 2011. Effectiveness of Brucella abortus lipopolysaccharide as an adjuvant for tuberculin PPD. *Biologicals* **39**: 23–28.

35. Allman, W. 2009. Cellular requirements for antibody production in a novel LPS-enhanced model of autoimmune myasthenia gravis. Dissertation, The University of Texas Medical Branch, Galveston, TX, USA.

Ann. N.Y. Acad. Sci. ISSN 0077-8923

ANNALS OF THE NEW YORK ACADEMY OF SCIENCES
Issue: *Myasthenia Gravis and Related Disorders*

Animal models of antimuscle-specific kinase myasthenia

David P. Richman,[1,2] Kayoko Nishi,[1] Michael J. Ferns,[2,3] Joachim Schnier,[1] Peter Pytel,[4] Ricardo A. Maselli,[1,2] and Mark A. Agius[1,2,5]

[1]Department of Neurology, Center for Neuroscience, [2]Center for Neuroscience, [3]Department of Physiology and Membrane Biology, University of California, Davis, California. [4]Department of Pathology, The University of Chicago, Chicago, Illinois. [5]Veterans Administration Northern California Health System, Sacramento, California

Address for correspondence: David P. Richman, Department of Neurology, University of California, 1515 Newton Court, Davis, CA 95616. dprichman@ucdavis.edu

Antimuscle-specific kinase (anti-MuSK) myasthenia (AMM) differs from antiacetylcholine receptor myasthenia gravis in exhibiting more focal muscle involvement (neck, shoulder, facial, and bulbar muscles) with wasting of the involved, primarily axial, muscles. AMM is not associated with thymic hyperplasia and responds poorly to anticholinesterase treatment. Animal models of AMM have been induced in rabbits, mice, and rats by immunization with purified xenogeneic MuSK ectodomain, and by passive transfer of large quantities of purified serum IgG from AMM patients into mice. The models have confirmed the pathogenic role of the MuSK antibodies in AMM and have demonstrated the involvement of both the presynaptic and postsynaptic components of the neuromuscular junction. The observations in this human disease and its animal models demonstrate the role of MuSK not only in the formation of this synapse but also in its maintenance.

Keywords: animal models; autoimmune; muscle-specific kinase; muscle wasting; MuSK; myasthenia; neuromuscular junction; synapse

Antimuscle-specific kinase myasthenia

Ninety percent of patients with generalized myasthenia gravis (MG) have measurable acetylcholine receptor (AChR) antibodies (Abs) circulating in blood. The remainder, referred to as having seronegative MG, have clinical characteristics that are similar, but not necessarily identical, to those with AChR Abs, that is, seropositive MG.[1] Vincent *et al.* and others have identified circulating Abs to the extracellular domain of antimuscle-specific kinase (anti-MuSK) in approximately 40% of seronegative patients.[2–7] This MuSK Ab-positive subgroup of seronegative patients, which we have referred to as anti-MuSK myasthenia (AMM), tends to differ from seropositive MG in demonstrating more focal muscle involvement (neck, shoulder, facial, and bulbar muscles), but with considerable variability from patient to patient.[2,3,6–9] Unlike symptoms in seropositive MG, many AMM patients have wasting of these muscles.[7,9–17] The data available, including

those from electrophysiologic studies of the involved muscles and a small number of histologic studies of (less involved) extremity muscles, have failed to show evidence of denervation but rather suggested a myopathic process, perhaps involving mitochondrial function.[8,11,15,18–23] Other differences from MG include poor response to treatment with cholinesterase inhibitors, intravenous Ig, or thymectomy.[3,6,24] Also, only a rare AMM patient has been found to have thymic lymphoid hyperplasia (commonly found in MG).[25–27] Histologic studies of the neuromuscular junction (NMJ) in AMM carried out to date[28–30] have observed[31] mild simplification of the EP pretzel architecture. Microelectrode analysis of two of these specimens revealed a mild decrease in miniature endplate potential (MEPP) amplitudes[29,30] and quantal content.[30]

Few studies[18,32–35] have addressed the pathogenesis of AMM. While it is a reasonable hypothesis that MuSK Abs represent the etiologic factor in AMM, until recently, the importance or precise role of these

doi: 10.1111/j.1749-6632.2012.06782.x

Ann. N.Y. Acad. Sci. 1274 (2012) 140–147 © 2012 New York Academy of Sciences.

Abs has been poorly understood. In fact, there have been a number of publications questioning their role in AMM, suggesting instead that they may occur secondary to some other process or even that they are an epiphenomenon.[29,36] However, recent experimental data have supported the above hypothesis with observations of weakness and NMJ changes in animals that had been actively[37–44] or passively immunized with MuSK.[33,34,42,45] A number of investigators have found both MuSK-activating (agonist) and MuSK-blocking (antagonist) effects of polyclonal serum MuSK Ab in muscle cell cultures, assaying both phosphorylation of various components of the downstream MuSK phosphorylation pathway (see below) and AChR clustering.[4,33,40,41,46,47] In addition, polyclonal human AMM serum added to muscle cultures appears to induce endocytic internalization of MuSK, leading to partial reduction in membrane MuSK.[33]

Role of MuSK in the NMJ

MuSK is a 100 kD transmembrane receptor tyrosine kinase. It is a single-pass integral membrane protein with an N-terminal extracellular domain followed by a short transmembrane domain and then a C-terminal cytoplasmic domain.[48–50] The extracellular domain, which appears to be required for interaction with agrin and low density lipoprotein receptor-related protein 4 (lrp4; see below), comprises three immunoglobulin (Ig)-like domains[51–54] and a cysteine-rich (frizzled-like) C6 box region.[48,49,53,55] The cytoplasmic domain contains the kinase activity and signaling components of the molecule that lead to the development of the postsynaptic apparatus.[56–58] Studies employing both rat and human MuSK have determined that it is only the extracellular domain of the molecule that is the target of the AMM Abs.[4,5] We have recently identified a splicing variant of MuSK, MuSK 60, containing an additional 20-residue domain located between Ig-2 and Ig-3 expressed primarily in adult muscle, which appears to be an important antigen in AMM.[59,60]

MuSK plays a major role in the development of the NMJ. The synapse begins to form when the axon growth cone of a developing motor neuron encounters a developing myotube and begins to secrete the glycoprotein agrin.[31,61–63] The secreted agrin induces dense clustering of AChRs in the postsynaptic endplate membrane, as well as the elaboration of this structure, including its pretzel-like topographic profile and the marked folding and specialization of the membrane at the ultrastructural level. Both the initial spontaneous AChR clustering[64] and the agrin-induced more extensive clustering require the presence of both MuSK and a second postsynaptic protein, lrp4.[51,54,65,66] However, the processes involved in further maturation of the NMJ and, in particular, the mechanisms involved in the maintenance of the mature NMJ—and the role of MuSK in these mechanisms—have been much less well delineated.[67–72]

NMJ histologic and electrophysiologic abnormalities in AMM

Histologic studies of the NMJ in AMM carried out to date have reported mild simplification of the EP pretzel architecture. Microelectrode analysis of two of these specimens revealed a mild decrease in MEPP amplitudes and, in one, reduced quantal content.[28–30] In contrast, an examination of a patient with very severe acute disease revealed simplified endplate membranes and poor registration between the nerve terminal and the abnormal endplate.[30]

Muscle wasting in AMM

Not only does the distribution of muscles involved in AMM differ from that of seropositive MG, but those muscles also are frequently wasted. The mechanism of the development of the prominent axial muscle wasting in these patients remains unclear. The data available, including those from electrophysiologic studies of the involved muscles and a small number of histologic studies of (less involved) extremity muscles, failed to show evidence of denervation but instead suggested a myopathic process, perhaps involving mitochondrial function.[8,11,15,18–23] Such myopathic changes support a role for MuSK in mediating trophic effects on muscle, perhaps through complex two-way communication between nerve and muscle at the NMJ. On the other hand, focal denervation with accompanying reinnervation, as suggested by the morphologic studies described the rat model of AMM (see later), might also lead to muscle wasting.

Rabbit and mouse models of AMM

In rabbits and mice repeatedly immunized with MuSK over extended periods of time weakness has

Table 1. Animal models of AMM

Immunization Type	Species	Strain	Mutation	Immunogen/number of immunizations/serum IgG transferred	Clinical severity	Muscle wasting	References
Active							
	Rabbit	NZW	No	Mouse ectodomain/3–4	Severe	No	41
	Mouse	A/J	No	Rat ectodomain ΔIg3/2–3	Mild-moderate	No	37
		BALBc6	No	Rat ectodomain ΔIg3/3	Mild-moderate	No	
	Mouse	C57BL/6	No	Rat ectodomain/3	Mild	Yes	43
	Mouse	A/WySnJ	C5 and BAFF-R deficient	Rat ectodomain/2	Moderate	No	39
	Mouse	C57BL/6	No	Human ectodomain/3	Mild (variable)	No	42
	Rat	Lewis	No	Mouse MuSK-60 ectodomain/1	Severe	Yes	72
Passive							
	Mouse/ human	C57BL/6	No	500–600 mg	Mild	No	34
	Mouse/ human	C57BL/6	No	250 mg	None	No	42

Ig = immunoglobulin-like domain; ΔIg3 = minus the Ig3 domain.

been observed[37–43] along with mild electrophysiologic evidence of disordered NMJ transmission (Table 1). NZW strain rabbits immunized with 100–400 µg of ectodomain of mouse MuSK, repeated times three, exhibited severe weakness.[41] Three immunizations of various mouse strains with the ectodomain of rat MuSK (minus the third Ig-like domain) produced mild to severe weakness and decremental responses, most severe in A/J and B6 strains but not in BALB/c mice. In additional mouse studies using either the same immunogen or intact rat ectodomain in C57BL/6 mice, 3–4 repeated immunizations resulted in mild disease.[39,42,43] In contrast, A/WySnJ mice, which are deficient in both complement C5 and BAFF receptor, injected twice with 20 µg of rat ectodomain developed severe weakness.[39]

In addition, in immunosuppressed mice passively injected with xenogeneic (human) AMM IgG repeatedly over 14 days (total of 0.68 g), mild-moderate weakness occurred in conjunction with reduced AChR staining and reduced registration between nerve terminals and EPs.[34] In a similar study using a total of 250 µg of AMM IgG, weakness was not observed, though microelectrode analysis re-

vealed reductions in both MEPP and endplate potential amplitudes.[42]

Experimental AMM: AMM model in Lewis rats

The strategy for the development of this model was to use a xenogeneic immunogen, mouse MuSK, that differed by a minor degree from the target of the autoimmune attack, native Lewis rat MuSK. In the course of purifying mouse MuSK for this purpose, we identified in adult mouse muscle a pair of new splice variants of this protein.[59,60] In fact, nearly half of the MuSK cDNAs cloned from adult mouse muscle encoded one of the variant isoforms, which we designated MuSK 60. We have found that MuSK 60 is expressed in progressively greater amounts during muscle differentiation, such that it represents on the order of 50% of the expressed MuSK in adult muscle.[59,60] Moreover, *in vitro* studies with this isoform demonstrated that it has a reduced ability to induce AChR clustering in response to the addition of agrin. Taken together, the latter two observations suggest that this "adult" form of MuSK has a distinct function from that of the other isoforms, which are found primarily in developing muscle.

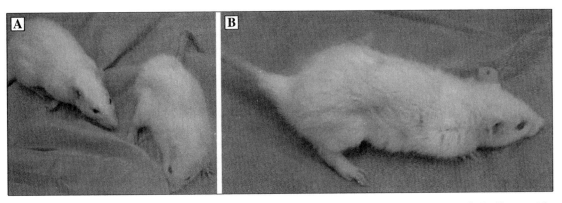

Figure 1. Clinical findings in EAMM. (A) Rat immunized with 100 μg of N-MuSK 60 (right), day 25, with significant weight loss, flank and neck muscle wasting, extremity weakness, kyphotic posture, and ruffled ungroomed fur. Adjuvant control (left) is normal. (B) Lateral view of N-MuSK 60–immunized rat from panel A (with permission from *Archives of Neurology*).

Immunization with the MuSK 60 isoform produced a very severe acute model of AMM resulting from a single injection in Lewis rats.[44] Unlike the disease induced in mice and rabbits, this severe form of experimental AMM (EAMM) reproduces all the major characteristics of the human disease: fatigable weakness, disordered neuromuscular transmission, and wasting of axial musculature. A single injection of 100 μg of the purified extracellular domain of the MuSK 60 isoform induces very high anti-MuSK Ab titers ($>1{:}10^6$) and severe weakness that is lethal by day 27 after immunization. Immunization with lower doses of this antigen produces a more chronic disease with lower anti-MuSK titers. Analysis of NMJ morphology in these animals suggests that Ab attack on MuSK affects both postsynaptic and presynaptic components of this synapse. The animals exhibit marked weight loss and axial muscle wasting not observed in other models of AMM or in EAMG. The ability of these animals to eat, drink, and chew is not observably abnormal until the last two days of life. As the disease progresses, the axial weakness/wasting leads to a striking kyphotic posture, eventually in association with the inability of the forelimbs to lift the chest from the floor of the cage (Fig. 1). Of note, similar posture and gait abnormalities have been observed in adult mice in which MuSK expression was abrogated using Cre recombinase-mediated MuSK gene deletion. The reproduction of all the characteristics of AMM in the current form of EAMM strongly supports the hypothesis that the autoimmune response to MuSK in AMM is pathogenically important in this disease, rather than it being an epiphenomenon. Moreover,

these observations highlight the potential usefulness of this model for studying the pathogenesis and future treatments of AMM. Moreover, the correlation between anti-N-MuSK 60 Ab titer and disease severity also supports the hypothesis that EAMM and AMM are the result of the action of the MuSK Abs.

The form of EAMM induced in this study is more severe than the forms induced in mice and rabbits by active immunization with rat or human MuSK and mouse MuSK, respectively. In those studies, relatively mild disease, as determined clinically and histologically, occurred only after three injections of antigen with adjuvant over an extended period, eight weeks. It is unclear why the present disease is so much more severe than that induced in those systems. One possibility is that the differences relate to species sensitivity to the anti-MuSK attack. For example, Lewis rats develop more severe EAMG—the animal model of seropositive MG induced by immunization with AChR—than do various mouse strains,[73] an observation previously ascribed to differences in the level of the safety factor of neuromuscular transmission, known to be quite high in mice.[74] A second possibility is that the Lewis rats are more prone to autoimmune disease induced by immunization with xenogeneic antigens. Such differences have been demonstrated for EAMG among various inbred mice strains, but in none of those strains is the EAMG as severe as it is in Lewis rats.[73,75] This possibility seems less likely to explain the differences in severity between the NZW strain rabbit and Lewis rat forms of EAMM because both strains develop equally severe EAMG when immunized with AChR.[76] A third possibility relates to the differences in the antigens used to induce the disease and, hence, the epitope targets of the disease-inducing Abs. The MuSK 60 isoform, used as immunogen in the current study, appears to be an adult form of the protein,[59,60] which may be an important target of the auto-Abs in EAMM and AMM. For the rabbit and mouse forms of EAMM, the immunogens have been either the fetal isoform or another splicing variant of the protein that is missing not only the 20 amino acid extra domain of MuSK 60 but also the entire third Ig domain.[37] The severe disease observed in adult animals resulting from Abs to an adult form of MuSK supports the possibility of a role for MuSK, perhaps through its MuSK 60 isoform, in the maintenance and functioning of the mature NMJ.[33]

Animals immunized with a lower dose of N-MuSK 60 experience a less severe form of EAMM, along with lower serum titers of MuSK Abs, suggesting that in EAMM Ab titer correlates with disease severity.[44] However, the animals receiving lower doses of N-MuSK 60 demonstrate higher degrees of diminished neuromuscular transmission, albeit at later times following the immunization. These observations suggest that the weakness, weight loss, and muscle wasting associated with rapidly fatal disease may not correlate with neuromuscular transmission per se. If true, then it is possible that interference with other physiologic activities at the NMJ is playing a role in AMM.

The histologic changes observed in this model support the hypothesis that factors other than reduced neuromuscular transmission play a role and suggest a possible mechanism by which this may occur. In particular, the animals receiving 100 μg of MuSK exhibit varying degrees of disruption of the normal NMJ architecture. The architecture of some endplates is disrupted, with terminal arbors and AChR clusters fragmented into smaller, discontinuous structures, with marked simplification of postsynaptic membranes. The nerve terminals at some NMJs are more severely affected, with complete or partial loss of these structures. In addition, some axons have an abnormal globular appearance and others exhibit local extension beyond the NMJ, or even frank terminal axon sprouting. In other NMJs there is misalignment between the presynaptic and postsynaptic portions of these synapses. The latter findings, some of which were also observed in the study of passive transfer of human AMM serum into

mice[34] and in one of the three studies of AMM,[30] suggest that there is abnormal signaling between nerve terminal and muscle endplate in both directions, independent of neuromuscular transmission, resulting in failure of maintenance of the mature synapse in these animals.

In addition, cholinesterase staining of teased muscle bundles from EAMM animals reveals abnormal dispersion of paraformaldehyde-resistant cholinesterase activity throughout the length of the muscle fibers. The observed segmented and dispersed cholinesterase-stained patches, away from the compact synaptic region (motor point),[44] is reminiscent of newly formed synapses, raising the possibility that the Ab attack leads first to frank denervation at some NMJs with subsequent and, possibly, ongoing attempts at reinnervation. The observation, also noted quantitatively in passively induced EAMM in mice,[33] that some NMJs are intact, while neighboring junctions are mildly disrupted and yet others are markedly abnormal, supports that possible scenario. It is of special note that severe damage to the endplate membrane, as is seen in acute forms of EAMG and MG, produces essentially no nerve terminal abnormalities and no denervation/reinnervation. Hence, the Ab attack on MuSK appears to have wider ranging effects on the NMJ, as described here and in passively induced EAMM,[33] than is seen with attack on the more abundant endplate AChRs.

The mechanism of the development of the prominent axial muscle wasting in these animals, not seen in EAMG and MG, also remains unclear. Both histologic and electrophysiologic studies in human AMM suggest that the muscle wasting is not the result of denervation but rather is the consequence of a primary myopathy.[10,11,15,18,20,30,32] Such myopathic changes support a role for MuSK in mediating trophic effects on muscle, perhaps through complex two-way communication between nerve and muscle at the NMJ. On the other hand, focal denervation with accompanying reinnervation, as suggested by the morphologic studies described above, might also lead to muscle wasting.

The observations in this model of AMM provide substantial support for the view that the Abs to MuSK play a major role in the pathogenesis of AMM. However, the molecular mechanisms by which the Abs induce the morphologic and physiologic changes are not yet understood. Data from EAMM passively induced in mice by repeated injections of very large quantities of serum IgG from AMM patients have demonstrated reduced quantities of MuSK (via internalization) and dispersion of AChR clusters in the endplate membrane.[33] However, the data obtained to date (including our own)[34,41,46] have failed to identify in EAMM a role for the major mechanism important in MG and EAMG, a wide-spread attack on the NMJ involving complement mediated mechanisms.

Finally, the observations presented here demonstrate that an immune attack on MuSK can result in weakness, muscle wasting, and severe disruption of the architecture of both the postsynaptic and presynaptic portions of the mature NMJ, thereby supporting the hypothesis that, in addition to its role in the developing NMJ, this protein plays a significant role in the maintenance and function of the mature structure.

Conflicts of interest

The authors declare no conflicts of interest.

References

1. Plested, C.P. *et al.* 2002. AChR phosphorylation and indirect inhibition of AChR function in seronegative MG. *Neurology* **59:** 1682–1688.
2. Evoli, A. *et al.* 1996. Clinical heterogeneity of seronegative myasthenia gravis. *Neuromuscul. Disord.* **6:** 155–161.
3. Evoli, A. *et al.* 2003. Clinical correlates with anti-MuSK antibodies in generalized seronegative myasthenia gravis. *Brain* **126:** 2304–2311.
4. Hoch, W. *et al.* 2001. Auto-antibodies to the receptor tyrosine kinase MuSK in patients with myasthenia gravis without acetylcholine receptor antibodies. *Nat. Med.* **7:** 365–368.
5. McConville, J. *et al.* 2004. Detection and characterization of MuSK antibodies in seronegative myasthenia gravis. *Ann. Neurol.* **55:** 580–584.
6. Sanders, D.B. *et al.* 2003. Clinical aspects of MuSK antibody positive seronegative MG. *Neurology* **60:** 1978–1980.
7. Vincent, A. *et al.* 2003. Seronegative generalised myasthenia gravis: clinical features, antibodies, and their targets. *Lancet Neurol.* **2:** 99–106.
8. Farrugia, M.E. *et al.* 2006. Single-fiber electromyography in limb and facial muscles in muscle-specific kinase antibody and acetylcholine receptor antibody myasthenia gravis. *Muscle Nerve.* **33:** 568–570.
9. Zhou, L. *et al.* 2004. Clinical comparison of muscle-specific tyrosine kinase (MuSK) antibody-positive and -negative myasthenic patients. *Muscle Nerve* **30:** 55–60.
10. Farrugia, M.E. *et al.* 2007. Magnetic resonance imaging of facial muscles. *Clin. Radiol.* **62:** 1078–1086.
11. Farrugia, M.E. *et al.* 2007. Quantitative EMG of facial muscles in myasthenia patients with MuSK antibodies. *Clin. Neurophysiol.* **118:** 269–277.
12. Farrugia, M.E. *et al.* 2006. MRI and clinical studies of facial and bulbar muscle involvement in MuSK antibody-associated myasthenia gravis. *Brain* **129:** 1481–1492.
13. Farrugia, M.E. & A. Vincent. 2010. Autoimmune mediated neuromuscular junction defects. *Curr. Opin. Neurol.* **23:** 489–495.
14. Guptill, J.T., D.B. Sanders & A. Evoli. 2011. Anti-MuSK antibody myasthenia gravis: clinical findings and response to treatment in two large cohorts. *Muscle Nerve.* **44:** 36–40.
15. Ishii, W. *et al.* 2005. Myasthenia gravis with anti-MuSK antibody, showing progressive muscular atrophy without blepharoptosis. *Intern. Med.* **44:** 671–672.
16. Zouvelou, V. *et al.* 2012. AchR-positive myasthenia gravis with MRI evidence of early muscle atrophy. *J. Clin. Neurosci.: Offic. J. Neurosurg. Soc. Austr.* **19:** 918–919.
17. Moon, S.Y., S.S. Lee & Y.H. Hong. 2011. Muscle atrophy in muscle-specific tyrosine kinase (MuSK)-related myasthenia gravis. *J. Clin. Neurosci.: Offic. J. Neurosurg. Soc. Austr.* **18:** 1274–1275.
18. Benveniste, O. *et al.* 2005. MuSK antibody positive myasthenia gravis plasma modifies MURF-1 expression in C2C12 cultures and mouse muscle *in vivo. J. Neuroimmunol.* **170:** 41–48.
19. Cenacchi, G. *et al.* 2011. Comparison of muscle ultrastructure in myasthenia gravis with anti-MuSK and anti-AChR antibodies. *J. Neurol.* **258:** 746–752.
20. Finsterer, J. 2007. Turn/amplitude analysis to assess bulbar muscle wasting in MuSK positive myasthenia. *Clin. Neurophysiol.* **118:** 1173–1174.
21. Martignago, S. *et al.* 2009. Muscle histopathology in myasthenia gravis with antibodies against MuSK and AChR. *Neuropathol. Appl. Neurobiol.* **35:** 103–110.
22. Zouvelou, V. *et al.* 2009. MRI evidence of early muscle atrophy in MuSK positive myasthenia gravis. *J. Neuroimaging* **21:** 303–305.
23. Lavrnic, D. *et al.* 2011. Proton magnetic resonance spectroscopy of the intrinsic tongue muscles in patients with myasthenia gravis with different autoantibodies. *J. Neurol. Sci.* **302:** 25–28.
24. Pasnoor, M. *et al.* 2010. Clinical findings in MuSK-antibody positive myasthenia gravis: a U.S. experience. *Muscle Nerve* **41:** 370–374.
25. Lauriola, L. *et al.* 2005. Thymus changes in anti-MuSK-positive and -negative myasthenia gravis. *Neurology* **64:** 536–538.
26. Leite, M.I. *et al.* 2005. Fewer thymic changes in MuSK antibody-positive than in MuSK antibody-negative MG. *Ann. Neurol.* **57:** 444–448.
27. Ponseti, J.M. *et al.* 2009. A comparison of long-term post-thymectomy outcome of anti-AChR-positive, anti-AChR-negative and anti-MuSK-positive patients with nonthymomatous myasthenia gravis. *Expert. Opin. Biol. Ther.* **9:** 1–8.
28. Shiraishi, H. *et al.* 2005. Acetylcholine receptors loss and postsynaptic damage in MuSK antibody-positive myasthenia gravis. *Ann. Neurol.* **57:** 289–293.

29. Selcen, D. *et al.* 2004. Are MuSK antibodies the primary cause of myasthenic symptoms? *Neurology* **62:** 1945–1950.

30. Niks, E.H. *et al.* 2010. Pre- and postsynaptic neuromuscular junction abnormalities in musk myasthenia. *Muscle Nerve* **42:** 283–288.

31. Hughes, B.W., L.L. Kusner & H.J. Kaminski. 2006. Molecular architecture of the neuromuscular junction. *Muscle Nerve* **33:** 445–461.

32. Boneva, N. *et al.* 2006. Major pathogenic effects of anti-MuSK antibodies in myasthenia gravis. *J. Neuroimmunol.* **177:** 119–131.

33. Cole, R.N. *et al.* 2010. Patient autoantibodies deplete post-synaptic Muscle Specific Kinase leading to disassembly of the ACh receptor scaffold and myasthenia gravis in mice. *J. Physiol* **588:** 3217–3229.

34. Cole, R.N. *et al.* 2008. Anti-MuSK patient antibodies disrupt the mouse neuromuscular junction. *Ann. Neurol.* **63:** 782–789.

35. ter Beek, W.P. *et al.* 2009. The effect of plasma from muscle-specific tyrosine kinase myasthenia patients on regenerating endplates. *Am. J. Pathol.* **175:** 1536–1544.

36. Lindstrom, J. 2004. Is "seronegative" MG explained by autoantibodies to MuSK? *Neurology* **62:** 1920–1921.

37. Jha, S. *et al.* 2006. Myasthenia gravis induced in mice by immunization with the recombinant extracellular domain of rat muscle-specific kinase (MuSK). *J. Neuroimmunol.* **175:** 107–117.

38. Mori, S. *et al.* 2012. 3,4-Diaminopyridine improves neuro-muscular transmission in a MuSK antibody-induced mouse model of myasthenia gravis. *J. Neuroimmunol.* **245:** 75–78.

39. Mori, S. *et al.* 2012. Antibodies against muscle-specific ki-nase impair both presynaptic and postsynaptic functions in a murine model of myasthenia gravis. *Am. J. Pathol.* **180:** 798–810.

40. Mori, S. *et al.* 2012. Divalent and monovalent autoantibodies cause dysfunction of MuSK by distinct mechanisms in a rabbit model of myasthenia gravis. *J. Neuroimmunol.* **244:** 1–7.

41. Shigemoto, K. *et al.* 2006. Induction of myasthenia by im-munization against muscle-specific kinase. *J. Clin. Invest.* **116:** 1016–1024.

42. Viegas, S. *et al.* 2012. Passive and active immunization mod-els of MuSK-Ab positive myasthenia: electrophysiological evidence for pre and postsynaptic defects. *Exp. Neurol.* **234:** 506–512.

43. Punga, A.R. *et al.* 2011. Muscle-selective synaptic disassem-bly and reorganization in MuSK antibody positive MG mice. *Exp. Neurol.* **230:** 207–217.

44. Richman, D.P. *et al.* 2012. Acute severe animal model of anti-muscle-specific kinase myasthenia: combined postsy-naptic and presynaptic changes. *Arch. Neurol.* **69:** 453–460.

45. Klooster, R. *et al.* 2012. Muscle-specific kinase myasthe-nia gravis IgG4 autoantibodies cause severe neuromuscular junction dysfunction in mice. *Brain* **135:** 1081–1101.

46. Hopf, C. & W. Hoch. 1998. Dimerization of the muscle-specific kinase induces tyrosine phosphorylation of acetyl-choline receptors and their aggregation on the surface of myotubes. *J. Biol Chem.* **273:** 6467–6473.

47. Xie, M.H. *et al.* 1997. Direct demonstration of MuSK in-volvement in acetylcholine receptor clustering through iden-tification of agonist ScFv. *Nat. Biotechnol.* **15:** 768–771.

48. Jennings, C.G., S.M. Dyer & S.J. Burden. 1993. Muscle-specific trk-related receptor with a kringle domain defines a distinct class of receptor tyrosine kinases. *Proc. Natl. Acad. Sci. USA* **90:** 2895–2899.

49. Valenzuela, D.M. *et al.* 1995. Receptor tyrosine kinase spe-cific for the skeletal muscle lineage: expression in embryonic muscle, at the neuromuscular junction, and after injury. *Neuron* **15:** 573–584.

50. Vincent, A. *et al.* 1997. Genes at the junction—candidates for congenital myasthenic syndromes. *Trends Neurosci.* **20:** 15–22.

51. Kim, N. *et al.* 2008. Lrp4 is a receptor for Agrin and forms a complex with MuSK. *Cell* **135:** 334–342.

52. Stiegler, A.L., S.J. Burden & S.R. Hubbard. 2006. Crystal structure of the agrin-responsive immunoglobulin-like do-mains 1 and 2 of the receptor tyrosine kinase MuSK. *J. Mol. Biol.* **364:** 424–433.

53. Stiegler, A.L., S.J. Burden & S.R. Hubbard. 2009. Crystal structure of the frizzled-like cysteine-rich domain of the receptor tyrosine kinase MuSK. *J. Mol. Biol.* **393:** 1–9.

54. Zhang, B. *et al.* 2008. LRP4 serves as a coreceptor of agrin. *Neuron* **60:** 285–297.

55. Hopf, C. & W. Hoch. 1998. Tyrosine phosphorylation of the muscle-specific kinase is exclusively induced by acetylcholine receptor-aggregating agrin fragments. *Eur. J. Biochem.* **253:** 382–389.

56. Hoch, W. 2003. Molecular dissection of neuromuscular junction formation. *Trends Neurosci.* **26:** 335–337.

57. Okada, K. *et al.* 2006. The muscle protein Dok-7 is essential for neuromuscular synaptogenesis. *Science* **312:** 1802–1805.

58. Strochlic, L., A. Cartaud & J. Cartaud. 2005. The synaptic muscle-specific kinase (MuSK) complex: new partners, new functions. *Bioessays* **27:** 1129–1135.

59. Nishi, K., M.A. Agius & D.P. Richman. 2008. Identification of a novel MuSK splicing variant. *Ann. N.Y. Acad. Sci.* **1132:** 362–362.

60. Nishi, K., M.A. Agius & D.P. Richman. 2008. Differentiation-dependent expression of a novel splicing variant of muscle-specific kinase, Vol. Neuroscience Meeting Planner, Online Program No. 10.8. 2008.

61. Burden, S.J. 2002. Building the vertebrate neuromuscular synapse. *J. Neurobiol.* **53:** 501–511.

62. Burden, S.J., C. Fuhrer & S.R. Hubbard. 2003. Agrin/MuSK signaling: willing and Abl. *Nat. Neurosci.* **6:** 653–654.

63. Sanes, J.R. & J.W. Lichtman. 2001. Induction, assembly, mat-uration and maintenance of a postsynaptic apparatus. *Nat. Rev. Neurosci.* **2:** 791–805.

64. Flanagan-Steet, H. *et al.* 2005. Neuromuscular synapses can form *in vivo* by incorporation of initially aneural postsynap-tic specializations. *Development* **132:** 4471–4481.

65. Weatherbee, S.D., K.V. Anderson & L.A. Niswander. 2006. LDL-receptor-related protein 4 is crucial for formation of the neuromuscular junction. *Development* **133:** 4993–5000.

66. Zhang, W. *et al.* 2011. Agrin binds to the N-terminal region of Lrp4 protein and stimulates association between Lrp4 and

the first immunoglobulin-like domain in muscle-specific kinase (MuSK). *J. Biol. Chem.* **286:** 40624–40630.

67. Kummer, T.T. *et al.* 2004. Nerve-independent formation of a topologically complex postsynaptic apparatus. *J. Cell Biol.* **164:** 1077–1087.

68. Kummer, T.T., T. Misgeld & J.R. Sanes. 2006. Assembly of the postsynaptic membrane at the neuromuscular junction: paradigm lost. *Curr. Opin. Neurobiol.* **16:** 74–82.

69. Amenta, A.R. *et al.* 2012. Biglycan is an extracellular MuSK binding protein important for synapse stability. *J. Neurosci.: Offic. J. Soc. Neurosci.* **32:** 2324–2334.

70. Kawakami, Y. *et al.* 2011. Anti-MuSK autoantibodies block binding of collagen Q to MuSK. *Neurology* **77:** 1819–1826.

71. Hesser, B.A., O. Henschel & V. Witzemann. 2006. Synapse disassembly and formation of new synapses in postnatal muscle upon conditional inactivation of MuSK. *Mol. Cell Neurosci.* **31:** 470–480.

72. Kong, X.C., P. Barzaghi & M.A. Ruegg. 2004. Inhibition of synapse assembly in mammalian muscle *in vivo* by RNA interference. *EMBO Rep.* **5:** 183–188.

73. Christadoss, P., M. Poussin & C. Deng. 2000. Animal models of myasthenia gravis. *Clin. Immunol.* **94:** 75–87.

74. Wood, S.J. & C.R. Slater. 2001. Safety factor at the neuromuscular junction. *Prog. Neurobiol.* **64:** 393–429.

75. Link, H. & B.G. Xiao. 2001. Rat models as tool to develop new immunotherapies. *Immunol. Rev.* **184:** 117–128.

76. Niemi, W.D. *et al.* 1981. Factors in the production of experimental autoimmune myasthenia gravis in acetylcholine receptor immunized rabbits. *Ann. N.Y. Acad. Sci.* **377:** 222–236.